This volume brings fully up to date the most recent scientific and clinical advances in gastrointestinal and liver immunology. An international team of authorities has summarised basic scientific advances in the area of the gut immune system and the immune abnormalities relevant to gastrointestinal and liver disease. It includes the latest developments in relation to organ transplantation of the liver and gut, HIV infection of the gut and the recently discovered disease *H. pylori* gastritis. Disorders of autoimmunity are also focussed upon as well as immunodeficiency. A feature of the volume is to highlight the relevance of such scientific advances to the clinical management of patients with immune gut and liver disorders. The volume will be an essential source of reference for all scientists interested in mucosal immunology, for clinical immunologists, gastroenterologists and hepatologists, transplant surgeons and paediatricians.

Gastrointestinal and hepatic immunology

CAMBRIDGE REVIEWS IN CLINICAL IMMUNOLOGY

Series editors:

D. B. G. OLIVEIRA
Lister Institute Research Fellow, University of Cambridge, Addenbrooke's Hospital, Cambridge.

D. K. PETERS
Regius Professor of Physic, University of Cambridge, Addenbrooke's Hospital, Cambridge.

A. P. WEETMAN
Professor of Medicine, University of Sheffield Clinical Sciences Centre.

Recent advances in immunology, particularly at the molecular level, have led to a much clearer understanding of the causes and consequences of autoimmunity. The aim of this series is to make these developments accessible to clinicians who feel daunted by such advances and require a clear exposition of the scientific and clinical issues. The various clinical specialities will be covered in separate volumes, which will follow a fixed format: a brief introduction to basic immunology followed by a comprehensive review of recent findings in the autoimmune conditions which, in particular, will compare animal models with their human counterparts. Sufficient clinical detail, especially regarding treatment, will also be included to provide basic scientists with a better understanding of these aspects of autoimmunity. Thus each volume will be self-contained and comprehensible to a wide audience. Taken as a whole the series will provide an overview of all the important autoimmune disorders.

Autoimmune Endocrine Disease   A. P. Weetman

Immunological Aspects of Renal Disease   D. B. G. Oliveira

Gastrointestinal and hepatic immunology

EDITED BY

RICHARD V. HEATLEY
Department of Medicine
St James's University Hospital
Leeds, UK

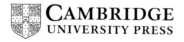

CAMBRIDGE
UNIVERSITY PRESS

Published by the Press Syndicate of the University of Cambridge
The Pitt Building, Trumpington Street, Cambridge CB2 1RP
40 West 20th Street, New York, NY 10011-4211, USA
10 Stamford Road, Oakleigh, Melbourne 3166, Australia

First published 1994

Printed in Great Britain at the University Press, Cambridge

A catalogue record for this book is available from the British Library

Library of Congress cataloguing in publication data

Gastrointestinal and hepatic immunology/edited by R. V. Heatley.
    p.   cm. — (Cambridge reviews in clinical immunology)
  Includes index.
    ISBN 0-521-44509-4
    1. Gastrointestinal system—Diseases—Immunological aspects.
2. Liver—Diseases—Immunological aspects.   I. Heatley, Richard.
II. Series.
    [DNLM: 1. Gastrointestinal Diseases—immunology.
2. Gastrointestinal   System—immunology. 3. Liver   Diseases—
immunology.   WI   100 G25823 1995]
RC802.9.G35   1995
616.3'3079—dc20
DNLM/DLC
for Library of Congress   94–1816 CIP

ISBN 0 521 44509 4

PN

Contents

List of contributors

DR J. BIENENSTOCK
Faculty of Health Sciences
McMaster University Room 2E1
1200 Main Street West
Hamilton
Ontario L8N 3Z5
Canada

DR H. DALTON
Department of Clinical Medicine
St James's University Hospital
Leeds
LS9 7TF, UK

DR M. H. DAVIES
Birmingham Liver Unit
Queen Elizabeth Hospital
Edgbaston
Birmingham
B15 2TH, UK

DR V. J. DJURIĆ
Faculty of Health Sciences
McMaster University
1200 Main Street West
Hamilton
Ontario L8N 3Z5
Canada

DR G. M. DUSHEIKO
University Department of Medicine
Royal Free Hospital
Pond Street
London
NW3 2QG, UK

DR H. C. GOOI
Blood Transfusion Service
Bridle Path
Leeds
LS15 7TW, UK

DR R. V. HEATLEY
Academic Unit of Medicine
Department of Clinical Medicine
St James's University Hospital
Leeds
LS9 7TF, UK

MRS CELIA INGHAM CLARK
Professorial Surgical Unit
St Bartholomew's Hospital
West Smithfield
London
EC1A 7BE, UK

PROFESSOR P. G. ISAACSON
Department of Histopathology
University College and
Middlesex School of Medicine
University Street
London
WC1E 6JJ, UK

DR D. JEWELL
Gastroenterology Unit
The Radcliffe Infirmary
Oxford
OX2 6HE, UK

PROFESSOR P. J. JOHNSON
Department of Clinical Oncology
Prince of Wales Hospital
Shatin
New Territories
Hong Kong

DR D. KELLEHER
Dept of Clinical Medicine
Trinity College
University of Dublin
Medical School Building
St James's Hospital
James's Street
Dublin 8

PROFESSOR T. T. MacDONALD
Department of Paediatric Gastroenterology
Suite 4.1 – Dominion House
St Bartholomew's Hospital
59 Bartholomew's Close
London
EC1A 7BE, UK

DR I. G. McFARLANE
Institute of Liver Studies
King's College School of
Medicine and Dentistry
Bessemer Road, London SE5 9PJ, UK

DR D. M. McKAY
Faculty of Health Sciences
McMaster University
1200 Main Street West
Hamilton
Ontario L8N 3Z5
Canada

DR J. NEUBERGER
The Liver and Hepatobiliary Unit
Queen Elizabeth Hospital
Edgbaston
Birmingham
B15 2TH, UK

DR C. A. OTTAWAY
Division of Gastroenterology
Department of Medicine
St Michael's Hospital
30 Bond Street
Toronto
Ontario M5B 1W8
Canada

DR J. PARKIN
Department of Immunology
The Medical College of
St Bartholomew's Hospital
West Smithfield
London
EC1A 7BE, UK

DR M. H. PERDUE
Faculty of Health Sciences
McMaster University
1200 Main Street West
Hamilton
Ontario L8N 3Z5
Canada

DR A. G. POCKLEY
Professorial Surgical Unit
The Medical College of
St Bartholomew's Hospital
West Smithfield
London
EC1A 7BE, UK

MR S. A. SADEK
Department of Surgery
Level 8
Clinical Sciences Building
St James's University Hospital
Leeds
LS9 7TF, UK

DR J. E. SMITHSON
Gastroenterology Unit
The Radcliffe Infirmary
Oxford OX2 6HE, UK

DR JO SPENCER
Department of Histopathology
University College and
Middlesex School of Medicine
University Street
London
WC1E 6JJ, UK

DR C. R. STOKES
Department of Veterinary Medicine
University of Bristol
Langford House
Langford
Bristol
BS18 7DU, UK

DR S. STROBEL
Department of Immunology
Institute of Child Health
309 Guilford Street
London
WC1N 1EH, UK

PROFESSOR D. G. WEIR
Dept of Clinical Medicine
Trinity College
University of Dublin
Medical School Building
St James's Hospital
James's Street
Dublin 8

PROFESSOR R. WOOD
Professorial Surgical Unit
St Bartholomew's Hospital
West Smithfield
London
EC1A 7BE, UK

DR A. WOTHERSPOON
Department of Histopathology
University College and
Middlesex School of Medicine
University Street
London
WC1E 6JJ, UK

PROFESSOR A. ZUCKERMAN
Royal Free Hospital
Pond Street
London
NW3 2QG, UK

Preface

The study of mucosal immunity has moved quickly in recent years, particularly in relation to gut and liver diseases. Our understanding of antigen handling, mucosal defences and cell traffic has increased dramatically. In parallel with this progress in basic scientific knowledge have come many significant clinical advances. Immunisation, immunosuppressive treatment and organ transplantation have over the last decade become everyday forms of treatment in hepatology. Sadly, in disorders of the gastrointestinal tract, similar progress has not been equally forthcoming. Immunosuppressive treatment has been used largely empirically in inflammatory bowel disease and intestinal transplantation remains at a developmental stage. One compensation for gastroenterologists has been the discovery of a 'new' disease – that of *H. pylori* gastritis. Developments in our understanding of the immune response to this organism are fascinating in terms of our knowledge of mucosal immunity and may one day lead to another disorder for which vaccine developments become necessary. The gut and liver are sites for apparently classical autoimmune disorders. Slowly, our understanding of these processes is increasing, and chronic hepatitis B infection must be a model envied by many immunologists.

As with any rapidly evolving field, a number of books have appeared on this topic over the years. In this volume, the aim has been to address the most recent developments in the basic scientific mechanisms and relate these, where applicable, to areas important to practising clinicians caring for patients with hepatic and gut disease. I am fortunate in being joined in this book by a group of colleagues, all recognised widely for their contributions to these fields. I am most grateful to them all, especially to those tackling the difficult task of trying to correlate the science with the clinical applications.

One omission is the contribution I had hoped to receive from David Triger, whose untimely death has deprived us all of an expert in his field and a valued colleague. James Neuberger stepped into the void at very short notice, and I am indebted to him.

I gratefully acknowledge the help and support of so many in bringing this volume to fruition, especially Peter Silver and his co-workers at Cambridge University Press and Tony Weetman and his colleagues for giving us all the opportunity to contribute to their developing series and for their help and encouragement in achieving this.

R. V. H.

Leeds

October 1993

–1–
Lymphoid cells and tissues of the gastrointestinal tract

THOMAS T. MacDONALD and JO SPENCER

Introduction

Mucosal immunology is of relevance to a large number of different biomedical sub-disciplines, as well as being of intrinsic interest for the study of the basic biology of the system. For efficiency, and a directed response, potential vaccines to enteric pathogens should be delivered by the oral route and generate specific mucosal immunity. Oral vaccination is also the preferred route to generate systemic immunity. In the developed world, the idiopathic inflammatory bowel disease and food-sensitive enteropathies are relatively common diseases, both of which have an immunological basis, and despite intense research in recent years, are still poorly understood.

It is still not widely appreciated that the gut-associated lymphoid tissue is the largest in the body. There is more organised lymphoid tissue in the gut than the rest of the body and there are more T cells in the gut epithelium than in the spleen. Furthermore, some cell types such as IgA2 secreting plasma cells and T cells using the gamma–delta T cell receptor are abundant in the gut, but less common elsewhere. It is the purpose of this chapter to detail the lymphoid tissues and cell types present in the gut, to delineate their unique features, and to briefly discuss how these cells interact with gut-derived antigen.

Peyer's patches

The organised lymphoid tissue of the small intestine was first described by de Peyer in 1667. Structurally, Peyer's patches are organised areas of lymphoid tissue in the mucosa overlying the muscularis mucosa. They usually contain follicle centres and well-defined cellular zonation into T and B cell zones with the former containing high endothelial venules. They are overlayed by a specialised lymphoepithelium (follicle associated epithelium–FAE) without crypts or villi. At birth, there are approximately 100 Peyer's patches with 5 follicles or more in human small intestine and the majority of these Peyer's

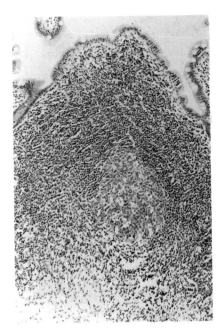

Fig. 1.1. Histology of a normal human Peyer's patch. Note the sparcity of goblet cells in the FAE (H&E original magnification ×32).

patches are in the distal small intestine (Cornes, 1965). The number of Peyer's patches increases to 225–300 in the whole small intestine by late adolescence and then decreases with increasing age, so that the small intestine from 90 year old individuals has roughly the same number of Peyer's patches as at birth (Cornes, 1965). The small bowel also contains thousands of isolated lymphoid nodules which almost certainly have the same function as the larger aggregates. In normal intestine, all organised mucosal follicles can be shown to have a FAE if the tissue is properly oriented for sectioning.

Histology and follicle associated epithelium in Peyer's patches

Histology of normal human Peyer's patches is shown in Fig. 1.1. The most prominent feature of Peyer's patches is the follicle centre, containing centrocytes and centroblasts. The follicle centre is surrounded by a mantle of small lymphocytes which merge into the mixed cell zone of the dome, underlying the epithelium. The dome area also contains plasma cells, dendritic cells, macrophages and small cells with cleaved nuclei (centrocyte-like cells), which infiltrate the overlying epithelium. These centrocyte-like cells can be identified immunohistochemically as B cells in frozen sections (Spencer, Finn & Isaacson, 1986a). B cells are rarely, if at all, seen in villus or crypt epithelium.

A characteristic of Peyer's patches is that the follicle is always associated with a specialised FAE. The epithelial cells overlying the follicle are derived from crypts of Lieberkuhn adjacent to the follicles. Follicle associated epithelium is different from columnar epithelium overlying the lamina propria, in that it is more cuboidal and contains few goblet cells; it does not contain secretory component (Bjerke & Brandtzaeg, 1988). In addition there are specialised 'M' cells, also derived from adjacent crypts (Bye, Allan & Trier, 1984), so-called because they have microfolds rather than microvilli on their surface (Owen & Jones, 1974). M-cells have a number of morphological and functional specialisations. They have attenuated processes to adjacent cells and are very closely associated with clusters of CD4+ lymphocytes (Bjerke, Brandtzaeg & Fausa, 1988).

It is clear from a large number of studies that M-cells can transport soluble molecules, inert particles, viruses and bacteria from the lumen into the epithelial intercellular space (Owen, 1977; Wolf et al., 1981; Sicinski et al. 1990; Trier, 1991). Access of these antigens to the lymphoid/myeloid elements of dome region from the epithelial paracellular space is relatively easy, since the basement membrane of the Peyer's patch epithelium is full of holes (McClugage, Low & Zimny, 1986). Whether the M-cell can process antigens is unclear. M-cells are low in cytoplasmic acid phosphatase and microvillus associated alkaline phosphatase (Owen, Apple & Bhalla, 1986). It is controversial whether M-cells express Class II MHC molecules, necessary to present peptides to CD4+ T cells. In man they appear to be Class II− or only very weakly positive (Bjerke & Brandtzaeg, 1988), but in the rat it has recently been demonstrated that they are Class II+ (Allan, Mendrick & Trier, 1993). Moreover, they also contain acidic endosomal and acid-phosphatase-containing prelysosomal and lysosomal compartments, which are necessary for processing of exogenous antigen (Allan, Mendrick & Trier, 1993).

Peyer's patches may also be a route by which environmental pollutants enter the body from the diet. Shepherd et al. (1987) detected pigment-filled macrophages in the basal aspect of the Peyer's patches, of all patients studied over 6 years of age. These macrophages were shown to contain aluminium, silicon and titanium.

Lymphoid/myeloid cells in Peyer's patches

Immunohistochemical staining of Peyer's patches with anti-CD3 monoclonal antibodies, shows T cells to be present in the greatest density in the areas surrounding the high endothelial venules (HEV) (Fig. 1.2(a)–(c)).

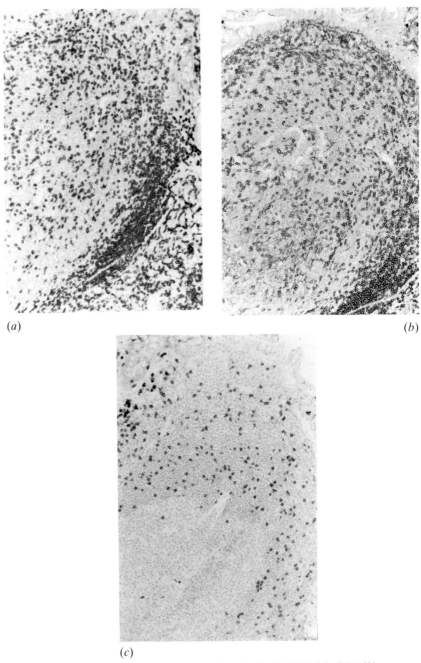

(a)

(b)

(c)

Fig. 1.2. Normal human Peyer's patch stained with CD3 (*a*), CD4 (*b*) or CD8 (*c*) (immunoperoxidase, original magnification ×32).

IL-2 receptor positive T cells are also present in this area. T cells are also present surrounding the follicle, in the mixed cell zone in the dome and in the lymphoepithelium (Spencer, Finn & Isaacson, 1986a). In man, in contrast to the mouse, the T cell zone extends between the follicle centre and the muscularis mucosa. Occasional T cells are seen in the follicle centre. The majority of the T cells are CD4+.

Human Peyer's patches contain large numbers of B cells. The narrow mantle zone surrounding the follicle centre is composed of cells expressing surface IgM and IgD. The B cells which surround the mantle zone, present in the mixed cell zone of the dome and infiltrate the epithelium do not express IgD but do express sIgM or sIgA (Spencer, Finn & Isaacson, 1986a). A major difference between rodent and human Peyer's patches is that in man, cells with surface IgD are restricted to a narrow zone around the follicle centre, whereas in the rat, the majority of the B cells surrounding the follicle centres, including those in the dome and dome epithelium, express sIgM and sIgD (Spencer, Finn & Isaacson, 1986b).

Most of the cells with abundant cytoplasmic immunoglobulin are in the dome area in human Peyer's patches. Most contain cytoplasmic (c) IgA, with fewer cIgM+ cells (Spencer, Finn & Isaacson, 1986a). Some workers have reported cIgG plasma cells are as abundant as cIgA cells in the dome (Bjerke & Brandtzaeg, 1986). There are also cells with cIgA in the T cell zone surrounding the HEV but the dense accumulation of IgA-containing immunoblasts around the high endothelial venules in rodents is not seen in man (Spencer, Finn & Isaacson, 1986b). A striking feature of cells with cIgG in the dome of Peyer's patches, is that less than half are J-chain+, in contrast to lamina propria cIgG+ cells which are 70–90% J-chain+ (Bjerke & Brandtzaeg, 1986). This might indicate that the J-chain-, cIgG+ cells in the dome are mature memory cell clones.

In man, B cells, activated T cells, dendritic cells, follicular dendritic cells, and macrophages, express Class II molecules necessary for antigen presentation to CD4+ T cells. All of these HLA-DR+ cell types are present in normal Peyer's patches (Fig. 1.3(a)).

Numerous, non-lymphoid HLA-DR+ cells with cytoplasmic processes, are present in the dome area of human Peyer's patches and in the T cell zones. The HLA-DR+ cells in the dome do not stain with anti-macrophage markers such as RFD7 or lysozyme (although these cells are abundant in adjacent lamina propria), but do stain with S-100 (Spencer, Finn & Isaacson, 1986a, Brandtzaeg & Bjerke 1990). These cells are probably dendritic cells but the HLA-DR+ cells between the follicles in the T cell zones are probably interdigitating cells. The dome epithelium itself is also HLA−DR+ (Spencer, Finn & Isaacson, 1986c) and may also be capable of presenting antigen to the numerous lymphoid cells in the epithelium. The presence of dendritic cells in the mixed cell zone of the dome, immediately

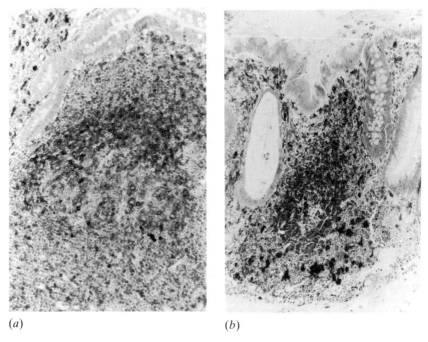

(*a*)   (*b*)

Fig. 1.3. Normal human Peyer's patch (*a*) or colonic lymphoid follicle (*b*) stained with anti-HLA-DR (immunoperoxidase, original magnification ×32).

underlying the M-cells, suggests that in Peyer's patches most antigen presentation takes place in the dome region.

Organised lymphoid tissue of the colon

Organised lymphoid tissue in human colon was first described in 1926 by Dukes and Bussey. They showed that in children there were eight follicles per square cm of colonic mucosa, which decreased to three per square cm in old age. More recent studies have shown that in the anorectal region of adults there are 20–30 follicles/cm^2 (Langman & Rowland, 1992). Aggregates of follicles akin to that seen in the multi-follicular Peyer's patches in the small bowel, are not seen in human colon. The bulk of the lymphoid tissue in colonic lymphoid follicles lies below the muscularis mucosa, the follicles producing points of discontinuity in the latter (Fig. 1.4, O'Leary & Sweeney, 1986). Unless colonic lymphoid tissue is properly orientated, it may appear as though it has no FAE. Serial sections however or re-oriented

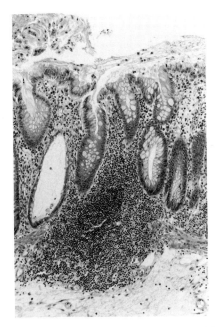

Fig. 1.4. Histology of a colonic lymphoid follicle. Note the discontinuity in the muscularis mucosa (H&E original magnification ×40).

blocks invariably reveals a FAE. Colonic FAE contains M-cells, identical to those seen in Peyer's patches (Jacob, Baker & Swaminathan, 1987, Fujimura, Hosobe & Kihara 1992). This may be the portal of entry for HIV during receptive homosexual intercourse, since it has been clearly shown that HIV is selectively taken up by M-cells in Peyer's patches (Amerongen *et al.*, 1991).

The colonic lymphoid follicles contain a central B cell zone, surrounded by a T cell zone, which contains interdigitating cells (O'Leary & Sweeney 1986). There are also large numbers of HLA-DR+ cells (Fig. 1.3(b)).

Lymphoid tissue of the stomach

The normal stomach mucosa is devoid of lymphoid tissue. There is a scattering of T cells in the lamina propria and a few in the epithelium. In the lamina propria, IgA plasma cells predominate over IgM and IgG cells. In chronic gastritis, there is an increase in plasma cells of all isotypes, but the increase in IgG cells is especially profound (Brandtzaeg, 1987). There is also an increase in epithelial T cells (Kazi *et al.*, 1989). A striking feature of the

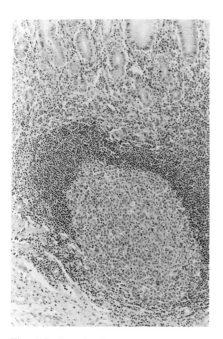

Fig. 1.5. Acquired MALT in the stomach of a patient with *H. pylori* (H&E original magnification ×32).

stomach, is the acquisition of organised lymphoid aggregates resembling Peyer's patches, in association with *Helicobacter pylori* infection (Fig. 1.5). In children this is especially striking and leads to antral nodularity which is visible at gastroscopy (Wyatt & Rathbone, 1988; Hassall & Dimmick, 1991). Whether this acquired lymphoid tissue functionally resembles Peyer's patches with FAE, remains to be seen. Wotherspoon *et al.* (1991), have observed that lymphoid tissue acquired in response to *H. pylori*, includes B cells infiltrating the epithelium, giving the appearance of a lymphoepithelium.

Organised lymphoid tissue at other mucosal sites – mucosa associated lymphoid tissue (MALT)

It is generally considered that the only other site in the body at which there is organised mucosa associated lymphoid tissue, is the upper respiratory tract, forming the so-called bronchus associated lymphoid tissue (BALT). This has been most thoroughly studied in rabbits, where nodules of lymphoid tissue have been described in the bronchial lamina propria at the junction of airways or between an artery and the bronchus (Bienenstock & Johnston, 1976). There is now, however, considerable doubt as to whether BALT is a constitutive feature of normal lung in man. Even in patients with severe bronchitis and bronchiectasis, BALT can only be identified in 8% of patients (Delventhal *et al.* 1992). BALT cannot be identified in some patients with diffuse panbronchiolitis (Sato *et al.*, 1992). In these patients in whom BALT has been identified, its anatomical location is similar to rabbits, and by immunohistochemistry, it resembles Peyer's patches. It also has a lympho-epithelium, although M-cells have not yet been identified (Sato *et al.*, 1992).

On the basis of this evidence, Pabst (1992) has argued forcibly that BALT is not a feature of normal human lung. By analogy with the stomach, it is likely that BALT is not constitutive in man, but is acquired as the result of chronic antigen stimulation in the lung. Yet more examples of this phenom-enon are the development of MALT in the salivary glands of patients with Sjogrens syndrome (Hyjek, Smith & Isaacson, 1988), the thyroid of patients with Hashimoto's thyroiditis (Hyjek & Isaacson, 1988), and, as mentioned above, in the stomach of patients with *H. pylori* infection. Acquisition of MALT in these tissues appears to be a prerequisite for the development of MALT lymphoma (Spencer & Isaacson, 1992).

The gut epithelium

Immunological role

The primary function of the gut is in nutrient digestion and absorption by the epithelium. The tight junctions at the apical aspects of epithelial cells in the bowel are the major barrier between the cells of the gut immune system and the large amounts of lumenal antigen. In particular, the lymphocytes which are dispersed basally in the epithelium between the enterocytes are particu-larly close to large amounts of antigen. Although for ease of discussion, it is convenient to consider the gut epithelium as a separate compartment, it should be remembered that processes from epithelial cells cross the basal lamina and protrude into the lamina propria, thereby providing a path by which epithelial cells could directly transport antigens into the lamina propria. Furthermore, sub-epithelial macrophages extend pseudopodia into the epithelium, where they may also pinocytose or phagocytose antigen in the inter-cellular space (Komuro, 1985; Hashimoto & Komuro, 1988).

The gut epithelium may also play an important immunoregulatory role. Villus epithelial cells in the small bowel express Class II (Fig. 1.6) and can present antigen (Scott *et al.*, 1980; Bland & Warren, 1986*a*,*b*; Mayer & Shlien, 1987). In addition, there is now increasing evidence that enterocytes may be an important source of mucosal cytokines, including TGFβ, IL-1,

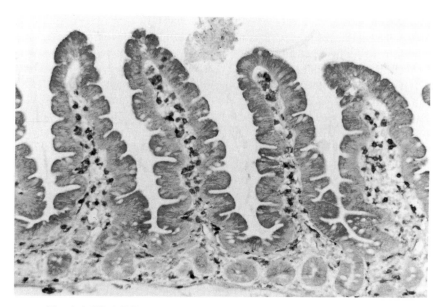

Fig. 1.6. HLA-DR expression in normal small bowel epithelium. Note that the bases of the crypts are HLA–DR− and that there are numerous HLA-DR+ cells in the lamina propria (immunoperoxidase, original magnification ×40).

IL-6 (Koyoma & Podolsky, 1989; Radema, Van Deventer & Cerami, 1991, Shirota *et al.*, 1990). However, enterocytes are lacking some important co-stimulatory molecules such as ICAM-1, the receptor for LFA-1 (Sturgess *et al.*, 1990) and B7, the receptor for CD28 (Sanderson & Walker, 1993*b*).

One of the most important roles of the epithelium (mainly the crypt epithelial cells), is in the transport of polymeric immunoglobulins from the lamina propria to the gut lumen. The polymeric immunoglobulin receptor (secretory component), is expressed on the basolateral aspect of the epi-thelial cells. It serves as a receptor for J-chain on polymeric immunoglobu-lins and the receptor–antibody complex is transcytosed across the epithelial cell and secreted into the lumen. For a recent, detailed review of this subject readers are referred to a recent article by Mestecky, Lue & Russell (1991).

The lymphoid cells of the intestinal epithelium

B cells and plasma cells are never found in the epithelium of the large or small bowel. The B cells present in preparations of human or animal intraepithelial lymphocytes (IEL) are derived from the lamina propria or FAE. IEL lie basally in the epithelium and characteristically are surrounded by a clear halo (Fig. 1.7(a)). Not all IEL are T cells since in some individuals many are CD3−, 7+ (Spencer *et al.*, 1989*a*). Of the CD3+ cells, the majority are CD8+ (Janossy *et al.*, 1980), with only around 10% being CD4+ (Fig. 1.7(b),(c),(d)). Most of the CD8+ cells use the CD8$\alpha\beta$ heterodimer (Jarry *et al.*, 1990). There are minor populations of CD3+, 4+, 8−; CD3+, 4−, 8− IEL in normal bowel epithelium (Spencer *et al*, 1989*a*). Most IEL in the small bowel also use the $\alpha\beta$ form of the T cell receptor (Brandtzaeg *et al.*, 1989), only a minority (approximately 10%) being $\gamma\delta$ TcR+ (Groh *et al.*, 1989; Spencer *et al.*, 1989*b*). Most of the latter are CD8− (Halstensen, Scott & Brandtzaeg, 1989). Slightly higher frequencies of $\gamma\delta$ TcR+ IEL have been reported in human colon (Trejdosiewicz *et al.*, 1989). There is no information in man as to whether IEL are the progeny of T cells activated in the Peyer's patches.

IEL in healthy individuals are rarely HLA-DR+, do not express IL-2 receptors (Choy *et al.* 1990*a*) and are non-dividing (Halstensen & Brandtzaeg, 1993). However, all human mucosal T cells express the activation antigen recognized by the monoclonal antibody HML-1 (Cerf-Bensussan *et al.*, 1987). Many normal IEL also express the activation marker VLA-1 (Choy *et al.*, 1990*b*). CD45R0 expression on T cells is associated with activation. Only 14–61% of normal $\alpha\beta$ TcR+ IEL express CD45R0 strongly. A somewhat higher frequency of $\gamma\delta$ TcR+ IEL are strongly CD45R0+ (Halstensen *et al.*, 1990). Taken together, these results would indicate that IEL are the progeny of activated cells, but that in normal individuals they are moving back to a resting stage. This is consistent with the fact that, by morphology, very few IEL are immunoblasts in healthy individuals (Marsh, 1985).

Lamina propria

T cells of the lamina propria

There have been a number of studies in which the phenotype of putative 'lamina propria' cells isolated from large segments of bowel has been studied. However, since these cells are almost certainly a mixture of follicular and lamina propria cells (Bull & Bookman, 1977), these results will not be discussed. By immunohistology, most lamina propria T cells are CD4+ (Fig. 1.7(c), Janossy *et al.*, 1980). They are non-dividing (Halstensen & Brantzaeg, 1993), HLA-DR− and the majority are HML1+ (Cerf-Bensussan *et al.*, 1987). Virtually all use the $\alpha\beta$ TcR+. Only about half express CD45R0 strongly and there are substantial numbers of CD45RA+ cells in the lamina propria (Halstensen *et al.*, 1990). Nearly all lamina propria CD4+ cells are Leu8− (L-selectin, the lymphocyte ligand for

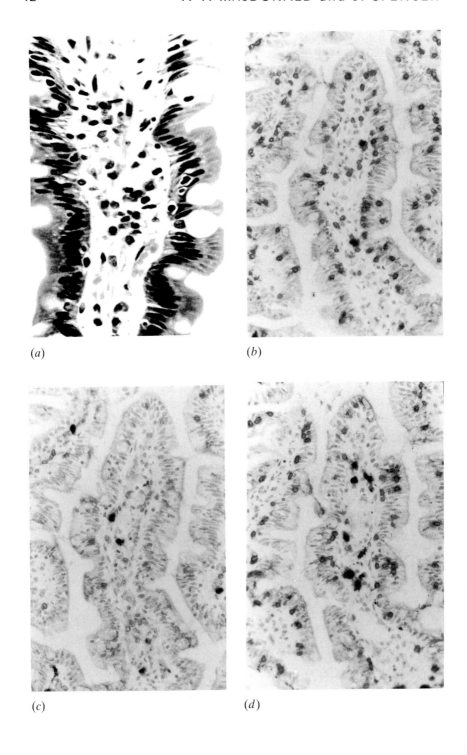

(a)

(b)

(c)

(d)

endothelial glycam-1, Berg *et al.*, 1991). The human fetal intestinal lamina propria contains large numbers of CD4+ cells, expressing HML1 and CD45R0, indicating that lumenal antigen is not necessary for the accumulation of cells in this compartment (Braegger, Spencer & MacDonald, 1992).

Accessory cells in the lamina propria

The lamina propria contains a dense population of HLA-DR+, DP+, DQ+ accessory cells (Selby *et al.*, 1983*a*). The majority of the HLA-DR+ cells in the lamina propria of the large and small intestine are macrophages and dendritic cells. It should be emphasised, however, that the distinction between these two cell types in the lamina propria is vague and controversial. It is virtually impossible to isolate these cells in any great number or purity (Pavli *et al.*, 1993) and so most studies have used immunohistologic and/or immunochemical techniques to characterise these cells.

The relative proportions of dendritic type cells to phagocytic type cells in human gut is unclear. Wilders *et al.* (1984) showed that, at the tops of the villi in normal intestine, there is a population of DR+, strongly acid phosphatase+ cells. These are probably phagocytic macrophages, identical to the population of 25F9+ cells (a marker of mature macrophages) identified in human small intestine (Hume *et al.*, 1987). Selby *et al.* (1983*b*) reported that in the normal human small intestine, 80–90% of the DR+ histiocytes were weakly acid phosphatase+, weakly non-specific esterase+, and strongly membrane ATPase+, suggesting that they are dendritic cells. In normal colon, Selby *et al.* (1983*b*) also reported that most of the DR+ cells were strongly acid phosphatase and esterase+ and were weakly ATPase+. This work would indicate that in the small bowel most of the DR+ accessory cells in the lamina propria are antigen-presenting cells whereas in the large bowel most are phagocytic.

Cells of the B cell lineage in the lamina propria

The lamina propria of normal human intestine contains abundant plasma cells. As first observed over 25 years ago, the major plasma cell isotype and

---

Fig. 1.7. Histological appearance of intraepithelial lymphocytes in a normal human small intestinal villus (*a*)) (H&E original magnification ×240). CD3+ cells (*b*), CD4+ cells (*c*) and CD8+ cells (*d*) are also shown. Note the sparcity of CD4+ cells in the epithelium (immunoperoxidase, original magnification × 50).

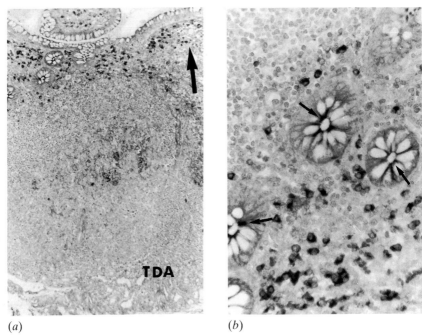

(a)   (b)

Fig. 1.8. IgA2+ plasma cells in and around a Peyer's patch. In 1.8(a), the IgA2 plasma cells in the dome region are arrowed. Note the absence of IgA2 plasma cells in the thymus dependent area (TDA) of the interfollicular zone. (Immunoperoxidase, original magnification ×32). In 1.8(b), lamina propria plasma cells containing IgA2 are shown. Note the dense apical staining (arrows) of IgA being transported into the lumen (immunoperoxidase, original magnification ×120).

hence the major immunoglobulin isotype in the intestinal secretions is IgA (Tomasi *et al.*, 1965; Crabbe & Heremans, 1966). IgA plasma cells make up 30–40% of the mononuclear cells in human intestinal lamina propria and small B cells make up 15–45% of the cells (MacDonald *et al.*, 1987). In the jejunum around 80% of the total plasma cells secrete IgA, around 18% secrete IgM and only 3% secrete IgG (Crabbe & Heremans, 1966; Brandt-zaeg, 1987). These same relative proportions are also seen in the ileum and the colon. IgD or IgE plasma cells are very uncommon. Most of the plasma cells regardless of isotype are found in the region around the crypts.

Slightly more than half of the IgA plasma cells in the gut secrete IgA2 (Fig. 1.8; Crago *et al.*, 1984), in contrast to tonsils and lymph nodes where most of the IgA is IgA1. In addition the majority of IgA secreted by the plasma cells is dimeric IgA; 100% of IgA2 immunocytes being J-chain positive and 88% of IgA1 immunocytes, J-chain positive (Kett, Brandtzaeg & Fausa, 1988).

Mechanisms of antigen uptake

It has been known for almost 60 years that dietary antigens can cross the gut epithelium and be detected in small but immunogenic amounts in serum (for review see Husby, 1988). M-cells are specialised to sample antigen from the gut, and when bacterial and dietary antigen first appears in the gut at birth, the primary follicles of the Peyer's patches and appendix develop germinal centres and the mucosal B cell (IgA) response is generated (Bridges *et al.*, 1959; Gebbers & Laissue, 1990). It then takes several years before mucosal IgA plasma cell numbers reach adult levels (Perkkio & Savilahti, 1980). It is more likely however that antigen from dietary products enters the circulation across villous or crypt epithelium. This could occur in two ways, either by intracellular transport through the enterocyte, or by a paracellular route through tight junctions. The former probably is more important and reflects a physiological process, which is important in the newborn for the uptake of growth factors from milk (Sanderson & Walker, 1993*a*). This would explain the very well-documented observation that antigen uptake is higher in the newborn and premature intestine than later in life (Robertson *et al.*, 1982; Weaver, Laker & Nelson, 1984). Importantly, this physiological uptake of macromolecules also decreases with age.

Paracellular transport of lumenal antigen in healthy intestine is not very high, since the pore size of the tight junction is too small to allow immunogenic polypeptides through. However, in disease where tight junction integrity is disrupted by neutrophils or interferon-gamma (Madara & Stafford, 1989; Nash *et al.*, 1991), larger molecules may pass through (the basis for intestinal permeability tests using large sugars). Indeed, Gruskay and Cooke (1955) showed higher serum levels of ovalbumin after oral challenge in infants recovering from gastroenteritis than controls. Once antigen has crossed the epithelium and basement membrane, it can readily enter the circulation through the relatively permeable endothelium of the subepithelial vascular arcade (Allan & Trier 1991). Although the subject has attracted a great deal of interest, it is not yet clear if increased uptake of macromolecules from the intestine as a result of mucosal infection or inflammation, is an important predisposing factor in the development of gastrointestinal disease.

Antigen-uptake by the gut

Immunological factors which control antigen-uptake

The phenomenon of immune exclusion documented by Walker and colleagues (Walker, Isselbacher & Bloch, 1972), is an obvious way by which secretory IgA, by complexing with antigen in the mucous layer above the epithelium, could inhibit uptake of immunogenic macromolecules. The relative importance of this mechanism is, however, unclear since it is difficult in man and animals to elicit a mucosal IgA response to non-replicating soluble antigens. Nevertheless, the finding of high levels of immune complexes in the serum of IgA-deficient patients (Cunningham-Rundles, 1987), indicates that IgA immune exclusion plays a role in man. More recently, a novel mechanism of immune exclusion has been proposed by Lamm and colleagues (Kaetzel *et al.*, 1991). They have shown in an *in vitro* model system that polymeric IgA complexed to its specific antigen can be transcytosed from the basolateral aspect of epithelial cells via the polymeric Ig receptor, to the epithelial cell surface. They propose that this is an important mechanism by which antigen which crosses the epithelium can be cleared from the lamina propria, back into the lumen.

What is clear, however, is that dietary proteins are highly immunogenic, especially in the infant. Virtually all bottle-fed infants have high levels of circulating IgG antibodies to cows' milk proteins (Rothberg & Farr, 1965, Scott *et al.*, 1985). Thus, in the presence of this serum antibody, any antigen crossing into the circulation would rapidly complex with serum antibody and be taken up by the Kupffer cells of the liver. What is perhaps of more interest, is the fact that despite the almost universal immunogenicity of cows' milk proteins in children, only 1–3% develop milk hypersensitivity. The factors which control the development of disease are complex and almost certainly include a substantial genetic component. However, there is evidence that by reducing both maternal milk consumption (to reduce cows' milk proteins in breast milk) and feeding infants a hydrolysed, less antigenic formula, that the incidence of atopy to cows' milk proteins can be reduced (Zeiger *et al.*, 1989; Vandenplas *et al.*, 1992).

Oral tolerance

The phenomenon of oral tolerance is widely perceived to play a role in down-regulating immune responses to dietary antigens and thereby preventing food hypersensitivity. Thus, healthy individuals maintain tolerance to dietary antigen, whereas in food-sensitive individuals, oral tolerance is broken. Most of the work has been done in experimental animals, mainly rodents. There is no doubt that after oral feeding of a specific antigen, upon systemic challenge, fed animals produce lower levels of antibody (of all isotypes), *in vitro* T cell proliferative responses and delayed-type hypersensitivity reactions than non-fed controls (reviewed by Challacombe & Tomasi, 1987). Oral tolerance has been demonstrated for a variety of soluble and particulate antigens. Multiple mechanisms appear to be important in the maintenance of oral tolerance. There is a wealth of data showing that T cells (suppressor cells?) and serum can adoptively transfer oral tolerance. The situation is, however, confused by the demonstration of contrasuppressor cells, which can break oral tolerance by inhibiting the activity of suppressor cells (Fujihashi *et al.*, 1992). It is obviously impossible to demonstrate such complex cell circuitry in man. However, it should be emphasised that there is considerable species variability in oral tolerance. Rodents fed soluble antigens rapidly become unresponsive and tend not to produce mucosal or serum antibodies, whereas rabbits and hamsters fed bovine serum albumin for example, produce vigorous antibody responses in serum and in the gut (Bienenstock & Dolezel, 1971; Peri & Rothberg, 1981).

Moreover, most experimental systems used to study oral tolerance have used systemic challenge after oral feeding, which is completely unphysiological.

Studies to address the question of oral tolerance in man are few. Controlled studies have shown that it is possible to reduce the incidence of food hypersensitivity, by avoiding food antigens or using hydrolysates (Zeiger *et al.*, 1989, Vandenplas *et al.*, 1992), but this probably reflects reduced antigen exposure rather than tolerance induced by so-called hypoallergenic formulae. Many years ago Korenblat *et al.* (1968) fed bovine serum albumen (BSA) to adult volunteers and measured serum anti-BSA antibody. There was a heterogeneous response. Individuals with pre-existing anti-BSA antibody showed a rise in antibody levels on feeding, whereas those without pre-existing antibody, made no response. On parenteral challenge of a sub-group of patients, individuals who were unresponsive to feeding BSA, were also unresponsive to parenteral challenge. More recently, Barnes *et al.* (1987), fed Rhesus antigens to men and then challenged them intravenously with Rh(D)+ cells. Most of the men fed antigen responded to oral challenge as did most of the controls. These are the only good studies on oral tolerance in man and as can be seen, the results are equivocal, although the systems used are very different.

Therapeutic effects of feeding antigens in man

While it may be the case that breakdown of oral tolerance or regulation of macromolecular uptake from the gut, is important in the development of some gut diseases (Sanderson & Walker, 1993a), the prospects for prophylactic use of the phenomenon to reduce gut diseases are dim. Instead, it may be possible to ameliorate ongoing immunity or inflammation by feeding antigen. This idea has been followed through in two situations in man. First, as an extension of the study on feeding Rh antigens mentioned above, they were also fed to mothers with pre-existing anti-Rh antibodies, as a possible way of reducing their anti-Rh antibody levels (Barnes *et al.*, 1987). However, instead of reducing anti-Rh antibody, it was boosted.

Oral administration of myelin basic protein (MBP) can effectively inhibit experimental autoimmune encephalitis, when given either before or after the induction of disease in rats (Higgins & Weiner, 1988). Inhibition is mediated by CD8+ cells and the key molecule in suppression appears to be TFGβ which is produced locally in the lesions and inhibits ongoing inflammation (Miller *et al.*, 1992). These results have now prompted a double-blind trial of the effects of oral tolerisation with myelin antigens in patients with multiple sclerosis (Weiner *et al.*, 1993). Preliminary results published recently, indicate that the treatment is safe and preliminary evidence indicates that oral tolerisation decreases both the frequency of exacerbations and the frequency of autoreactive T cells.

Conclusions

In recent years, with the development of monoclonal antibodies and the widespread use of immunohistology, a great deal of information has been gained about the basic organisation and cells of the mucosal immune system and the changes in disease states. There has, however, not yet been much progress in extrapolating this knowledge to practical application in gut disease or the generation of mucosal vaccines. This is probably because there is as yet little understanding of the molecular interactions between cells of the immune system, epithelial and stromal elements in the gut wall, and their interactions with enteric antigens and pathogens. Nevertheless there is now some progress on several key areas, notably the potential of targeting M-cells to facilitate oral immunisation and identification of the host epithelial surface molecules used by pathogens for initial binding. It is to be hoped that the increasing interest in mucosal immunology will facilitate progress, and that the gut immune system will eventually be as well understood as the systemic immune system.

References

Allan, C. H. & Trier, J. S. (1991). Structure and permeability differ in subepithelial villus and Peyer's patch follicle capillaries. *Gastroenterology*, **100**, 1172–9.

Allan, C. H., Mendrick, D. L. & Trier, J. S. (1993). Rat intestinal M cells contain acidic endosomal–lysosomal compartments and express Class II major histocompatibility complex determinants. *Gastroenterology*, **104**, 698–707.

Amerongen, H. M., Weltzin, R., Farnet, C. M., Michetti, P., Hasaltine, W. A. & Neutra, M. (1991). Transepithelial transport of HIV-1 by intestinal M cells: a mechanism for transmission of AIDS. *Journal of Acquired Immunodeficiency Syndrome*, **4**, 760–5.

Barnes, R. M. R., Duguid, J. K. M., Roberts, F. M. *et al*. (1987). Oral administration of erythrocyte membrane antigen does not suppress anti-Rh(D) antibody responses in humans. *Clinical and Experimental Immunology*, **67**, 220–6.

Berg, M., Murakawa, Y., Camerini, D. & James, S. P. (1991). Lamina propria lymphocytes are derived from circulating cells that lack the Leu-8 lymph node homing receptor. *Gastroenterology*, **101**, 90–9.

Bienenstock, J. & Dolezel, J. (1971). Peyer's patches: lack of specific antibody-containing cells after oral and parenteral immunization. *Journal of Immunology*, **106**, 938–45.

Bienenstock, J. & Johnston, N. (1976). A morphological study of rabbit bronchial lymphoid aggregates and lymphoepithelium. *Laboratory Investigations*, **35**, 343–8.

Bjerke, K. & Brandtzaeg, P. (1986). Immunoglobulin- and J chain-producing cells associated with lymphoid follicles in the human appendix, colon and ileum, including Peyer's patches. *Clinical and Experimental Immunology*, **64**, 432–41.

Bjerke, K. & Brandtzaeg, P. (1988). Lack of relation between expression of HLA-DR and secretory component (SC) in follicle-associated epithelium of human Peyer's patches. *Clinical and Experimental Immunology*, **71**, 502–7.

Bjerke, K., Brandtzaeg, P. & Fausa, O. (1988). T cell distribution is different in follicle-associated epithelium of human Peyer's patches and villous epithelium. *Clinical and Experimental Immunology* **74**, 270–5.

Bland, P. W. & Warren, L. G. (1986*a*). Antigen presentation by epithelial cells of the rat small intestine. 1. Kinetics, antigen specificity and blocking by anti-Ia antisera. *Immunology*, **58**, 1–7.

Bland, P. W. & Warren, L. G. (1986*b*). Antigen presentation by epithelial cells of the rat small intestine. 2. Selective induction of suppressor T cells. *Immunology*, **58**, 9–14.

Braegger, C. P., Spencer, J. & MacDonald, T. T. (1992). The mucosal immune response: ontogenetic aspects. *International Journal of Clinical and Laboratory Research*, **22**, 1–4.

Brandtzaeg, P. (1987). The B cell system. *In Food Allergy and Intolerance*, ed. J. Brostoff and S. B. Challacombe, pp. 11–155. London: Baillière Tindall.

Brandtzaeg, P., Bosnes, V., Halstensen, T. S., Scott, H., Sollid, L. M. & Valnes, K. N. (1989). T lymphocytes in human gut epithelium express preferentially the α/β antigen receptor and are often CD45/UCHL1-positive. *Scandinavian Journal of Immunology*, **30**, 123–8.

Brandtzaeg, P. & Bjerke, K. (1990). Immunomorphological characteristics of human Peyer's patches. *Digestion*, **46**(Suppl. 2), 262–73.

Bridges, R. A., Condie, R. M., Zak, S. J. & Good, R. A. (1959). The morphologic basis of antibody formation development during the neonatal period. *Journal of Laboratory and Clinical Medicine*, **53**, 331–59.

Bull, D. M. & Bookman, M. A. (1977). Isolation and functional characterisation of human intestinal mucosal lymphoid cells. *Journal of Clinical Investigation*, **59**, 966–74.

Bye, W. A., Allan, C. H. & Trier, J. S. (1984). Structure, distribution, and origin of M cells in Peyer's patches of mouse ileum. *Gastroenterology*, **86**, 789–801.

Cerf-Bensussan, N., Jarry, A., Brousse, N., Lisowska-Grospierre, B., Guy-Grand, D. & Griscelli, C. (1987). A monoclonal antibody (HML1) defining a novel membrane molecule present on human intestinal lymphocytes. *European Journal of Immunology*, **17**, 1279–85.

Challacombe, S. J. & Tomasi, T. B. (1987). Oral tolerance. *In Food Allergy and Intolerance*, edited by J. Brostoff and S. B. Challacombe, pp. 255–268. London: Baillière Tindall.

Choy, M-Y., Richman, P. I., Walker-Smith, J. A. & MacDonald, T. T. (1990*a*). Differential expression of CD25 on lamina propria T cells and macrophages in the intestinal lesions in Crohn's disease and ulcerative colitis. *Gut*, **31**, 1365–70.

Choy, M-Y., Richman, P. I., Horton, M. E. & MacDonald, T. T. (1990*b*). Expression of the VLA family of integrins in human intestine. *Journal of Pathology*, **160**: 35–40.

Cornes, J. S. (1965). Number, size, and distribution of Peyer's patches in the human small intestine. Part 1. The development of Peyer's patches. *Gut*, **6**: 225–9. Part 2. The effect of age on Peyer's patches. *Gut*, **6**: 230–3.

Crabbe, P. A. & Heremans, J. F. (1966). The distribution of immunoglobulin containing cells along the human gastrointestinal tract. *Gastroenterology*, **51**, 305–16.

Crago, S. S., Kutteh, W. H., Moro, I., Allansmith, M. R., Radl, J., Haaijman, J. J. & Mestecky, J. (1984). Distribution of IgA1-IgA2-, and J chain-containing cells in human tissues. *Journal of Immunology*, **132**, 16–18.

Cunningham-Rundles, C. (1987). Failure of antigen exclusion. In *Food Allergy and Intolerance*, ed. J. Brostoff and S. B. Challacombe, pp. 223–236. London: Baillière Tindall.

Delventhal, S., Brandis, A., Ostertag, H. & Pabst, R. (1992). Low incidence of bronchus-associated lymphoid tissue (BALT) in chronically inflamed human lungs. *Virchow's Archiv B Cell Pathology*, **62**: 271–4.

Dukes, C. & Bussey, H. J. R. (1926). The number of lymphoid follicles of the human large intestine. *Journal of Pathology and Bacteriology*, **29**: 111–16.

Fujihashi, K., Taguchi, T., Aicher, W. K. (1992). Immunoregulatory functions for murine intraepithelial lymphocytes: γδ T cell receptor-positive (TCR+) T cells abrogate oral tolerance, while αβ TCR+ T cells provide B cell help. *Journal of Experimental Medicine*, **175**, 695–707.

Fujimura, Y., Hosobe, M. & Kihara, T. (1992). Ultrastructural study of M cells from colonic lymphoid follicles obtained by colonoscopic biopsy. *Digestive Diseases Sciences*, **37**, 1089–98.

Gebbers, J.-O. & Laissue, J. A. (1990). Post-natal immunomorphology of the gut. In *Inflammatory Bowel Disease and Coeliac Disease in Children*, ed. F. Hadziselimovic, B. Herzog, A. Burgin-Wolff, pp. 3–42. Dordrecht: Kluwer Academic Publishers.

Groh, V., Porcelli, S., Fabbi, M. (1989). Human lymphocytes bearing the T cell receptor γ/δ are phenotypically diverse and evenly distributed throughout the lymphoid system. *Journal of Experimental Medicine*, **169**, 1277–94.

Gruskay, F. L. & Cooke, R. E. (1955). Gastrointestinal absorption of unaltered protein in normal infants and in infants recovering from diarrhea. *Pediatrics*, **16**, 763–9.

Halstensen, T. S., Scott, H. & Brandtzaeg, P. (1989) Intraepithelial T cells of the TcRγ/δ+ CD8− and Vδ1/Jδ1+ phenotypes are increased in coeliac disease. *Scandinavian Journal of Gastroenterology*, **30**, 665–72.

Halstensen, T. S., Farstad, I. N., Scott, H., Fausa, O. & Brandtzaeg, P. (1990). Intraepithelial TcR α/β+ lymphocytes express CD45R0 more often than the TcR γδ+ counterparts in coeliac disease. *Immunology*, **71**, 460–6.

Halstensen, T. S. & Brandtzaeg, P. (1993) Activated T cells in the celiac lesion: non-proliferative activation (CD25) of CD4+ αβ cells in the lamina propria but proliferation (Ki-67) of αβ and γδ cells in the epithelium. *European Journal of Immunology*, **23**, 505–10.

Hashimoto, Y. & Komuro, T. (1988). Close relationships between the cells of the immune system and the epithelial cells in the rat small intestine. *Cell Tissue Research*, **254**, 41–47.

Hassall, E. & Dimmick, J. E. (1991). Unique features of *Helicobacter pylori* disease in children. *Digestive Diseases Sciences*, **36**, 417–23.

Higgins, P. J. & Weiner, H. L. (1988). Suppression of experimental autoimmune encephalitis by oral administration of myelin basic protein and its fragments. *Journal of Immunology*, **140**, 440–5.

Hume, D. A., Allan, W., Hogan, P. G. & Doe, W. F. (1987). Immunohistochemical characterisation of macrophages in human liver and gastrointestinal tract, Expression of CD4, HLA-DR, OKM1, and the mature macrophage marker 25F9 in normal and diseased tissue. *Journal of Leukocyte Biology*, **42**, 474–84.

Husby, S. (1988). Dietary antigens: uptake and humoral immunity in man. *Acta Pathologica Microbiologica Immunologica Scandinavica*, **96** (Suppl. 1), 1–40.

Hyjek, E. & Isaacson, P. G. (1988). Primary B cell lymphoma of the thyroid and its relationship to Hashimoto's thyroiditis. *Human Pathology*, **19**, 1315–26.

Hyjek, E., Smith, W. J. & Isaacson, P. G. (1988). Primary B-cell lymphoma of salivary glands and its relationship to myoepithelial sialadenitis. *Human Pathology*, **19**, 766–76.

Jacob, E., Baker, S. J. & Swaminathan, S. P. (1987). 'M' cells in the follicle-associated epithelium of the human colon. *Histopathology*, **11**, 941–52.

Janossy, G., Tidman, N., Selby, W. S. *et al.* (1980). Human T lymphocytes of inducer and suppressor type occupy different microenvironments. *Nature*, **288**, 81–4.

Jarry, A., Cerf-Bensussan, N., Brousse, N., Selz, F. & Guy-Grand, D. (1990). Subsets of CD3+ T cell receptor ($\alpha\beta$ or $\gamma\delta$) and CD3-lymphocytes isolated from normal human gut epithelium display phenotypical features different from their counterparts in peripheral blood. *European Journal of Immunology*, **20**, 1097–104.

Kaetzel, C. S., Robinson, J. K., Chintalacharuvu, K. R., Vaerman, J-P. & Lamm, M. E. (1991). The polymeric immunoglobulin receptor (secretory component) mediated transport of immune complexes across epithelial cells: a local defense function for IgA. *Proceedings of the National Academy of Sciences, USA*, **88**, 8796–800.

Kazi, J. I., Sinniah, R., Jaffrey, N. A. *et al.* (1989). Cellular and humoral immune responses in *Campylobacter pylori*-associated chronic gastritis. *Journal of Pathology*, **159**, 231–7.

Kett, K., Brandtzaeg, P. & Fausa, O. (1988). J-chain expression is more prominent in immunoglobulin A2 than in immunoglobulin A1 colonic immunocytes and is decreased in both subclasses associated with inflammatory bowel disease. *Gastroenterology*, **94**, 1419–25.

Komuro, T. (1985). Fenestrations of the basal lamina of intestinal villi in the rat. *Cell Tissue Research*, **239**, 183–8.

Korenblat, P. E., Rothberg, R. M., Minden, P. & Farr, R. S. (1968). Immune responses of human adults after oral and parenteral exposure to bovine serum albumin. *Journal of Allergy*, **41**, 226–35.

Koyoma, S. & Podolsky, D. K. (1989). Differential expression of transforming growth factors α and β in rat intestinal epithelial cells. *Journal of Clinical Investigation*, **83**, 1768–73.

Langman, J. M. & Rowland, R. (1992). Density of lymphoid follicles in the rectum and anorectal junction. *Journal of Clinical Gastroenterology*, **14**, 81–4.

MacDonald, T. T., Spencer, J, Viney, J. L., Williams, C. B. & Walker-Smith, J. A. (1987). Selective biopsy of Peyer's patches during ileal endoscopy. *Gastroenterology*, **93**, 1356–62.

Madara, J. L. & Stafford, J. (1989). Interferon-γ directly affects barrier function of cultured intestinal epithelial monolayers. *Journal of Clinical Investigation*, **83**, 724–7.

Marsh, M. N. (1985). Studies of intestinal lymphoid tissue V. Functional and structural aspects of the epithelial lymphocyte, with implications for coeliac disease and tropical sprue. *Scandinavian Journal of Gastroenterology*, **20** (Suppl. 114), 55–75.

Mayer, L. & Shlien, R. (1987). Evidence for function of Ia molecules on gut epithelial cells in man. *Journal of Experimental Medicine*, **166**, 1471–83.

McClugage, S. G., Low, F. N. & Zimny, M. L. (1986). Porosity of the basement membrane overlying Peyer's patches in rats and monkeys. *Gastroenterology*, **91**, 1128–33.

Mestecky, J., Lue, C. & Russell, M. W. (1991). Selective transport of IgA. *Gastroenterology Clinics of North America*, **20**, 441–71.

Miller, A., Lider, O., Roberts, A. B., Sporn, M. B. & Weiner, H. L. (1992). Suppressor T cells generated by oral tolerization to myelin basic protein suppress both in vitro and in vivo immune responses by the release of transforming growth factor β after antigen-specific triggering. *Proceedings of the National Academy of Sciences, USA*, **89**, 421–5.

Nash, S., Parkos, C., Nusrat, A., Delp, C. & Madara, J. L. (1991). In vitro model of intestinal crypt abscess. *Journal of Clinical Investigation*, **87**, 1474–7.

O'Leary, A. D. & Sweeney, E. C. (1986). Lymphoglandular complexes of the colon, structure and distribution. *Histopathology*, **10**, 267–83.

22 T. T. MacDONALD and J. SPENCER

Owen, R. L. & Jones, A. L. (1974). Epithelial cell specialization within human Peyer's patches, an ultrastructural study of intestinal lymphoid follicles. *Gastroenterology*, **66**, 189–203.

Owen, R. L. (1977). Sequential uptake of horseradish peroxidase by lymphoid follicle epithelium of Peyer's patches in normal unobstructed mouse intestine, an ultrastructural study. *Gastroenterology*, **72**, 440–51.

Owen, R. L., Apple, R. T. & Bhalla, D. K. (1986). Morphometric and cytochemical analysis of lysosomes in rat Peyer's patch follicle epithelium, their reduction in volume fraction and acid phosphatase content in M cells compared to adjacent enterocytes. *Anatomical Record*, **216**, 521–7.

Pabst, R. (1992) Is BALT a major component of the human lung immune system? *Immunology Today*, **13**, 119–22.

Pavli, P, Hume, D. A., Van de Pol, E. & Doe, W. F. (1993). Dendritic cells, the major antigen presenting cells of the human colonic lamina propria. *Immunology*, **78**, 132–41.

Peri, B. A. & Rothberg, R. M. (1981). Specific suppression of antibody production in young rabbit kits after maternal ingestion of bovine serum albumin. *Journal of Immunology*, **127**, 2520–5.

Perkkio, M. & Savilahti, E. (1980). Time of appearance of immunoglobulin-containing cells in the mucosa of the neonatal intestine. *Pediatric Research*, **14**, 953–5.

Radema, S. A., Van Deventer, S. J. H. & Cerami, A. (1991). Interleukin 1β is expressed predominately by enterocytes in experimental colitis. *Gastroenterology*, **100**, 1180–6.

Robertson, D. M., Paganelli, R., Dinwiddie, R. & Levinsky, R. J. (1982). Milk antigen absorption in the preterm and term neonate. *Archive of Diseases of Childhood*, **57**, 369–72.

Rothberg, R. M. & Farr, R. S. (1965). Anti-bovine serum albumin and anti-alpha lactalbumin in the serum of children and adults. *Pediatrics*, **35**, 571–88.

Sanderson, I. R. & Walker, W. A. (1993a). Uptake and transport of macromolecules by the intestine: possible role in clinical disorders (an update). *Gastroenterology*, **104**, 622–39.

Sanderson, I. R. & Walker, W. A. (1993b). Expression of B7 in the gut epithelium. *Immunology*, **79**, 434–8.

Sato, A., Chida, K., Iwata, M. & Hayakawa, H. (1992). Study of bronchus-associated lymphoid tissue in patients with diffuse pan bronchiolitis. *American Review Respiratory Diseases*, **146**, 473–478.

Scott, H., Solheim, B. G., Brandtzaeg, P. & Thorsby, E. (1980). HLA-DR-like antigens in the epithelium of the human small intestine. *Scandinavian Journal of Immunology*, **12**, 77–82.

Scott, H., Rognum, T. O., Midtvedt, T. & Brandtzaeg, P. (1985). Age-related changes of human serum antibodies to dietary and colonic bacterial antigens measured by an enzyme-linked immunosorbent assay. *Acta Pathologica Microbiologica Immunologica Scandinavica* Sect. C, **93**, 65–70.

Selby, W. S., Janossy, G., Mason, D. Y. & Jewell, D. P. (1983a). Expression of HLA-DR antigens by colonic epithelium in inflammatory bowel disease. *Clinical Experimental Immunology*, **53**, 614–18.

Selby, W. S., Poulter, L. W., Hobbs, S., Jewell, D. P. & Janossy, G. (1983b). Heterogeneity of HLA-DR-positive histiocytes in human intestinal lamina propria, a combined histochemical and immuno histological analysis. *Journal of Clinical Pathology*, **36**, 379–84.

Shepherd, N. A., Crocker, P. R., Smith, A. P. & D. Levison, D. A. (1987). Exogenous pigment in Peyer's patches. *Human Pathology*, **18**: 50–4.

Shirota, K., LeDuy, L., Yuan, S. & Jothy, S. (1990). Interleukin-6 and it's receptor are expressed in human intestinal epithelial cells. *Virchow's Archiv B Cell Pathology*, **58**, 303–8.

Sicinski, P., Rowinski, J., Warchol, J. B. *et al.* (1990). Poliovirus type 1 enters the human host through intestinal M cells. *Gastroenterology*, **98**, 56–8.

Spencer, J., Finn, T. & Isaacson, P. G. (1986a). Human Peyer's patches, an immunohisto-chemical study. *Gut*, **27**, 405–10.

Spencer, J. Finn, T. & Isaacson, P. G. (1986*b*). A comparative study of the gut-associated lymphoid tissue of primates and rodents. *Virchow's Archive [Cell Pathology]*, **51**, 509–19.

Spencer, J., Finn, T. & Isaacson, P. G. (1986*c*). Expression of HLA-DR antigens on epithelium associated with lymphoid tissue in the human gastrointestinal tract. *Gut*, **27**, 153–7.

Spencer, J., MacDonald, T. T., Diss, T. C., Walker-Smith, J. A., Ciclitira, P. J. & Isaacson, P. G. (1989*a*). Changes in intraepithelial lymphocyte sub-populations in coeliac disease and enteropathy associated T cell lymphoma (malignant histiocytosis of the intestine). *Gut*, **30**, 339–46.

Spencer, J., Isaacson, P. G., Diss, T. C. & MacDonald, T. T. (1989*b*). Expression of disulphide linked and non-disulphide linked forms of the T cell receptor gamma/delta heterodimer in human intestinal intraepithelial lymphocytes. *European Journal of Immunology*, **19**, 1335–9.

Spencer, J. & Isaacson, P. G. (1992). Immunology of gastrointestinal lymphoma. In *Immunology of Gastrointestinal Disease*, edited by T. T. MacDonald, pp. 193–208, Kluwer Academic Publishers, Dordrecht.

Sturgess, R. P., Macartney, J. C., Makgoba, M. W., Hung, C.-H., Haskard, D. O. & Ciclitira, P. J. (1990). Differential upregulation of intercellular adhesion molecule-1 in coeliac disease. *Clinical Experimental Immunology*, **82**, 489–92.

Tomasi, T. B., Tan, E. M., Soloman, E. A. & Prendergast, R. A. (1965). Characterisation of an immune system common to certain external secretions. *Journal of Experimental Medicine*, **121**, 101–24.

Trejdosiewicz, L. K., Smart, C. J., Oakes, D. J. *et al.* (1989). Expression of T-cell receptors TcR1 ($\gamma\delta$) and TcR2 ($\alpha\beta$) in the human intestinal mucosa. *Immunology*, **68**, 7–12.

Trier, J. S. (1991). Structure and function of intestinal M cells. *Gastroenterology Clinics of North America*, **20**, 531–48.

Vandenplas, Y., Hauser, B., Van den Borre, C., Sacre, L. & Dab, I. (1992). Effect of a whey hydrolysate prophylaxis on atopic disease. *Annals of Allergy*, **68**, 419–24.

Walker, A. W., Isselbacher, K. J. & Bloch, K. J. (1972). Intestinal uptake of macromolecules: effect of oral immunization. *Science*, 608–10.

Weaver, L. T., Laker, M. F. & Nelson, R. (1984). Intestinal permeability in the newborn. *Archives of Diseases of Childhood*, **59**, 236–41.

Weiner, H. L., Mackin, G. A., Matsui, M. *et al.* (1993). Double-blind trial of oral tolerization with myelin antigens in multiple sclerosis. *Science*, **259**, 1321–4.

Wilders, M. M., Drexhage, H. A., Kokje, M., Verspaget, H. & Meuwissen, G. M. (1984). Veiled cells in chronic idiopathic inflammatory bowel disease. *Clinical Experimental Immunology*, **55**, 377–87.

Wolf, J. L., Rubin, D. H., Finberg, R., Kauffman, R. S., Sharpe, A. H., Trier, J. S. & Fields, B. N. (1981). Intestinal M cells, A pathway for entry of reovirus into host. *Science*, **212**, 471–2.

Wotherspoon, A. C., Ortiz-Hitalgo, C., Falzon, M. R. & Isaacson, P. G. (1991). *Helicobacter pylori*, associated gastritis and primary B-cell gastric lymphoma. *Lancet*, **338**, 1175–6.

Wyatt, J. I. & Rathbone, B. J. (1988). Immune response of the gastric mucosa to *Campylobacter pylori*. *Scandinavian Journal of Gastroenterology*, **23** (Suppl. 142), 44–9.

Zeiger, R. S., Heller, S., Mellon, M. H. *et al.* (1989). Effect of combined maternal and infant food-allergen avoidance on development of atopy in early infancy: a randomized study. *Journal of Allergy and Clinical Immunology*, **84**, 72–89.

–2–
Lymphocyte migration to the gut mucosa

CLIFFORD A. OTTAWAY

Introduction

Populations of T and B cells in the lymphoid compartments of the intestine are continuously remodelled by selective migration of lymphocytes. Although many aspects of this migration have been well reviewed elsewhere (Reynolds, 1988; Ottaway, 1990; Salmi & Jalkanen, 1991; Picker & Butcher, 1992; Ottaway & Husband, 1992), there have been rapid changes recently in our understanding of these processes, especially as they apply to the human intestine. The purposes of this chapter are to provide a brief overview of the physiological basis of lymphocyte migration in the intestine, to highlight some emerging concepts of its regulation at the cellular and molecular level and to examine aspects of these processes that relate to our understanding of immune and inflammatory events in the intestine.

Physiology of lymphocyte migration to the intestine

A substantial proportion of the 10^{11} to 10^{12} lymphocytes that exit the thoracic duct to enter the subclavian vein each day (Pabst, 1988), will have passed through the intestine. Three distinct lymphoid domains are present in the intestine (Fig. 2.1). The aggregated gut associated lymphoid tissues (GALT) include the Peyer's patches (PP), the appendix, the lymphoid nodules of the colon, the rectum and the pharynx. In response to luminal antigen, the GALT tissues generate activated B and T cells which can populate the effector lymphoid domains of the mucosa (Brandtzaeg et al., 1991). The mucosal effector compartments include the epithelial layer, where intraepithelial lymphocytes (IEL) are interposed between approximately every fifth to fifteenth epithelial cell (Cerf-Bensussan & Guy-Grand, 1991) and the lamina propria, the volume of which is up to 50% lymphoid (Lee, Schiller & Fordtran, 1988).

The constitutents of the mucosal lymphoid compartments differ. GALT tissues such as Peyer's patches have fewer T cells and more B cells than do other secondary lymphoid tissues (Fig. 2.2), but T cells predominate within

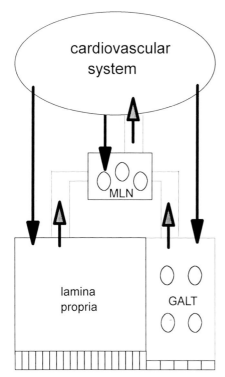

Fig. 2.1. Principal pathways of lymphoid cell migration in the intestine. Solid arrowheads indicate blood-borne cells; hatched arrowheads indicate lymph-borne cells. GALT = gut associated lymphoid tissue; MLN = mesenteric lymph nodes.

the lamina propria and the epithelium (Fig. 2.3). Physiological continuity between these compartments is provided, in large part, by the migration of lymphocytes from one site to another by means of the blood, but the lymphocyte populations of the intestine are not simple filtrates of those available in the blood (Fig. 2.2, 2.3).

What factors regulate the assembly of lymphocytes in these intestinal compartments? Several organising concepts can be used to describe our current understanding of lymphocyte migration and accumulation in the intestine (Table 2.1). First, the extent of migration of lymphocytes through the intestine differs in regions containing GALT tissues compared to regions of absorptive mucosa. For example, the rate at which lymphocytes exit the intestine, via the lymphatics in Peyer's patch-containing regions, is approximately ten-fold higher than it is in lymphatics draining the absorptive mucosa (Baker, 1933; Steer; 1988). Moreover, if resting lymphocytes are obtained from thoracic duct lymph (TDL), intestinal (pre-nodal) lymph, or

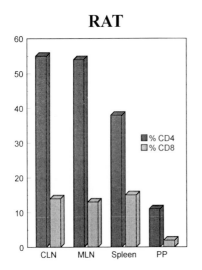
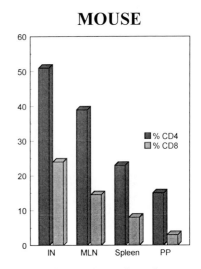

Fig. 2.2. T cell constituents of secondary lymphoid tissues. Data adapted from Koornstra *et al.* (1993) for the rat, and Ottaway (1989) for the mouse. CLN = cervical lymph nodes; MLN = mesenteric lymph nodes; PP = Peyer's patch; IN = inguinal lymph nodes.

Table 2.1. *General features of lymphocyte migration to the intestine*

Migration differs in GALT vs. lamina propria.
Migration varies with the state of activation of lymphocytes.
Migration depends on phenotype of lymphocytes (i.e. B vs CD4 vs CD8).
Lymphocytes interact with endothelial cells in post-capillary venules.
Lymphocytes interact with stroma.
Adhesion receptor-counter receptor interactions dominate the interaction of
  lymphocytes with the endothelium and the stroma.
Migration and adhesion interactions vary with immune and inflammatory events.

from mesenteric lymph nodes (MLN) or the Peyer's patches (Gowans & Knight, 1964; Hall, Parry & Smith, 1972; Hall, Scollay & Smith, 1976; Smith & Ford, 1983; Ottaway, 1982), they will after infusion into the blood stream, accumulate more rapidly in Peyer's patches than they will in adjacent regions of the absorptive intestine. In contrast, if rapidly dividing lymphocytes (lymphoblasts) which have been activated *in vivo* are obtained from the TDL, Peyer's patch, or the MLN and infused into the blood stream, these cells accumulate rapidly within the lamina propria (Hall *et al.*, 1976; Smith, Martin & Ford, 1980; Guy-Grand, Griscelli & Vassalli, 1974; Rose,

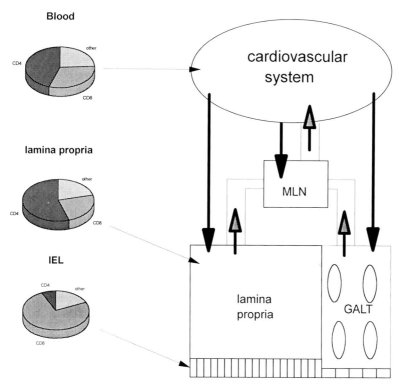

Fig. 2.3. Lymphocyte constituents of human blood and lamina propria and epithelial layer of the intestine. Data adapted from Schiefferdecker *et al.* (1992) for lamina propria and blood, and from Cerf-Bensussan & Guy-Grand (1991) for the intraepithelial lymphocytes. Each pie chart represents the proportions of T cell subsets and other lymphocytes in that compartment.

Parrott & Bruce, 1976*a,b*) and at least some of them can reach the epithelial compartment (Guy-Grand, Griscelli & Vassalli, 1978).

Net accumulation depends upon the balance of the rate at which migrating cells are admitted from the blood and the rate at which they depart from the tissue and both admission and departure depend upon the phenotype of the lymphocytes involved. For example, the accumulation of MLN lymphoblasts in the lamina propria results largely from prolonged retention of these cells in the tissue compared to small lymphocytes, rather than a difference in admission (Ottaway, 1982; Ottaway, Bruce & Parrott, 1983). In contrast, the retention of small lymphocytes is greater in GALT tissues than it is in the absorptive mucosa (Smith & Ford, 1983; Ottaway, 1988).

In general, the ability of T and B cells to migrate through GALT structures is similar in many species. In sheep, labelled B or T lymphocytes

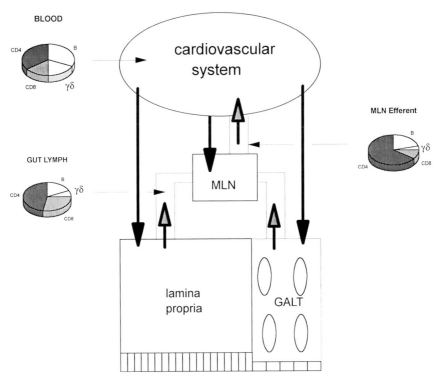

Fig. 2.4. Lymphocyte constitutents in cardiovascular and lymphatic spaces in the sheep. Each pie chart represents the proportions of T and B cell types in the compartment indicated. Data adapted from Mackay *et al.* (1990, 1992), and from Washington *et al.* (1988) and Kimpton *et al.* (1989).

obtained from intestinal lymph and transfused intravenously reappear in mesenteric or intestinal lymph at a similar rate (Reynolds, 1988; Cahill *et al.*, 1977) and, in rats, B and T cells from the thoracic duct accumulate equivalently in Peyer's patches (Fossum, Smith & Ford, 1983*a*,*b*). There are, however, differences in GALT migration for the major T cell subsets examined. In mice, the rate of admission of CD4 T cells into Peyer's patches from the blood is twice as great as that for the admission of CD8 T cells (Fisher and Ottaway, 1991). A very similar difference in the entry of blood-borne CD4 and CD8 cells has been inferred from the distribution of T cell subsets between the blood and the lymph draining the ileocaecal regions of the sheep (Washington, Kimpton & Cahill, 1988; Kimpton, Washington & Cahill, 1989). The distribution of T and B cells in the blood and intestinal lymph of sheep (Fig. 2.4) shows that CD4 and CD8 T cells are more concentrated in lymph draining the normal intestine than they are in the blood, while B cells and $\gamma\delta$ T cells are not (Mackay *et al.*, 1992). These steady-state differences reflect variation in the admission rates of these different cell types into the absorptive mucosa.

A lymphocyte in the blood can leave the intact blood stream by one of two routes. Either it reaches the splenic artery and enters the specialised lymphatic spaces surrounding the terminal branches of splenic arterioles (Pabst, 1988) or, in non-splenic tissues it migrates across the endothelial surface of postcapillary venules (PCV) (Ottaway, 1988). Thus, to reach lymphoid domains in the intestine, a blood-borne lymphocyte must arrive in the mesenteric vasculature and then attach to and cross the PCV endothelium in the GALT or in the lamina propria. In GALT organs, PCV are most prominent in the paracortical T cell areas of the lymphoid tissue, whereas in the lamina propria, PCV are most dense in the periglandular mucosa surrounding the crypts. The PCV endothelium of the GALT and lymph nodes is different from that which serves the lamina propria and permits much more lymphocyte attachment and transfer. The marked ability of lymphocytes to bind to the PCV endothelial cells in the GALT has been demonstrated in histological sections of Peyer's patches, after intravenous transfer of labelled lymphocytes (Gowans & Knight, 1964), at *in vivo* microscopy of fluorescent lymphocytes in Peyer's patch venules (Bjerknes, Cheng & Ottaway, 1986) by *in vitro* assays of lymphocyte attachment to rodent (Stamper & Woodruff, 1976, Gallatin, Weissman & Butcher, 1983), in human GALT tissues (Salmi & Jalkanen, 1991) and in cultures of Peyer's patch endothelial cells (Chin, Cai & Johnson, 1990). The attachment of migrating lymphocytes to the endothelium depends upon the interaction of different types of adhesion molecules at the surface of these cells.

Cellular and molecular biology of lymphocyte migration to the intestine

Four major groups of molecular determinants have been implicated in complementary adhesive interactions between lymphocytes and endothial cells. Those on lymphocytes include integrins, a leukocyte specific selectin and specific carbohydrate determinants (Table 2.2). Those on endothelial cells include members of the immunoglobulin-like super-family of cell adhesion molecules, site-specific mucin-like glycoprotein adhesins or addressins and endothelial selectins (Table 2.3).

Integrin and immunoglobulin-like adhesion molecules

Integrins are a diverse family of surface molecules that facilitate adhesion in many cell types (Haynes, 1992, Dustin & Springer, 1991). They consist of

Table 2.2. *Lymphocyte surface molecules involved in localization of lymphocytes in the intestine*

Molecule	Other names	Ligand(s)	Remarks
$\alpha_4\beta_1$ Integrin	VLA4	VCAM-1 MadCAM-1 Fibronectin	T and B cells
$\alpha_4\beta_7$ Integrin	LPAM	VCAM-1 MadCAM-1 Fibronectin	T and B cells
$\alpha_e\beta_7$ Integrin	HML-1	unknown	CD8 T cells
$\alpha_L\beta_2$ Integrin	LFA-1 CD11a/CD18	ICAM-1 ICAM-2	T and B cells
L-Selectin	Mel-14, Leu-8 determinant	MECA-79 determinant GlyCAM-1 others?	T and B cells
Sialyl Lewis X	CLA	E-selectin	T cells

dimers of α and β subunits, each of which occur in a variety of forms. Several integrins on lymphocytes contain β_1 chains and collectively these are referred to as the VLA (*very late after activation*) antigens (Hemler, 1990). Despite this name, many VLA proteins are expressed constitutively and alterations following activation can occur quickly.

One form of VLA, $\alpha_4\beta_1$, is very important in the interactions of lymphocytes with intestinal tissues. Fibronectin (Wayner *et al.*, 1989) is one ligand for $\alpha_4\beta_1$, so that this integrin may play an important role in lymphocyte interactions with the intestinal stroma, but $\alpha_4\beta_1$ can also participate in lymphocyte–endothelial interactions. Antibodies to the α_4 chain inhibit the binding of lymphocytes to the specialised PCV endothelium of murine Peyer's patches *in vitro* (Holzmann, McIntyre & Weissman, 1989) and inhibit the *in vivo* accumulation of lymphocytes in Peyer's patches in rats (Issekutz, 1991). In intact animals, either pretreatment of transferred lymphocytes, or systemic treatment of the recipients with anti-α_4, decreases the accumulation of lymphocytes in Peyer's patches by approximately 95%, but has no effect on the accumulation of migrating lymphocytes in subcutaneous lymph nodes (SCLN) (Issekutz, 1991). The $\alpha_4\beta_1$ integrin can bind to the vascular immunoglobulin-like cell adhesion molecule VCAM-1, on activated endothelium (Elices *et al.*, 1990; Issekutz & Wykretowicz, 1991), but this is not its usual ligand in the intestine. VCAM-1 is not normally expressed on the endothelium of either GALT or lamina propria PCV (Mackay *et al.*, 1992, Rice *et al.*, 1991). A mucosal endothelial adhesion cell

Table 2.3. *Endothelial surface molecules involved in localization of lymphocytes in the intestine*

Molecule	Other names	Ligand(s)	Remarks
MadCAM-1	Mucosal addressin MECA-367 determinant	$\alpha_4\beta_1$ Integrin $\alpha_4\beta_7$ Integrin $\alpha_L\beta_2$ Integrin?	Constitutive expression on Peyer's patch and lamina propria venules
GlyCAM-1		L-selectin	Constitutive expression on SCLN and Peyer's patch venules
PLN addressin	MECA 79 determinant	L-selectin	Constitutive expression on SCLN and Peyer's patch venules and in venules in colonic nodules
ICAM-2		$\alpha_L\beta_2$ Integrin	Constitutive expression on endothelia
ICAM-1	CD54	$\alpha_L\beta_2$ Integrin	Inducible by inflammation
VCAM-1	INCAM-110	$\alpha_4\beta_1$ Integrin $\alpha_4\beta_7$ Integrin	Inducible by inflammation
E-selectin	ELAM	Siayl Lewis X	Inducible by inflammation

molecule (i.e. MadCAM-1), recognised by the antibody MECA 367 (*murine* endothelial cell antibody (Streeter *et al.*, 1988; Nakache *et al.*, 1989), has been cloned and has two immunoglobulin-like extracellular domains: one with homology to human VCAM-1 and the rat intercellular adhesion molecule ICAM-1, and the other with homology to mouse VCAM-1 (Briskin, McEvoy & Butcher, 1993). Antibody to the α_4 chain inhibits the binding of lymphocytes to purified MadCAM-1 *in vitro* (Mackay & Imhof, 1993) and this molecule is likely the major ligand for α_4-containing integrins in the intestine.

The α_4 integrin chain can associate with another β chain designated by β_7 (previously βp) (Parker *et al.*, 1992; Holzmann & Weissman, 1989) and both the $\alpha_4\beta_7$ and $\alpha_4\beta_1$ participate in MadCAM-1-mediated adhesion of lymphocytes to the PCV endothelium in sections of Peyer's patches *in vitro* (Holtzmann and Weissman, 1989). Antibody to β_7, also inhibits lymphocyte binding to MadCAM-1 (Mackay & Imhof, 1993) and antibody to MadCAM-1 (i.e. MECA 367), inhibits the binding of lymphocytes to sections of Peyer's patches *in vitro* by approximately 90% (Streeter *et al.*, 1988). *In vivo*, pretreatment of recipient animals with anti-MadCAM-1 antibody, inhibits the localisation of tranferred lymphocytes in Peyer's patches by more than 95%, but does not alter the localisation of those cells in SCLN in the same animals (Streeter *et al.*, 1988). The localisation of migrating lymphocytes, in the MLN of anti-MadCAM-1 treated animals, is disturbed to a lesser extent than that to Peyer's patches (Streeter *et al.*, 1988).

Immunohistochemically, MadCAM-1 is expressed strongly by endothelial cells in PCV of Peyer's patches, more heterogeneously by those in the mesenteric nodes, but not by PCV in SCLN (Streeter *et al.*, 1988). PCV in the periglandular regions of the lamina propria of both the small and large intestine also express this determinant, although less intensely than does the endothelium in Peyer's patches (Streeter *et al.*, 1988).

A determinant called MLA (mucosal lymphocyte antigen), recognized by the antibodies HML-1 or BerACT 8 in humans (Cerf-Bensussan *et al.*, 1987; Picker *et al.*, 1990) and RGL-1 in rat (Cerf-Bensussan *et al.*, 1986) and M290 in mouse (Kilshaw & Murant, 1990), is expressed by approximately 40% of lamina propria lymphocytes, but only a small proportion of peripheral blood lymphocytes (Cerf-Bensussan *et al.*, 1987; Schiefferdecker *et al.*, 1992). This member of the integrins contains the β_7 subunit in association with an α chain designated as α_e (Parker *et al.*, 1992). The expression of $\alpha_e\beta_7$ appears not to be involved in lymphocyte endothelial interactions, but may be a key participant in the interaction of intraepithelial lymphocytes with epithelial cells. The migration of lymphocytes into the lamina propria or the intraepithelial compartment, is not affected in rats by treatments with the antibody RGL-1 (Cerf-Bensussan *et al.*, 1988) and the binding of human IELs to cytokine-activated endothelium, is not inhibited in the presence of BerACT antibodies (Cepek *et al.*, 1993). In contrast, the binding of human IELs to monolayers of intestinal epithelial cells is inhibited by about 75% in the presence of anti-$\alpha_e\beta_7$ antibodies (Cepek *et al.*, 1993). Thus, the expression of $\alpha_e\beta_7$ permits the adherence of IELs to some, as yet, unknown ligand on epithelial cells.

A further class of integrins use a chain designated as β_2. One of these, LFA-1 (lymphocyte function-associated antigen), has a unique α chain (α_L) and acts as an accessory molecule for the adhesion of lymphocytes to PCV endothelia. Antibodies to either α_L or β_2 inhibit the binding of human T cells *in vitro* to sections of lymph nodes, tonsils or appendix (Pals *et al.*, 1988) and antibodies to α_L inhibit the binding of murine lymphocytes to lymph node sections (Hamann *et al.*, 1988). Furthermore, when lymphocytes are transferred to recipient mice in conjunction with anti-α_L antibody, the accumulation of cells in both Peyer's patches and lymph nodes (subcutaneous or mesenteric) is reduced by approximately 50% compared to similar transfers in the absence of the antibody (Hamann *et al.*, 1988). Treatment with anti-α_L antibodies also disrupts the recruitment of lymphocytes into sites of immune reaction *in vivo*. For example, intraperitoneal administration of

anti-α_L to mice, prior to challenge with a contact sensitising agent, significantly decreased the subsequent delayed type hypersensitivity (DTH)
response and inhibited the normal increase in the mass and cellular content
of the lymph nodes draining the sensitised skin (Scheynius, Camp & Pure,
1993).

There are two known endothelial counter-ligands for the $\alpha_L\beta_2$ integrin,
both of which are also members of the immunoglobulin-like super-family of
adhesion molecules. ICAM-1 can be induced on endothelial cells in response to inflammatory cytokines (Dustin et al., 1986; Simmons, Makgoba
& Seed, 1988; Staunton et al., 1988) and treatment of animals with
antibodies to ICAM-1 can prolong renal allograft survival (Cosimi et al.,
1990), or partially inhibit the development of contact sensitisation reactions
(Scheynius et al., 1993) in vivo. A shorter, homologous molecule known as
ICAM-2 (Staunton, Dustin & Springer, 1989), is constitutively expressed on
normal endothelium and may be a predominant ligand for $\alpha_L\beta_2$ in the
absence of inflammatory stimulation cells. The finding that MadCAM-1
contains an ICAM-1-like region, however, suggests that this determinant
may also be a constitutive ligand for $\alpha_L\beta_2$ in mucosal PCVs.

Selectin and carbohydrate adhesion molecules

An important class of adhesion proteins that is involved in lymphocyte
migration is referred to as selectins. This name signifies their lectin-like
nature and their selective distribution. The prototype is L-selectin, which is
expressed by both B and T lymphocytes. Other names by which it has been
known include LECAM-1, LAM-1, gp90^{mel}, and Leu-8 antigen in humans
and the antigen recognised by the monoclonal Mel-14 in mice (Bevilacqua et
al., 1991; Spertini et al., 1991; Picker & Butcher, 1992; Bevilacqua, 1993). L-
selectin is a major contributor to the adhesion of lymphocytes to the
specialised endothelium of the PCV of lymph nodes. Although originally
viewed as a specific adhesion molecule for lymphocyte binding in SCLN
(Gallatin et al., 1983), L-selectin also participates in the in vivo attachment of
lymphocytes to the PCV of Peyer's patches. In mice, anti-L-selectin antibody treatment markedly inhibits the localisation of lymphocytes in subcutaneous lymph nodes and produces partial inhibition of Peyer's patch
lymphocyte accumulation (approximately 50%), when the Fab fragment of
the Mel-14 antibody is used (Hamann et al., 1991).

Two endothelial ligands for L-selectin have been identified. One, the
determinant recognised by the antibody MECA 79, is referred to as the
peripheral lymph node addressin (Streeter, Rouse & Butcher, 1988; Berg et
al., 1991a). This is expressed on endothelium of PCV in subcutaneous lymph
nodes and mesenteric lymph nodes, in small quantities in Peyer's patches
and in the PCV of colonic lymphoid nodules (Bargatze, Streeter & Butcher,

1990). MECA 79 is not expressed, however, by endothelia in PCV of the lamina propria (Picker & Butcher, 1992). The other known ligand for L-selectin is a sulphated mucin-like cell adhesion molecule (GlyCAM-1) (Lasky et al., 1992). Up to 70% of the expressed molecule consists of o-linked carbohydrate and some portion(s) of this carbohydrate-containing region permits the binding of L-selectin (Lasky et al., 1992). GlyCAM-1 is expressed on the PCV endothelium of subcutaneous lymph nodes and mesenteric lymph nodes at high levels and at lower levels on the endo-thelium of Peyer's patches (Lasky et al., 1992). It is also of interest that MadCAM-1 contains a mucin-like region and, therefore, may be able to engage in the binding of selectin molecules (Briskin et al., 1993).

Specific oligosaccharide structures on lymphocytes can also participate in lymphocyte–endothelial interactions. Sialylated Lewis determinants have been identified as ligands for two selectin molecules that are expressed by endothelial cells (i.e. E-selectin and P-selectin) (Bevilacqua, 1993). Only a small proportion of circulating lymphocytes react with antibodies to these carbohydrate determinants, but one monoclonal antibody (HECA 452) reacts with a subset of T cells, with an apparent propensity to be recruited into the skin (Picker et al., 1991; Berg et al., 1991b). The endothelial ligand for this so-called cutaneous lymphocyte antigen (CLA) is E-selectin, which is induced on endothelial cells by inflammatory mediators (Picker et al., 1991; Bevilacqua et al., 1987).

The effect of immune and inflammatory events on lymphocyte migration to the intestine

B and T cells, that have not previously encountered antigen, express fairly uniform levels of the $\alpha_4\beta_1$ and $\alpha_L\beta_2$ integrins and L-selectin and recirculate extensively through the secondary lymphoid tissues. Following stimulation, two populations of daughter cells result: rapidly dividing lymphoblasts and a population of recirculating, antigen-specific memory cells that facilitate subsequent encounters to the same antigen (Fig. 2.5).

Lymphoblasts

Lymphoblasts migrate from their sites of stimulation into the blood stream and then to other tissues, to seed the local populations of plasma cells or T effector cells. Lymphoblasts have limited life-spans (hours to days) and tend not to recirculate after tissue arrival. The site at which B and T cells experience antigen stimulation, however, influences the accumulation sites

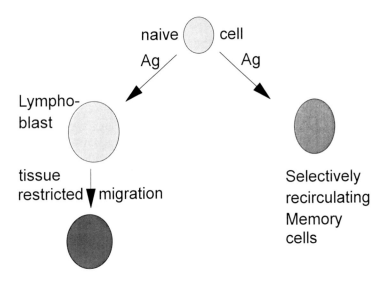

Fig. 2.5. Naive and antigen-experienced lymphocytes migrate in different patterns. Antigen activation in the intestine can lead to lymphoblasts
that accumulate in the lamina propria and recirculating memory cells
that have a biased recirculation through the intestine. See text for
details.

of their lymphoblast daughters. Lymphoblasts generated in subcutaneous
lymph nodes (LN) will accumulate in skin sites, but do not accumulate well
in the intestine (Hall *et al.*, 1972; Rose *et al.*, 1976*a,b*). In contrast,
lymphoblasts from the thoracic duct, MLN, or intestinal lymph accumulate
readily in the gut mucosa after transfers (Hall *et al.*, 1972; Smith *et al.*, 1980;
Rose *et al.*, 1976*a,b*; Guy-Grand *et al.*, 1974). The tendency of B lymphoblasts to colonise particular regions of the mucosa depends, as well, on their
regional origin within the intestine. For example, the transfer of thoracic
duct lymphoblasts from rats immunised with cholera toxin presented via the
colon, resulted in a greater density of antitoxin plasma cells in the colon than
in the duodenum of recipient animals (Pierce & Cray, 1982). In contrast, if
donor immunisation occurred at duodenal sites, the density of antitoxin
producing cells in lymphoblast recipients was greater in the duodenum than
in the colon (Pierce & Cray, 1982). These, and allied observations, have led
to the concept that lymphoblasts undergo specific changes in adhesion
behaviour, during activation, that encodes properties of the local stimulatory environment. The mechanisms underlying this process, however, are
still incompletely understood.

Murine MLN, or thoracic duct lymphoblasts accumulation in the intestine, is inhibited by anti-MadCAM-1 treatment of recipients animals. The degree of inhibition achieved is only about one half of that which affects the accumulation of small lymphocytes into the GALT tissues of similarly treated recipients (Picker & Butcher, 1992), suggesting that accessory mechanisms may be even more important than they are in the GALT. Activation of B and T cells *in vitro* leads to increased expression of $\alpha_L\beta_2$ and changes its activation (Haynes, 1992). For example, cross-linking of the T cell receptor strengthens the adhesiveness of $\alpha_L\beta_2$ to ICAM-1 *in vitro* (van Kooyk *et al.*, 1989; Dustin & Springer, 1991). Antigen activation generally also leads to increased expression of β_1 integrins (Hemler, 1990; Haynes, 1992). These include $\alpha_4\beta_1$, but also the forms $\alpha_2\beta_1$, $\alpha_5\beta_1$ and $\alpha_6\beta_1$ which provide binding sites for collagens, fibronectin and laminin respectively. These β_1 integrins can also be activated. For example, phorbol ester or antigen stimulation of T cells leads to activation of ligand binding by each of the above β_1 dimers *in vitro* (Shimizu *et al.*, 1990; Chan *et al.*, 1991; Wilkins *et al.*, 1991).

Integrin alterations may contribute to the enhanced retention of gut-derived lymphoblasts in the intestinal mucosa, but we do not yet understand the molecular basis for the exquisite intra-intestinal specificity of accumulation of gut programmed lymphoblasts.

Memory cells

Following resolution of an initial immunisation event, populations of lymphocytes are maintained in an animal that facilitate a rapid and pronounced response to secondary antigen exposure. An important concept that has emerged is that the lymphocytes that mediate this memory, also migrate differently to naive cells. At present, this notion is best established for T cells.

Memory is a functional rather than a physical property, but the expression of different isoforms of the leukocyte-common antigen CD45 (Thomas, 1989; Vitetta *et al.*, 1991; Gray, 1993) distinguishes populations of T cells that appear to be in fundamentally different physiological states and provides an heuristic marker of whether a T cell has had previous antigen experience. CD45 isoforms are generated by alternative splicing of several exons and those isoforms that are restricted in their expression on T cells, depending upon antigen experience, are referred to as CD45R determinants. In general, the isoforms that are expressed on antigen-experienced cells are smaller in molecular weight (MW) than those expressed by naive or inexperienced cells. For example, with human T cells, those that express a high MW form, CD45RA, can be distinguished from those T cells expressing a lower MW form, CD45R0, by their relatives with the monoclonal antibodies 2H4 and UCHL1 respectively (Thomas, 1989; Smith *et al.*, 1986; Terry, Brown & Beverley, 1988; Merckenschalger *et al.*, 1988; Akbar *et al.*, 1988).

These two T cell populations are in different physiological states. CD45R0-positive cells respond *in vitro* to recall antigens, whereas CD45RA-positive cells do not. Although both populations are much longer lived than lymphoblasts, CD45R0-positive cells have a mean lifetime *in vivo* of about 9 months, while that for CD45RA-positive cells is approximately 30 months (Mitchie *et al.*, 1992). At birth, virtually all peripheral blood T cells are CD45RA-positive, but the proportion of circulating CD45R0-positive cells increases steadily with age to reach a level of approximately 50% by young adulthood (Sanders *et al.*, 1988) and, *in vitro*, CD45RA bearing cells lose this marker and become CD45R0-positive upon activation in culture (Akbar *et al.*, 1988). Similar features of CD45R expression have been identified in rodents and sheep. Although at least some T cells bearing low MW isoforms of CD45R are able to revert to the expression of high MW forms *in vivo* in humans and rats (Mitchie *et al.*, 1992; Bell & Sparshott, 1990; Sparshott, Bell & Sarawar, 1991), the proposition that T cells expressing high MW forms such as CD45RA represent naive cells and that T cells expressing lower MW forms, such as CD45R0, have been previously activated and serve memory function, has found wide utility across species.

There are marked differences in the representation of CD45R phenotypes within the lymphoid domains of the human intestine. A large proportion of the T cells resident in the lamina propria are CD45R0-positive (Harvey, Jones & Wright, 1989; Janossy *et al.*, 1989) and 85–95% of the T cells isolatable from the lamina propria are of the CD45R0 phenotype (James *et al.*, 1986; Berg *et al.*, 1991c; Schiefferdecker *et al.*, 1992). Within the epithelium, IEL are approximately 90% CD45R0-positive (Cerf-Bensussan & Guy-Grand, 1991), but approximately 50% of T cells in GALT lymphoid nodules and as few as one-third of T cells in the parocortical regions of tonsillar lymphoid tissue, are CD45R0-positive (Janossy *et al.*, 1989).

In sheep, the partition of T cells between the blood and lymph compartments varies with CD45R phenotypes (Mackay, Marston & Dudler, 1990; Mackay *et al.*, 1992). Approximately 40% of blood T cells in sheep express a low MW form of CD45R and function like memory cells (Mackay *et al.*, 1990). In afferent lymph draining skin the T cells are almost entirely of the low MW CD45R phenotype, but in the lymph efferent from the node serving that area, approximately 80% of the T cells express the high MW isoform associated with naive cells (Mackay *et al.*, 1990; Mackay *et al.*, 1992). These observations imply that the ability of antigen-experienced T cells to migrate across the venules of the skin, is at least an order of magnitude greater than that of naive cells, whereas the ability of naive T cells to migrate into the subcutaneous lymph node is of the order of fourfold greater than that of the antigen experienced cells. Segregation on the basis of CD45R expression is not as extreme, however, in gut compartment T cells leaving the intestine in prenodal lymph which is made up of almost equal proportion of naive and memory cells (Mackay *et al.*, 1992). This suggests that, to a first approximation, the ability of T cells to exit from the blood across the PCVs serving the lamina propria, is similar for naive and memory cells. This need not be the case, however, if the memory cells have previously experienced the intestinal environment.

In sheep, lymphocytes emigrating from the gut show a preferential, but by no means exclusive, ability to recirculate through the intestine after reinfusion in the blood (Scollay, Hopkins & Hall, 1976; Cahill *et al.*, 1977; Chin & Hay, 1980). Mackay and co-workers re-examined this phenomenon in light of CD45R expression and found that when lymphocytes draining from the gut lymph were labelled fluorescently and reinfused, a proportion of the cells clearly showed an enhanced ability to reappear in the intestinal lymph and these were enriched for memory-like T cells (Mackay *et al.*, 1992). Interestingly, the relative proportion of the returning cells, that were CD4 or CD8 T cells, was unchanged from the original infusate, so that both of these subpopulations appear to share this ability. Thus, although memory cells do not appear to dominate the lymphocyte migration through the intestine to the same degree as they do in the skin, there is a small subset of antigen-experienced T cells that display definite enterotropic behaviour.

The altered pattern of adhesion molecules expressed by antigen-experienced T cells depends, in part, on the site of activation. During the transition of T cells to memory phenotype in lymph nodes and appendix, there is an equivalent increase in the expression of the integrin $\alpha_L\beta_2$ in both sites, but L-selectin expression is down-regulated on T cells activated in the appendix, but not on those activated in subcutaneous lymph nodes (Picker *et al.*, 1992). Circulating memory T cells also demonstrate selective patterns of expression of other integrins. Although CD45RA-positive T cells have homogenous and low levels of the α_4, α_6 and β_1 integrin subunits, the CD45R0-positive population contains subsets with heterogeneity in these markers (Horgan *et al.*, 1992). Some memory T cells express high levels of α_6 and β_1, some express high levels of α_4 and β_1, while others express high α_4 but low levels of β_1 (Horgan *et al.*, 1992). The constituents of the latter group may include $\alpha_4\beta_7$-bearing memory T cells previously activated in the intestine. In this regard, it is noteworthy that comparison of the CD45R0-positive cells in blood and lamina propria, shows a relative depletion of the expression of the β_1 integrin subunit in the mucosa (Fig. 2.6). Among the recirculating memory T cells in the sheep, those in gut prenodal lymph have high expression of α_4, but low expression of the α_6 and β_1 subunits, while those in skin lymph have high expression of each of these chains (Mackay *et al.*, 1992).

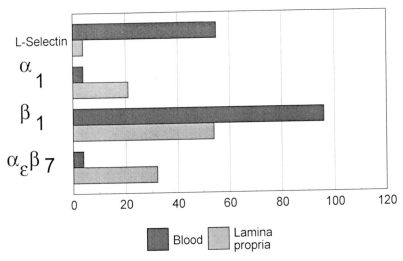

Fig. 2.6. Adhesion molecules on antigen-experienced T cells in human lamina propria and peripheral blood. Bars represent the percentage of CD45RA-positive T cells in each compartment expressing L-selectin and the indicated integrin subunits. Data adapted from Schiefferdecker *et al.* (1992).

Inflammatory events

The entry and retention of lymphocytes in the intestine can be regulated by inflammatory cytokines. Tumour necrosis factor-α (TNF-α) induces the expression of E-selectin (Bevilacqua *et al.*, 1987, 1989), ICAM-1 (Dustin *et al.*, 1986; Pober *et al.*, 1986) and VCAM-1 on endothelial cells (Rice & Bevilacqua, 1989; Rice, Munro & Bevilacqua, 1990; Schwartz *et al.*, 1990). Interleukin-1 (IL-1) has a similar profile of effects, though it is less potent, but other cytokines show more selectivity. For example, interferon-γ (IFNγ) does not include E-selectin of VCAM-1 expression directly, but augments the effect of TNF-α on E-selectin (Doukas & Prober, 1990, Leeuwenberg *et al.*, 1990). IFNγ also induces endothelial ICAM-1 expression (Dustin *et al.*, 1986, Pober *et al.*, 1986), but does not have an effect on VCAM-1 expression. Infusion of IFNγ into rats enhances the entry of T and B lymphocytes into many tissues and also promotes prolongation of their residence after entry (Westermann *et al.*, 1993).

The precise contribution of such effects in the diseased intestine is largely undetermined, but both E-selectin and ICAM-1 expression has been reported in the venules of the lamina propria of patients with Crohn's disease and ulcerative colitis (Ohtani *et al.*, 1992; Nakamura *et al.*, 1991).

Further assessments of the distribution of the other endothelial adhesion molecules during inflammatory diseases of the intestine are expected.

Several studies suggest that the specialized endothelium of the GALT structures also participates in the response to inflammation. Treatment of cultures of the specialised endothelial cells, from the PCV of Peyer's patches of rats with TNF-α, enhances their binding of lymphocytes (Chin et al., 1990). A similar response is seen with IFNγ treatment, but simultaneous treatment of the cultures with either IFNγ or TNF-α in the presence of transforming growth factor-β (TGF-β), abrogates the enhanced adhesion (Chin et al., 1992). Peyer's patch endothelial cell cultures also respond to IL-4 treatment with increased lymphocyte adhesiveness (Chin et al., 1991), but this effect is not blocked by TGF-β (Chin, Cai & Xu, 1992). Human endothelial cells can be induced to express VCAM-1 by stimulation with IL-4 (Thornhill & Haskard, 1990) and this may be the mechanism involved in the rat Peyer's patch endothelial cells, since the increased adhesiveness induced by IL-4 is blocked by antibody to the α_4 integrin chain (Chin et al., 1992). It will be important, however, to determine what effect cytokine signals can have on the expression of the polyvalent MadCAM-1 in both the GALT and the lamina propria.

Modulation of the effects of inflammation on lymphocyte migration is an important potential target for therapy. Corticosteroids affect the accumulation of lymphocytes in most tissues, including the mucosa (Walzer et al., 1984). Systemic treatment of experimental animals with pharmacological doses of corticosteroids impairs the ability of lymphocytes to migrate from the blood into lymphoid tissues (Cox & Ford, 1982), but alteration in the endothelial cells, rather than alterations in the adhesiveness of the lymphocytes, appear to be the major cause of this disturbance (Chung, Samlowski & Daynes 1986). Corticosteroid treatment alters the cytokine response of human subjects (Barber et al., 1993) and inhibits the production of endothelial E-selectin and ICAM-1 in response to cytokine stimulation (Cronstein et al., 1992).

Summary

The assembly of migrating lymphocytes in intestinal compartments results from a highly regulated set of eclectic processes. Selection of particular lymphocytes occurs at admission and by selective retention of appropriate cells. The cellular mechanisms involved respond to immune and inflammatory events in the intestine and some of the mechanisms are intestinally specific. The molecular basis for lymphocyte–endothelial interactions is beginning to be understood in fine detail, and a number of important groups of adhesion molecules have been identified. To date, the interactions of lymphocyte integrins such as $\alpha_4\beta_1$ and $\alpha_4\beta_7$ with the polyvalent endothelial adhesion molecule MadCAM are the best understood, but other contributors are likely to play important roles. Unlike the skin, which is very highly restrictive in admitting antigen-experienced cells, the intestine is a more open system. Both naive and experienced cells can enter the intestine, but in the lamina propria there is selective retention of antigen-experienced cells. A small, but important proportion of the T cells admitted to the intestine appear to represent an enterotropic population of memory T cells. Therapeutic interventions alter lymphocyte accumulation in the intestine and are likely to be an important area for further development. Although corticosteroids have important, but largely neglected, effects in this regard, agents that could more selectively interfere with adhesion events between lymphocytes, the endothelium and lymphocytes and the intestinal stroma, would be of great therapeutic benefit.

References

Akbar, A., Terry, L., Timms, A., Beverley, P. & Jannossy, G. (1988). Loss of CD45R and gain of UCHL 1 reactivity is a feature of primed T cells. *Journal of Immunology* **140**, 2171–8.

Baker, R. (1933). The cellular content of chyle in relation to lymphoid tissue and fat transportation. *Anatomical Record,* **55**, 207–21.

Barber, A., Coyle, S., Marano, M. *et al.* (1993). Glucocorticoid therapy alters hormonal and cytokine responses to endotoxin in man. *Journal of Immunology,* **150**, 1999–2006.

Bargatze, R., Streeter, P. & Butcher, E.C. (1990). Expression of low levels of peripheral lymph node-associated vascular addressin in mucosal lymphoid tissues: possible relevance to the dissemination of passaged AKR lymphomas. *Journal of Cell Biochemistry,* **42**, 1–9.

Bell, E. & Sparshott, S. (1990). Interconversion of CD45R subsets of CD4 T cells *in vivo.* *Nature,* **348**, 163–6.

Berg, E., Robinson, M., Warnock, R. & Butcher, E. C. (1991a). The human peripheral lymph node addressin is a ligand for LECAM-1, the peripheral lymph node homing receptor. *Journal of Cell Biology,* **114**, 343–9.

Berg, E., Robinson, M., Mansson, O., Butcher, E. & Magnami, J. (1991b). A carbohydrate domain common to sialyl Lea and sialyl Lex is recognized by the endothelial cell leukocyte adhesion molecule ELAM-1. *Journal of Biological Chemistry,* **23**, 14869–72.

Berg, M., Murakawa, Y., Camerini, D. & James, S. (1991c). Lamina propria lymphocytes are derived from circulating cells that lack the Leu-8 lymph node homing receptor. *Gastroenterology,* **101**, 90–9.

Bevilacqua, M., Pober, J., Mendrick, D., Cotran, R. & Gimbrone, M. (1987). Identification of an inducible endothelial–leukocyte adhesion molecule. *Proceedings of the National Academy of Science, USA,* **84**, 9238–42.

Bevilacqua, M., Stengelin, S., Gimbrone, M. & Seed, B. (1989). Endothelial leukocyte adhesion molecule-1: an inducible receptor for neutrophils related to complement regulatory proteins and lectins. *Science,* **243**, 1160–5.

Bevilacqua, M., Butcher, E. C., Furie, B. *et al.* (1991). Selectins: a family of adhesion receptors. *Cell* **67**, 233–4.

Bevilacqua, M. P. (1993). Endothelial–leukocyte adhesion molecules. *Annual Reviews in Immunology,* **11**, 767–804.

Bjerknes, M., Cheng, H. & Ottaway, C. A. (1986). Dynamics of lymphocyte endothelial interactions *in vivo*. *Science*, **231**, 402–5.

Brandtzaeg, P., Nilssen, D. E., Rognum, T. O. & Thrane, P. S. (1991). Ontogeny of the mucosal immune system and IgA deficiency. *Gastroenterology Clinics of North America*, **20**, 397–439.

Briskin, M., McEvoy, L. & Butcher, E. C. (1993). MadCAM-1 has homology to immuno-globulin and mucin-like adhesion receptors and to IgA1. *Nature*, **363**, 461–4.

Cahill, R., Poskitt, D., Frost, H. & Trnka, Z. (1977). Two distinct pools of recirculating T lymphocytes: migratory characteristics of nodal and intestinal T lymphocytes. *Journal of Experimental Medicine*, **145**, 420–6.

Cepek, K. L., Parker, C., Madara, J. & Brenner, M. B. (1993). Integrin mediates adhesion of T lymphocytes to epithelial cells. *Journal of Immunology*, **150**, 3459–70.

Cerf-Bensussan, N., Guy-Grand, D., Lisowska-Grospierre, B., Griscelli, C. & Bhan, A. (1986). A monoclonal antibody specific for rat intestinal lymphocytes. *Journal of Immunology*, **136**, 76–82.

Cerf-Bensussan, N. & Guy-Grand, D. (1991). Intestinal intraepithelial lymphocytes. *Gastroenterology Clinics of North America*, **20**, 549–76.

Cerf-Bensussan, N., Jarry, A., Brousse, N., Lisowska-Grospierre, B., Guy-Grand, D. & Griscelli, C. (1987). A monoclonal antibody (HML-1) defining a novel membrane molecule present on human intestinal lymphocytes. *European Journal of Immunology*, **17**, 1279–85.

Cerf-Bensussan, N., Jarry, A., Gneragbe, T. *et al.* (1988). Monoclonal antibodies specific for intestinal lymphocytes. *Monographs of Allergy*, **24**, 167–72.

Chan, B., Wong, J., Rao, A. & Hemler, M. (1991). T cell receptor-dependent antigen-specific stimulation of the murine T cell clone induces a transient VLA-protein-mediated binding to extracellular matrix. *Journal of Immunology*, **147**, 398–404.

Chin, W. & Hay, J. (1980). Comparison of lymphocyte migration through intestinal lymph nodes, subcutaneous lymph nodes and chronic inflammatory sites of sheep. *Gastroenterology*, **79**, 1231–9.

Chin, Y. H. Cai, J. & Johnson, K. (1990). Lymphocyte adhesion to cultured Peyer's patch high endothelial venules cells is mediated by organ specific homing receptors and can be regulated by cytokines. *Journal of Immunology*, **145**, 3669–77.

Chin, Y. H., Cai, J. & Xu, X. (1992). Transforming growth factor-beta 1 and IL4 regulate the adhesiveness of Peyer's patch high endothelial venule cells for lymphocytes. *Journal of Immunology*, **148**, 1106–12.

Chin, Y. H., Cai, J. & Xu, X. (1991). Tissue specific homing receptor mediates lymphocyte adhesion to cytokine stimulated lymph node high endothelial venule cells. *Immunology*, **74**, 478–83.

Chung, H., Samlowski, W. & Daynes, R. (1986). Modification of the murine immune system by glucorticosteroids: alterations of the tissue localization properties of circulating lympho-cytes. *Cellular Immunology*, **101**, 571–85.

Cosimi, A., Conti, D., Delmonico, F. *et al.* (1990). *In vivo* effects of monoclonal antibody to ICAM-1 (CD54) in nonhuman primates with renal allografts. *Journal of Immunology*, **144**, 4604–12.

Cox, J. & Ford, W. (1982). The migration of lymphocytes across specialized vascular endothelium IV. Prednisolone acts at several points on the recirculation pathway of lymphocytes. *Cellular Immunology*, **66**, 407–19.

Cronstein, B., Kimmel, S., Levin, R., Martiniuk, F. & Weissmann, G. (1992). A mechanism for the anti-inflammatory effects of corticosteroids: the glucocorticoid receptor regulates leukocyte adhesion to endothelial cells and expression of endothelial-leukocyte adhesion molecule 1 and intercellular adhesion molecule. *Proceedings of the National Academy of Sciences, USA*, **89**, 9991–5.

Doukas, J. & Prober, J. (1990). IFN-gamma enhances endothelial activation induced by tumor necrosis factor but not IL-1. *Journal of Immunology*, **145**, 1727–33.

Dustin, M. L., Rothlein, R., Bhan, A., Dinarello, C. & Springer, T. A. (1986). Induction by IL-1 and interferon: tissue distribution, biochemistry, and function of a natural adherence molecule (ICAM-1). Journal of Immunology, **137**, 245–52.

Dustin, M. L. & Springer, T. A. (1991). Role of lymphocyte adhesion receptors in transient interactions and cell locomotion. *Annual Reviews in Immunology*, **9**, 27–66.

Elices, M., Osborn, L., Takada, Y., Crouse, C., Luhowskyj, S., Hemler, M. & Lobb, R. R. (1990). VCAM-1 on activated endothelium interacts with the leukocyte integrin VLA-4 at a site distant from the VLA/fibronectin binding site. *Cell*, **60**, 577–83.

Fisher, L. & Ottaway, C. A. (1991). The kinetics of migration of murine CD4 and CD8 lymphocytes *in vivo*. *Regulation Immunology*, **3**, 156–62.

Fossum, S., Smith, M. & Ford, W. (1983a). The migration of lymphocytes across specialized vascular endothelium VII. The migration of T and B lymphocytes in the athymic rat. *Scandinavian Journal of Immunology*, **17**, 539–49.

Fossum, S., Smith, M. & Ford, W. (1983b). The recirculation of T and B lymphocytes in the athymic rat. *Scandinavian Journal of Immunology*, **17**, 551–7.

Gallatin, W. M., Weissman, I. L. & Butcher, E. C. (1983). A cell surface molecule involved in organ-specific homing of lymphocytes. *Nature*, **304**, 30–4.

Gowans, J. & Knight, E. (1964). The route of recirculation of lymphocytes in the rat. *Proceedings of the Royal Society (B)*, **59**, 257–82.

Gray, D. (1993). Immunological memory. *Annual Reviews in Immunology*, **11**, 49–77.

Guy-Grand, D., Griscelli, C. & Vassalli, P. (1974). The gut associated lymphoid system: nature and properties of the large dividing cells. *European Journal of Immunology*, **4**, 435–41.

Guy-Grand, D., Griscelli, C. & Vassalli, P. (1978). The mouse gut T lymphocyte: a novel type of T cell. *Journal of Experimental Medicine*, **148**, 1661–77.

Hall, J. G., Parry, D. & Smith, M. (1972). The distribution and differentiation of lymph-borne immunoblasts after intravenous transfer into syngeneic recipients. *Cell Tissue Kinetics*, **5**, 269–72.

Hamann, A., Jablonski-Westrich, D., Duijvestijn, A. *et al.* (1988). Evidence for an accessory role of LFA-1 in lymphocyte–high endothelium interaction during homing. *Journal of Immunology*, **140**, 693–9.

Hamann, A., Jablonski-Westrich, D., Jonas, P. & Thiele, H. (1991). Homing receptors reexamined: mouse LECAM-1 (Mel-14 antigen) is involved in lymphocyte migration into the gut associated lymphoid tissue. *European Journal of Immunology*, **21**, 2925–9.

Harvey, J., Jones, D. & Wright, D. (1989). Leucocyte common antigen expression on T cells in normal and inflamed human gut. *Immunology*, **68**, 13–17.

Haynes, R. O. (1992). Integrins: versatility, modulation and signalling in all adhesion. *Cell*, **69**, 11–25.

Hemler, M. E. (1990). VLA proteins in the integrin family: structures, functions and their role on leukocytes. *Annual Reviews in Immunology*, **8**, 365–400.

Holzmann, B., McIntyre, B. & Weissman, I. L. (1989). Identification of a murine Peyer's patch-specific lymphocyte homing receptor as an integrin molecule with an alpha chain homologous to human VLA-a. *Cell*, **56**, 37–46.

Holzmann, B. & Weissman, IL. (1989). Peyer's patch specific lymphocyte homing receptors consist of a VLA-4-like alpha chain associated with either of two integrin beta chains, one of which is novel. *EMBO Journal*, **8**, 1735.

Horgan, K., Ginther-Luce, G., Tanaka, Y. *et al.* (1992) Differential expression of VLA-alpha4 and VLA-beta-1 discriminates multiple subsets of CD4CD45R0 memory T cells. *Journal of Immunology*, **149**, 4082–7.

Issekutz, T. B. & Wykretowicz, A. (1991). Effect of a new monoclonal antibody, TA-2, that inhibits adherence to cytokine stimulated endothelium in the rat. *Journal of Immunology*, **147**, 109–14.

Issekutz, T. B. (1991). Inhibition of *in vivo* lymphocyte migration to inflammation and homing to lymphoid tissues by the TA-2 monoclonal antibody: a likely role for VLA-4 *in vivo*. *Journal of Immunology*, **147**, 4178–84.

James, S., Fiocchi, C., Graeff, A. & Strober, W. (1986). Phenotypic analysis of lamina propria lymphocytes. *Gastroenterology*, **91**, 1483–9.

Janossy, G., Bofill, M., Rowe, D., Muir, J. & Beverley, P. (1989). The tissue distribution of T lymphocytes expressing different CD45 polypeptides. *Immunology*, **66**, 517–25.

Kilshaw, P. & Murant, S. J. (1990). A new surface antigen on intraepithelial lymphocytes in the intestine. *European Journal of Immunology*, **20**, 2201–7.

Kimpton, W., Washington, E. & Cahill, R. (1989). Recirculation of lymphocyte subsets through gut and peripheral lymph nodes. *Immunology*, **66**, 69–75.

Koornstra, P., Duijvestijn, A., Viek, L., Marres, E. & van Breda Vriesman, J. (1993). Tonsillar (Waldyer's ring equivalent) lymphoid tissue in the rat: lymphocyte subset binding to high endothelial venules and in situ distribution. *Regulation Immunology*, **4**, 401–8.

Lasky, L. A., Singer, M., Dowbenko, D. *et al.* (1992). An endothelial ligand for L-selectin is a novel mucin-like molecule. *Cell*, **69**, 927–38.

Lee, E. Schiller, L. R. & Fordtran, J. S. (1988). Quantification of colonic lamina propria cells by means of a morphometric point-counting method. *Gastroenterology*, **94**, 409–14.

Leeuwenberg, J., von Asmuth, E., Jeunhomme, T. & Buurman, W. (1990). IFN-gamma regulates the expression of the adhesion molecule ELAM-1 and IL-6 production by human endothelial cells *in vitro*. *Journal of Immunology*, **145**, 2110–14.

Mackay, C., Marston, W. & Dudler, L. (1990). Naive and memory T cells show distinct pathways of lymphocyte recirculation. *Journal of Experimental Medicine*, **171**, 801–17.

Mackay, C., Marston, W., Dudler, L., Spertini, O., Tedder, T. & Hein, W. (1992). Tissue specific migration pathways by phenotypically distinct subpopulations of memory T cells. *European Journal of Immunology*, **22**, 887–95.

Mackay, C. & Imhof, B. (1993). Cell adhesion in the immune system. *Immunology Today* **14**, 99–102.

Merkenschalger, M. Terry, L., Edwards, R. & Beverley, P. (1988). Limiting dilution analysis of proliferative responses in human lymphocyte population defined by the antibody UCHL1: implications for differential CD45 expression in T cell memory formation. *European Journal of Immunology*, **18**, 1653–61.

Mitchie, C., McLean, A., Alcock, C. & Beverley, P. (1992). Lifespan of human lymphocyte subsets defined by CD45 isoforms. *Nature*, **360**, 264–6.

Nakache, M., Berg, E., Streeter, P. & Butcher, E. C. (1989). The mucosal vascular addressin is a tissue-specific endothelial cell adhesion molecule for circulating lymphocytes. *Nature*, **337**, 179–81.

Nakamura, S., Ohtani, H., Fukushima, K. *et al.* (1991). Immunohistochemical study of the distribution of cell adhesion molecules in inflammatory bowel disease. *Shokaki to Men'eki (Japan)* **25**, 110–14.

Ohtani, H., Nakamura, S., Watanabe, Y. *et al.* (1992). Light and electron microscopic immunolocalization of endothelial leukocyte adhesion molecule-1 in inflammatory bowel disease. *Virchow's Archiv A Pathology Anatomy*, **420**, 403–9.

Ottaway, C. A. (1990). Migration of lymphocytes within the mucosal immune system. In *Immunology and Immunopathology of the Liver and Gastrointestinal Tract*, ed. S. Targan & F. Shanahan, pp. 49–69. New York: Igaku-Shoin.

Ottaway, C. A., Bruce, R. & Parrott, D. (1983). The *in vivo* kinetics of lymphoblast localization in the small intestine. *Immunology*, **49**, 641–8.

Ottaway, C. A. & Husband, A. J. (1992). Central nervous system influences on lymphocyte migration. *Brain, Behavior and Immunity,* **6,** 97–116.

Ottaway, C. A. (1982). The efficiency of entry of lymphoid cells into lymphoid and nonlymphoid tissues. *Advances in Experiments in Medicine Biology,* **149,** 219–24.

Ottaway, C. A. (1989). Neurophysiological events and lymphocyte migration and distribution *in vivo.* In *Neuroimmune Networks: Physiology and Diseases,* ed. E. Goetzl & N. Spector, pp. 235–241. New York: Alan R. Liss, Inc.

Ottaway, C. A. (1988). Dynamic aspects of lymphoid cell migration. In *Migration and Homing of Lymphoid Cells,* vol II, ed. A. J. Husband, pp. 167–194. Boca Raton: CRC Press.

Pabst, R. (1988). Lymphocyte migration, *Immunology Today,* **9,** 43–5.

Pals, S. T., den Otter, A., Miedma, F. *et al.* (1988). Evidence that leukocyte function-associated antigen-1 is involved in recirculation and homing of human lymphocytes via high endothelial cells. *Journal of Immunology,* **140,** 1851–3.

Parker, C. M., Cepek, K., Russel, G. *et al.* (1992). A family of beta-7 integrins on human mucosal lymphocytes. Proceedings of National Academy of Sciences, USA, **89,** 1924–8.

Picker, L., Terstappen, L., Rott, L., Streeter, P., Stein, H. & Butcher, E. C. (1990). Differential expression of homing-associated adhesion molecules by T cell subsets in man. *Journal of Immunology,* **145,** 3247–55.

Picker, L., Kishimoto, T., Smith, C., Warnock, R. & Butcher, E. C. (1991). ELAM-1 is an adhesion molecule for skin-homing T cells. *Nature,* **349,** 796–9.

Picker, L., Treer, J., Ferguson-Darnell, B., Collins, P., Buck, D. & Terstappen, W. (1992). Control of lymphocyte recirculation in man. I. Differential regulation of the peripheral lymph node homing receptor L-selectin on T cells during the virgin to memory cell transition. *Journal of Immunology,* **150,** 1105–21.

Picker, L. J. & Butcher, E. C. (1992). Physiological and molecular mechanisms of lymphocyte homing. *Annual Reviews in Immunology,* **10,** 561–91.

Pierce, N. & Cray, S. (1982). Determinants of localization, magnitude and duration of a specific IgA plasma cell response in enterically immunized rats. *Journal of Immunology,* **128,** 1311–16.

Pober, J., Gimbrone, M., Lapierre, L., Mendrick, D., Fiers, W., Rothlein, R. & Springer, T. (1986). Overlapping patterns of activation of human endothelial cells by interleukin 1, tumor necrosis factor and immuno-interferon. *Journal of Immunology,* **137,** 1893–6.

Reynolds, J. (1988). Lymphocyte traffic associated with the gut: a review of studies in the sheep. In *Migration and Homing of Lymphoid Cells,* vol II, ed. A. J. Husband, pp. 113–179. Boca Raton: CRC Press.

Rice, G., Munro, J. & Bevilacqua, M. (1990). Inducible cell adhesion molecule 110 (INCAM110) is an endothelial receptor for lymphocytes. A CD11/CD18-independent adhesion mechanisms. *Journal of Experimental Medicine,* **171,** 1369–74.

Rice, G. & Bevilacqua, M. (1989). An inducible endothelial cell surface glycoprotein mediates melanoma adhesion. *Science,* **246,** 1303–6.

Rice, G. E., Munro, J. Colrless, C. & Bevilacqua, M. (1991). Vascular and nonvascular expression of the INCAM-110. A target for mononuclear leukocyte adhesion in normal and inflamed human tissues. *American Journal of Pathology,* **138,** 385–93.

Rose, M., Parrott, D. & Bruce, R. (1976a). Migration of lymphoblasts to the small intestine. I. Effect of *Trichinella spiralis* infection on the migration of mesenteric lymphoblasts in syngeneic mice. *Immunology,* **31,** 723–30.

Rose, M., Parrott, D. & Bruce, R. (1976b). Migration of lymphoblasts to the small intestine II Divergent migration of mesenteric and peripheral immunoblasts to sites of inflammation in the mouse. *Cell Immunology,* **27,** 36–45.

Salmi, M. & Jalkanen, S. (1991). Regulation of lymphocyte traffic to mucosa-associated lymphatic tissues. *Gastroenterology Clinics of North America,* **20,** 495–510.

Sanders, M., Makgoba, M., Sharrow, S., Springer, T., Yound, H. & Shaw, S. (1988). Human memory T cells express increased levels of three cell adhesion molecules (LFA-3, CD2 and LFA-1) and three other molecules (UCHL1, CDw29 and Pgp-1) and have enhanced IFN-gamma production. *Journal of Immunology*, **140**, 1401–7.

Scheynius, A., Camp, R. & Pure, E. (1993). Reduced contact sensitivity reactions in mice treated with monoclonal antibodies to leukocyte function-associated molecule-1 and intracellular adhesion molecule-1. *Journal of Immunology*, **150**, 655–63.

Schiefferdecker, H. L., Ullrich, R., Hirseland, H. & Zeitz, M. (1992). T cell differentiation antigens on lymphocytes in the human intestinal lamina propria. *Journal of Immunology*, **149**, 2816–22.

Schwartz, B., Wayner, E., Carlos, T., Ochs, H. & Harlan, J. (1990). Identification of surface proteins mediating adherence of CD11/CD18 deficient lymphoblastoid cells to cultured human endothelium. *Journal of Clinical Investigation*, **82**, 2019–22.

Scollay, R., Hopkins, J. & Hall, J. (1976). Possible role of surface Ig in nonrandom migration of small lymphocytes. *Nature*, **260**, 528–34.

Shimizu, Y., van Seventer, G., Horgan, K. & Shaw, S. (1990). Regulated expression and binding of three VLA integrin receptors on T cells. *Nature*, **345**, 250–3.

Simmons, D., Makgoba, M. & Seed, B. (1988). ICAM, an adhesion ligand of LFA-1 is homologous to the neural cell adhesion molecule NCAM. *Nature*, **331**, 624–6.

Smith, M. & Ford, W. (1983). The recirculating lymphocyte pool of the rat: a systematic description of the migratory behaviour of recirculating lymphocytes. *Immunology*, **49**, 83–92.

Smith, M., Martin, A. & Ford, W. (1980). Migration of lymphoblasts in the rat. *Monographs in Allergy*, **16**, 203–31.

Smith, S., Brown, M., Rowe, D., Callard, R. & Beverley, P. (1986). Functional subsets of helper-inducer cells defined by a new monoclonal antibody UCHL1. *Immunology*, **58**, 63–70.

Sparshott, M., Bell, M. & Sarawar, S. (1991). CD45R CD4 T cell subset reconstituted nude rats: subset dependent survival of recipients and bidirectional isoform switching. *European Journal of Immunology*, **21**, 993–1000.

Spertini, O., Kansas, G., Reimann, K., Mackay, C. & Tedder, T. (1991). Function and evolutionary conservation of distinct epitopes on the leukocyte adhesion molecule-1 (TQ-1, Leu-8) that regulate leukocyte migration. *Journal of Immunology*, **147**, 942–9.

Stamper, H. & Woodruff, J. J. (1976). Lymphocyte homing into lymph nodes: *In vitro* demonstration of the selective affinity of recirculating lymphocytes for the high endothelial venules. *Journal of Experimental Medicine*, **144**, 828–31.

Staunton, D., Marlin, C., Stratowa, C., Dustin, M. & Springer, T. A. (1988). Primary structure of ICAM-1 demonstrates interaction between members of the immunoglobulin and integrin supergene families. *Cell*, **52**, 925–31.

Staunton, D., Dustin, M. & Springer, T. A. (1989). Functional cloning of ICAM-2, a cell adhesion ligand for LFA-1 homologous to ICAM-1. *Nature*, **339**, 61–73.

Steer, H. (1988). Analysis of the lymphocyte content of rat lacteals. *Journal of Immunology*, **125**, 1845–8.

Streeter, P., Rouse, B. & Butcher, E. C. (1988). Immunohistologic and functional characterization of a vascular addressin involved in lymphocyte homing into peripheral lymph nodes. *Journal Cell Biology*, **107**, 1853–62.

Streeter, P., Berg, E. L., Rouse, B., Bargatze, R. & Butcher, E. C. (1988). A tissue specific endothelial cell molecule involved in lymphocyte homing. *Nature*, **331**, 41–7.

Terry, L., Brown, M. & Beverley, P. (1988). The monoclonal antibody UCHL1 recognizes a 180 000 MW component of the human leucocyte–common antigen CD45. *Immunology*, **64**, 331–6.

Thomas, M. L. (1989). The leukocyte–common antigen family. *Annual Reviews in Immunology*, **7**, 579–99.

Thornhill, M. & Haskard, D. (1990). IL4 regulates endothelial cell activation by IL1, tumor necrosis factor of IFN-gamma. *Journal of Immunology*, **145**, 865–72.

van Kooyk, Y., van de Wiel-van Kamenade, P., Weder, P., Kuipers, T. & Figdor, C. (1989). Enhancement of LFA-1 mediated cell adhesion by triggering through CD2 and CD3 on T lymphocytes. *Nature*, **342**, 811–13.

Vitetta, E., Berton, M., Burger, C., Kepron, M., Leed, W. & Yin, X. M. (1991). Memory B and T cells. *Annual Reviews in Immunology*, **9**, 193–217.

Walzer, P., LaBine, M., Redinton, T. & Cushion, M. (1984). Lymphocyte changes during chronic administration and withdrawal from corticosteroids. Relation to *Pneumocystis carinii* pneumonia. *Journal of Immunology*, **133**, 2502–8.

Washington, E., Kimpton, W. & Cahill, R. (1988). CD4 lymphocytes are extracted from the blood by peripheral lymph nodes at different rates from other T cell subsets and B cells. *European Journal of Immunology*, **18**, 2093–6.

Wayner, E. E., Garcia-Pardo, A., Humphries, M., McDonald, J. & Carter, W. (1989). Identification and characterization of the lymphocyte adhesion receptor for an alternative cell attachment domain in plasma fibronectin. *Journal of Cell Biology*, **109**, 1321–30.

Westermann, J., Person, S., Matyas, J., van der Meide, P. & Pabst, R. (1993). IFN-gamma influences the migration of thoracic duct B and T lymphocyte subsets *in vivo*. *Journal of Immunology*, **150**, 3848–52.

Wilkins, J., Stupack, D., Stewart, S. & Caixaia, S. (1991). Beta-1 integrin-mediated lymphocyte adherence to extracellular matrix is enhanced by phorbol ester treatment. *European Journal of Immunology*, **21**, 517–22.

–3–
Regulating factors affecting gut mucosal defence

D. M. McKAY, V. J. DJURIĆ, M. H. PERDUE
and J. BIENENSTOCK

Introduction

The traditional view of functionally independent compartmentalised bio-logical systems has, during the last decade, largely been surpassed by an awareness of the co-operation of diverse cell types to achieve a common goal. This new theme of 'interactive systems' is exemplified by a consider-ation of the intestinal nervous and immune systems. A large body of data has been amassed showing that messenger molecules are shared by these two systems and are active in both systems. Indeed, it is more realistic to consider the nervous and immune systems as extreme ends of the neuroendocrine-immune continuum.

With the exception of lesions in the skin, antigen gains access to the body by oral intake or inhalation and the significance of this becomes apparent when we consider that the human mucosal surface area equals ~ 400 m^2 as compared to ~ 2 m^2 of skin. In light of this constant antigenic insult, it should come as no surprise that with 10^{10} plasma cells/m^2, the intestine is the largest lymphoid tissue in the body (Beagley & Elson, 1992). This gut-associated lymphoid tissue (GALT) can be divided into three compartments: aggre-gates in follicles and Peyer's patches; diffuse elements of the lymphoid and reticuloendothelial network; intraepithelial lymphocytes. When antigen enters the intestinal submucosa/mucosa a variety of immune (of lymphoid and myeloid origin) and non-immune (epithelial, stromal) cells interact to remove the noxious stimulus and thus maintain a constant interstitial environment. When this homeostatic mechanism is compromised, or inap-propriately exaggerated, pathophysiological reactions can occur and disease may develop (Fig. 3.1).

Neurones are classified as enteric if their cell bodies reside within the gastrointestinal tract (Cooke, 1986). The processes of these nerve cells form an anastomosing network that ramifies throughout the mucosa and contain an array of neurotransmitters and putative neuroregulatory molecules (Table 3.1). The enteric nervous system (ENS), although integrated with the central nervous system (CNS), can function independently of central

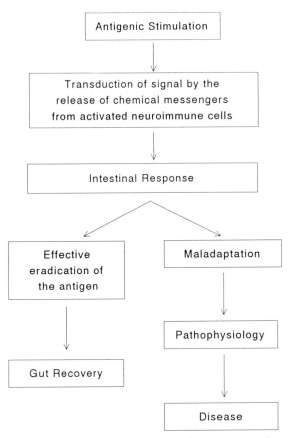

Fig. 3.1. Flow diagram showing the general pathway that leads to disease or an adaptive gut response and antigen loss following antigenic stimulation.

control. Furthermore, it has been estimated that this peripheral 'little brain' consists of 10^8 cell bodies, a number equal to that of the spinal cord (Costa & Furness, 1989). The discovery of the neurosecretory neurone has eroded the traditional standpoint of functionally discrete nervous and endocrine systems, which are now recognised as opposite ends of the neuroendocrine system. The recognition of more than 20 peptidergic putative neurotransmitters has imparted a degree of sophistication on neuronal control of physiological events that was unappreciated only 15 years ago (Costa & Furness, 1989). As a cautionary note, it must be added that many of these neuropeptides are also synthesised by gut enteroendocrine cells (Table 3.2) (Polak, 1989). The apical plasma membrane of the enteroendocrine cell is

Table 3.1. *Neurotransmitter/neuromodulator diversity in enteric neurones*

1) *Cholinergic*
2) *Aminergic*
   histamine, serotonin (5-hydroxytryptamine), noradrenaline
3) *Purinergic*
4) *GABAergic* (γ-amino-butyric acid)
5) *Peptidergic*
   calcitonin, calcitonin gene-related peptide (CGRP), cholecystokinin,
   dynorphin, enkephalins, galinin, gastrin inhibitory peptide (GIP), gastrin
   releasing peptide (GRP), neuromedin U (NMU), neuropeptide Y (NPY),
   neurotensin (NT), peptide histidine isoleucine (PHI), somatostatin (SOM),
   substance P (SP), vasoactive intestinal peptide (VIP)

Table 3.2. *Neuroendocrine localisation of enteric neuropeptides*

Neuropeptide	Neuronal localisation	Enteroendocrine cell type and location
CCK	+	'I' cell – duodenum/jejunum
Enteroglucagon	–	'EG' cell – ileum/colon
Gastrin	–	'G' cell – gastric mucosa
GIP	+	'K' cell – duodenum
GRP	+	—
Motilin	+	'M' cell – duodenum/jejunum
NPY	+	—
NT	+	'N' cell – ileum
Peptide YY		
(PYY)	–	'EG' cell – ileum/colon
PHI	+	—
SOM	+	'D' cell – GI tract
SP	+	'EG' cell – GI tract
VIP	+	—

exposed to the lumen and thus these cells may act as 'sensory' cells and affect
the underlying submucosal cells by the release of amines and/or neuropeptides that act in a paracrine fashion. Given the enormity of the ENS
(estimated at 2 m linear length of fibre/mm^3 tissue in human bowel (Ferri *et
al.*, 1984)) and the abundance of immune cells in the restricted space of the
mucosa, there is ample opportunity for these cells to meet and for the bi-
directional exchange of information (estimated that 99% of mucosal mass is
within 13 μm of a nerve fibre (Ferri *et al.*, 1984). In addition, enteric nerves
possess numerous varicosities which are believed to be sites of *en passant*

release of neuroactive substances and thus information can be disseminated along the length of the fibre. Furthermore, it has been suggested that nerve fibres in the submucosa are continually being degraded and new ones assembled (nerve remodelling) (Stead, 1992). This dynamic aspect of the ENS implies that nerve–immune cell associations may be transient and therefore may occur in response to environmental cues (e.g. antigen, chemotactic gradients, bacterial tripeptides).

Thus, our aim is to illustrate neuroimmune interactions in the intestinal mucosae, emphasise how these events may regulate the coordinated cellular responses to antigen and finally to draw attention to the complexity of this system, the subtleties of which we are only beginning to appreciate.

Relationship to nerves

Morphological studies

Using standard histochemical methodologies for the recognition of mucosal mast cells (MCs) and immunocytochemical techniques to identify peptidergic nerve fibres, the spatial associations of these two cell types have been examined in detail in rats and humans (Yonei et al., 1985). Rats infected with the enteric nematode parasite *Nippostrongylus brasiliensis* display an initial loss of granulated MCs (presumably due to activation) and then a mastocytosis reaction between days 35–42 post-infection, some 2–3 weeks after the parasitic burden has been expelled (Befus, Johnston & Bienenstock, 1979). Examination of jejunal segments from normal and nematode-infected rats revealed that ~50% and 66% of MCs were juxtaposed to peptidergic (substance P (SP), calcitonin gene-related peptide (CGRP)), unmyelinated nerve fibres, respectively (Fig. 3.2) (Stead et al., 1987). Of these associations, 4–8% showed membrane-to-membrane contacts with the MCs actually extending pseudopodial projections around the nerve fibre. Similarly, in human small and large intestine and appendix MC–nerve associations occurred at an incidence of 47–77% (Stead et al., 1989). More recently, these observations have been extended to include spatial associations between eosinophils and lymphocytes with mucosal nerve fibres (Arizono et al., 1990).

Within biological systems, anatomical relationships are most often indicative of some functional interaction and there is now a compelling body of evidence illustrating neuro-immune interactions. Indeed, in their histological studies Stead and co-workers observed that MCs juxtaposed to nerve fibres often display characteristics of degranulation and the nerve fibre can appear degenerate ('ballooning') (Stead, 1992). Neurones with this ballooned phenotype occur with higher frequency in the mucosa of patients

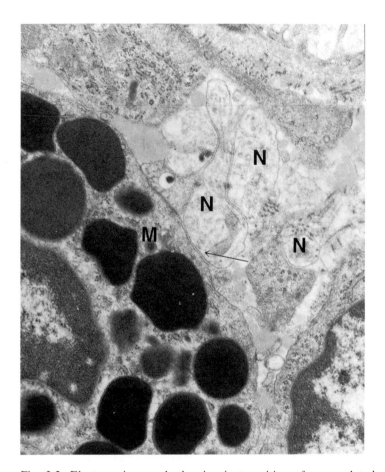

Fig. 3.2. Electronmicrograph showing juxtaposition of a granulated mucosal mast cell (M) and a nerve fibre (N) in the jejunal lamina propria of a rat, 49 days after infection with *N. brasiliensis*. Note the membrane-to-membrane association between the two cells (arrow). Original magnification = 12 000. (Courtesy of Dr R. Stead, McMaster University, reprinted with permission).

with inflammatory bowel disease (IBD), which can also contain increased numbers of MCs (Dvorak & Monahan, 1983). This led the authors to speculate that MC activation may evoke neuronal degeneration and that this is a contributory event in the pathophysiology of IBD.

These observations in intestinal tissue have been complemented by studies that have described co-culture systems of murine sympathetic nerves with rat basophilic leukaemia (RBL) cells or isolated MCs. The nerves rapidly formed contacts with the RBLs that were maintained for more than 12 h and during this time RBL membrane conductance increased in a manner that could only be mimicked by the exogenous application of SP (Blennerhassett, Tomioka & Bienenstock, 1991).

Functional studies

Epithelial function

Representing the interface between the internal and external worlds, the epithelium is one of the first lines of defence against invading antigen/ pathogens. The primary roles of this single cell layer are 1) transport of nutrients, electrolytes (ions) and water and 2) to serve as a barrier to the entry of antigen. Both of these functions are elements of the host's defence mechanism. The transepithelial electrogenic flux of chloride (Cl^-) into the lumen creates an osmotic driving force and water moves passively into the lumen. It is generally accepted that this 'washer' event serves to flush antigen from the epithelium. Active ion secretion across a tissue can be measured by mounting the preparation, under voltage-clamped conditions in Ussing chambers and monitoring short-circuit current (Isc, current required to maintain zero voltage) (Schultz & Zalusky, 1964). Subsequent electrical transmural stimulation (TS) of enteric nerves evokes an increase in Isc, that is sensitive to atropine and tetrodotoxin, implicating cholinergic and non-cholinergic neurones in the mediation of this event (Crowe, Sestini & Perdue, 1990). Application of exogenous sources of neuropeptides can elicit increased (with SP, vasoactive intestinal peptide (VIP) (Perdue, Galbraith & Davison, 1987; Waldman et al., 1977)) or decreased (with neuropeptide Y (NPY) (Cox et al., 1988), water secretion into the lumen. These neuropeptides may affect the epithelium directly or indirectly by releasing secretagogues from nerves, MCs or other immunocytes (see below).

   Mast cells are a granulated, heterogenous population that in the rat can be classified as connective tissue MCs (CTMC) or mucosal MC (MMCs) on the basis of their mediator, protease and proteoglycan content (Befus, Bienenstock & Denburg, 1986). However, a more appropriate view of these cells may be as extreme ends of a continuum of MC types (Tainsh & Pearce, 1992). The classification of MCs is less clear in humans, although the cells are equally diverse in character. The immunological activation of MCs by cross-linkage of membrane receptor-bound IgE causes the release of stored (histamine, proteases), rapidly synthesised (eicosanoids, platelet-activating factor (PAF)) and more slowly formed (cytokines) mediators. These mediators are then available to modulate a range of immune related events, such as increasing luminally directed Cl^- secretion. Nitric oxide (NO) is a recently recognised neurotransmitter that is formed from L-arginine by the nitric oxide synthase (NOS) (Moncada, Palmer & Higgs, 1991). This

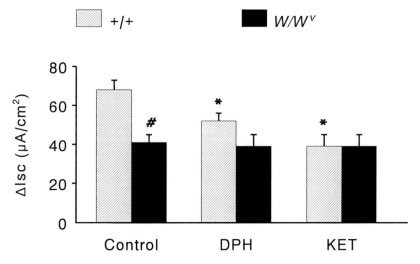

Fig. 3.3. Histogram showing intestinal short-circuit current (Isc) responses to electrical transmural stimulation of enteric nerves in mid-ileal segments from mast cell-deficient mice (W/W^v) or their congenic normal littermates $(+/+)$ in the presence of an anti-histamine (diphenhydramine (DPH), $10^{-5}M$) or the serotonin receptor antagonist, ketanscerin (KET, $10^{-5}M$). (Data are mean $\pm$ SEM; $n = 16$; *, $p < 0.05$ as compared with $+/+$; #, $p < 0.05$ for W/W^v compared with $+/+$; after Perdue *et al.*, 1991).

molecule is also produced by macrophages (where constitutive and inducible forms of NOS occur) and MCs, and has been implicated as a causative agent in inflammatory reactions and tissue destruction (Hogaboam *et al.*, 1993; Grisham & Yamada, 1992). The full spectrum of the bioactivity of NO is currently unknown, but its dual cellular location and its role as neurotransmitter and inflammatory mediator highlights the link between nerve and immune cells.

MC activation is central to immediate hypersensitivity reactions to secondary antigen challenge. The role of MCs in immunophysiological regulation of epithelial function has recently been reviewed (McKay & Perdue, 1993). Electrical transmural stimulation (TS) can elicit MC degranulation (Bani-Sacchi *et al.*, 1986), and Ussing chamber studies with MC-deficient mice (W/W^v) have provided additional evidence of a direct functional link between MCs and nerves. TS stimulation of ileum from W/W^v mice caused an increase in Isc that was ~50% of the magnitude of TS-induced ΔIsc in control tissue from normal $(+/+)$ littermates (Perdue *et al.*, 1991). Furthermore, the Isc response in $+/+$ mice was partially blocked by pretreatment with antagonists of MC-mediators; this was not true of the W/W^v response to TS (Fig. 3.3). Thus, assuming that nerves in W/W^v mice are functionally normal, then nerve stimulation can directly cause anion secretion and also indirectly by eliciting the release of inflammatory mediators from MCs. This intimate MC-nerve relationship is typified by the ability of neuropeptides to degranulate MC. Neurotensin (NT), somatostatin (SOM), SP, and VIP have all been shown to degranulate CTMC; however, only SP was effective in causing MMC activation (Shanahan et al., 1985; Sagi-Eisenberg et al., 1983). Moreover, a SP-receptor has yet to be described on MCs and this has led to the current speculation that this neuropeptide may function by the direct interaction with G-proteins located in the plasmalemma (Church, El-Lati & Caulfield, 1991). Neuropeptide release of MC mediators (e.g. histamine and adenosine) can also lead to changes in nerve function. For example, in the guinea-pig colon, occupation of the neuronal histamine-2 (H_2) receptor causes a long lasting cyclical pattern of secretion and parallel muscle contractility (Cooke, 1992) and activation of the adenosine A_2 receptor elicits a slow depolarisation of submucosal neurones (Barajas-Lopez, Surprenant & North, 1991).

   In contrast to the wealth of data on neuroimmune regulation of ion secretion, there is a paucity of information on a putative involvement of the ENS in the regulation of epithelial permeability. Equivocal data have been presented to suggest that in the rat cholinergic stimulation in vivo can enhance the movement of macromolecules from the lumen into the submucosa (Phillips, Phillips & Neutra, 1987) and that neuronal blockade may regulate paracellular permeability (Crowe et al., 1993). These data require confirmation and the field in general is deserving of greater research efforts.

Mucus and IgA secretion

Mucus is a viscous gel-like composite secreted by goblet cells and consists of glycoproteins, glycolipids and immunoglobulins. Mucus forms a protective layer over the epithelium, trapping antigen and pathogens and thus denying them access to the epithelium. Mucus also acts as a lubricant, and in conjunction with increased peristalsis, can facilitate the expulsion of trapped antigenic material. Classical neurotransmitters, such as serotonin (5-hydroxytryptamine), histamine and carbachol (acetylcholine agonist) have been shown to induce mucus secretion in the rat colon in vivo (Phillips, 1992; Neutra, O'Malley & Specian, 1982) or from monolayers of the human differentiated epithelial cell line, HT-29 (Cl.16E) (Augeron et al., 1992). The latter study also demonstrated increased mucus secretion by the exogenous application of the neuropeptides, VIP, NT and neuromedin N (NN). The ability of these agents to regulate mucus secretion has clear ramifications for defence against antigens.

   The major immunoglobulin isotype secreted by the intestinal mucosa is IgA and in humans up to 30 mg/Kg of IgA can be deposited into the gut lumen per day (Brandtzaeg *et al.*, 1988). Production of IgA and IgM precedes that of antigen-specific IgG and is a primary mucosal defence mechanism. Dimeric IgA and pentameric IgM are translocated across the epithelium following conjugation of the J-chain of the antibody to trans-membrane secretory component. Once released into the lumen the anti-bodies can 'mop-up' antigen, coat the surface of unicellular or metazoan fauna and target them for phagocytosis. Antibody synthesis by plasma cells, *in vivo* and *in vitro*, is influenced by neuropeptides in an isotype, organ specific manner (see below). Additionally, neuropeptides have been impli-cated in the control of the secretion of immunoglobulins into the gut lumen. Freier and co-workers have reported that intravenous injection of cholecys-tokinin (CCK) evokes an increase in immunoglobulin, particularly IgA and IgM, in rodents and humans. Treatment with the cholinergic agonist, pilocarpine, and SP elicited similar events (Freier, Eran & Alon, 1989). The mechanism behind these events has not been fully defined; however, studies with blockers of Cl^- secretion diminished CCK-evoked immunoglobulin secretion. Thus, a hypothesis has been proposed where neuropeptides and cholinergic agonists stimulate active Cl^- secretion and immunoglobulin is deposited into the lumen as a result of a solvent-drag mechanism (Freier *et al.*, 1991).

Neuropeptides

One of the first clues that neuropeptides were involved with immune events and disease was the demonstration that tissue and serum levels of these molecules were altered in patients with IBD (Kock, Carney & Go, 1987; Bishop *et al.*, 1980) and in animal models of inflammation and parasitic infection (Swain *et al.*, 1992; McKay *et al.*, 1991). The identification of neuropeptide receptors on immune cells revealed that these neuroactive messengers could bind to the surface and trigger intracellular changes in immunocytes (Table 3.3). However, it is difficult to generalise about neuropeptide effects on immune cells, as many studies have shown that these reactions are time, dose and tissue/cell specific. These data highlight the complexity of the system and also allude to our lack of appreciation of the intricacies of neuroimmune events.

Although more than 20 neuropeptides have been identified, the majority of immunological studies have focused on SP, VIP and SOM and more recent studies have provided data on the immune effects of nerve growth factor (NGF). The following discussion outlines the current status of our knowledge of neuropeptide-regulated immune events and thus reflects this bias toward SP, SOM and VIP (see Stanisz, 1993; Ottaway, 1991).

Table 3.3. *Immune activity, receptor localisation and leucocyte synthesis of neuropeptides*

	Influence on immunocytes	Receptor	Synthesis
SOM	decreased and increased, dose-dependent lymphocyte proliferation decreased NK activity decreased and increased IgA synthesis increased rat T cell cytotoxicity	T and B lymphocytes monocytes cell lines	rat basophils eosinophils lymphocytes
SP	increased lymphocyte proliferation increased IgA>IgM>IgG synthesis increased NK activity increased traffic through lymph nodes macrophage chemotaxis macrophage cytokine production increased neutrophil phagocytosis	T and B lymphocytes macrophages peripheral blood monocytes cell lines	eosinophils macrophages
VIP	decreased lymphocyte proliferation affects T cell homing decreased NK activity decreased or increased, organ specific, Ig synthesis	T and B lymphocytes monocytes cell lines	neutrophils* mast cells* macrophages

*VIP produced is not structurally identical to the neuronal form of the neuropeptide (for literature citations see text; Ottaway, 1991).

Substance P (SP) This 11 amino-acid residue peptide is the original member of the tachykinin family that share sequence homology in their C-terminal pentapeptide. SPergic nerve fibres have been immunocytochemically identified throughout the intestinal mucosa and submucosa. Pharmacological studies have defined three tachykinin receptors (NK_{1-3}). Ligand-binding studies have shown SP receptors on human and murine T and B cells and on lymphoblast cells (Stanisz *et al.*, 1987; Payan, Brewster & Goetzl, 1984). SP has been found to enhance B lymphocyte proliferation and to stimulate murine immunoglobulin synthesis. This event is isotype and organ specific, such that IgA is preferentially produced over IgM>IgG and Peyer's patch cells are more responsive to SP, than splenic lymphocytes (Stanisz, Befus & Bienenstock, 1986). The specificity of these results was

confirmed by experiments with an anti-SP antibody and the use of SP
antagonists (Spandide). T cell proliferation is also increased by SP and
isolated murine intraepithelial lymphocytes display enhanced NK activity in
the presence of this peptide (Croitoru et al., 1990; Scicchitano, Bienenstock
& Stanisz, 1988). In the same study SP was found to have no effect on the
killer function of splenic lymphocytes and this implies specific effects of this
neuropeptide on different classes of lymphocytes. Support for this hypothesis comes from receptor studies that illustrated twice as many SP-receptors
on CD4+ helper T cells as compared to CD8+ cytotoxic/suppressor cells
(Payan et al., 1984). Furthermore, macrophage eicosanoid (e.g. prostaglandin E_2) and superoxide (O_2^-) production is enhanced by SP and this may
exacerbate inflammatory reactions (Hartung & Toyka, 1983). In addition,
SP promotes endothelial expression of leucocyte adhesion molecules
(ELAM-1) (Matis, Lavker & Murphy, 1990) and a recent report, using
confluent monolayers of a human endothial cell line (HUVEC), has shown
that SP and CGRP can increase neutrophil adherence to endothelial cells
(Zimmerman, Anderson & Granger, 1992). Thus, SP may affect local
immunity by influencing neutrophil migration and activation (Hafstrom et
al., 1989).

Increased levels of SP are often concomitant with inflammation (Masson
et al., 1990; Swain et al., 1992), where the peptide is considered pro-
inflammatory by virtue of its ability to activate neutrophils and macrophages. Finally, SP and the related tachykinin neurokinin A (NKA =
substance K) are known to be potent and specific stimuli for the release of
inflammatory cytokines (ILs 1 and 6, TNFα) from macrophages (Lotz,
Vaughan & Carson, 1988).

Vasoactive intestinal peptide (VIP)   First identified as a potent vasodilatory
peptide, VIP has been isolated and structurally characterised as a 28 amino-
acid residue peptide and has been identified in an extensive network
throughout the intestine (Costa & Furness, 1989). Subsequently, VIP
receptors were described on human and murine lymphocytes and transformed cell lines (O'Dorisio et al., 1989; Ottaway & Greenberg, 1984). In
comparison with SP, one third more VIP-receptors have been shown on
CD4+ cells as compared to CD8+ cells (Ottaway, Lay & Greenberg, 1990).
In terms of immunoregulation, VIP inhibits proliferation of mitogen-
stimulated murine splenic, mesenteric lymph node and Peyer's patch lymphocytes. The same study illustrated the pleiotrophic nature of VIP by
demonstrating that it inhibited IgA synthesis in Peyer's patch cells, while
slightly increasing production from splenic and lymph node lymphocytes
(Stanisz, Befus & Bienenstock, 1986). Similarly, VIP increased IgM synthesis in lymphocytes isolated from Peyer's patches only. Depending on the
dose of VIP used, decreases and increases in human lymphocyte NK activity

in vitro have been recorded (Rola-Pleszczynski, Bulduc & St. Pierre, 1985). Elegant studies by Ottaway and co-workers have shown that down-regulation of the expression of VIP receptors on lymphocytes, reduces their ability to localise to the gut (Ottaway, 1984). This loss of 'homing' ability could retard mucosal immune reactions, by reducing the number of immunocompetent cells that enter the mucosa. In addition, VIP has been implicated in the regulation of lymphocyte traffic through ovine lymph nodes (Moore, Spruck & Said, 1988). The respiratory burst, and by implication the production of inflammatory reactive oxygen metabolites in human monocytes, is inhibited by VIP, possibly via a cAMP-mediated mechanism (Wiik *et al.*, 1989). Also, VIP has been shown to evoke the production of interferon α/β (IFNα/β) from the human colonic HT-29 cell line (Chelbi-Alix *et al.*, 1991), and this cytokine has anti-inflammatory properties. VIP also reduces and delays the production of IL-2 (T cell growth factor) from cultured murine lymphocytes (Ottaway, 1987). Therefore, in contrast to SP, VIP exerts a more inhibitory influence over immune and inflammatory events and these messenger molecules may act antagonistically.

Somatostatin (SOM)   Intestinal SOM-positive nerve fibres are less extensive and dense than either the distribution of SPergic and VIPergic fibres. This 14 amino-acid peptide generally exerts an inhibitory influence on immune events, by specific receptor-mediated mechanisms (Hiruma *et al.*, 1990; Scicchitano *et al.*, 1988). Thus, SOM has been shown to inhibit mitogen-proliferation of T cell lines, human colonic and murine splenic and mucosal lymphocytes (Elitsur & Luk, 1990; Stanisz, Befus & Bienenstock, 1986; Payan, Hess & Goetzl, 1984). However, at high SOM concentrations, some enhancement of proliferation has been noted. SOM ablated lymphocyte NK activity in cells isolated from the spleen and Peyer's patches; the effect being more pronounced in the Peyer's patch cells (Agro, Padol & Stanisz, 1991). Also, *in vitro* and *in vivo* studies have shown that SOM diminishes the synthesis of IgA, IgG and IgM (Stanisz, Befus & Bienenstock, 1986). Ligand binding studies have revealed receptors for SOM and VIP on human lymphoid cell lines (Jurkat, U266) (Finch, Sreedharan & Goetzl, 1989) and if these cells are a reflection of the normal cell *in vivo*, then this intimates that multiple neuropeptides can influence the physiology of individual cell types.

Nerve growth factor (NGF)   This neurotrophic polypeptide is composed of α, β and γ subunits, with the functional unit being a homodimeric cleavage product of the β subunit (designated β-NGF or 2.5S NGF) (Greene & Shooter, 1980). Receptors for NGF have been localised on human lymphoid cells and splenic mononuclear cells (Chesa *et al.*, 1988). Receptors have also been found on follicular dendritic cells in germinal centres in human tonsils, intestine and appendix and this may intimate that NGF has some regulatory role in antigen presentation (Pezzati *et al.*, 1992). NGF can elicit pro-inflammatory reactions by enhancing survival, phagocytosis and superoxide production by murine neutrophils, promoting the growth of granulocytes and evoking MC degranulation (Kannan *et al.*, 1991; Matsuda *et al.*, 1988; Pearce & Thompson, 1986). Recently, data have been reported that describe NGF-induced CTMC and MMC hyperplasia (Marshall *et al.*, 1990) and this has obvious implications for the regulation of immune function (see above). It has also been reported that NGF evokes changes in platelet morphology (most likely related to activation), increases DNA synthesis in spleen cells and may induce the expression of IL-2 receptors on cultured human lymphocytes (Stepien *et al.*, 1991; Thorpe, Werbach-Perez & Perez-Polo, 1987; Gudat *et al.*, 1981). Finally, it should be emphasised that fibroblasts can secrete NGF (Murase *et al.*, 1992) and thus a new system, that of stromal cells, has been added to the mechanism(s) of controlling immune responses. Moreover, fibroblasts can also synthesise an array of cytokines, such as IL-1 and granulocyte–macrophage colony stimulating factor (GM-CSF).

Other neuropeptides   CGRP has been found to reduce macrophage presentation of antigen and to diminish the production of hydrogen peroxide by these cells (Nong *et al.*, 1989). The amphibian analogue of gastrin-releasing peptide (GRP), bombesin can enhance the release of antigen-specific IgA and IgM from rat plasma cells (Jin, Guo & Houston, 1989). The same study also reported that pentagastrin and CCK caused an increase in the recovery of IgG and IgM in intestinal perfusates. Neuropeptide Y (NPY) has been shown to inhibit the proliferation of guinea-pig lymph node lymphocytes (Soder & Hellstrom, 1987). The lack of data concerning any immunological roles for the majority of neuropeptide species appears as an obvious gap in the current state of our knowledge.

It is now known that leucocytes can synthesise their own neuropeptides (Table 3.3), which are essentially structurally identical to their counterparts isolated from nervous tissue (Weinstock *et al.*, 1988; Goetzl *et al.*, 1985; O'Dorisio *et al.*, 1980). The role(s) of these neuropeptides is unclear but it has been suggested that they may stimulate the cell of origin in an autocrine fashion (Pascual & Bost, 1990) or that low levels of neuropeptide synthesis and release is required for maintenance of surface receptors. An alternative postulate suggests that leucocyte-derived neuropeptides may in some way regulate cytokine release. Before concluding this section it is important to emphasise one cautionary note. The information relating to neuropeptide alteration of mucosal immune events has mostly been derived from *in vivo* experiments with normal animals or *in vitro* tests with cells obtained from normal animals and/or people. However, during disease states both neuro-peptide levels and neuropeptide receptor expression are significantly elev-ated or decreased and this may give rise to an additional series of events that are absent or below the level of detection under normal (disease-free) circumstances (Kock, Carney & Go, 1987; Manty *et al.*, 1989).

Psychoneuronal influences

A putative involvement of the central nervous system (CNS) adds a new and vast dimension to the regulation of gut mucosal defence. Different types of psychological experience may have a modulating effect on the already existing CNS–PNS-immune system axis and thus may be contributing factors in some observed, and yet not fully understood gastrointestinal disorders. For instance, early reports illustrated that central anaesthetic agents can protect animals against fatal anaphylactic shock (Banzhaf & Famulener, 1910) and a consideration of the putative role of the CNS in mediating anaphylactic reactions in a variety of animal models has led to the coining of the term psychoneuroimmunology (Ader, 1981). It now seems plausible to assume that signals originating from MC-peripheral nerve interactions are forwarded to the CNS where they can be processed and orchestrated with other incoming signals to elicit the appropriate response. Thus, vagotomy prevents the stress-induced reduction in tissue levels of histamine (possibly MC-derived) (Ganguly & Gopinath, 1979). Since their recognition, the aetiology of the inflammatory bowel diseases has remained enigmatic and it has recently been postulated that there may be a genetic predisposition for these disorders. We would also contend that psychologi-cal variables are likely to be involved in at least modulating the course of these diseases (also see Whitehead, 1992).

The laboratory rat is a particularly good model for studying neurological factors of immediate hypersensitivity in the gastrointestinal tract (see above). In addition, evidence for a connection between psychological variables and immediate hypersensitivity was obtained utilising the same system. Succinctly put, susceptibility to anaphylaxis has so far been related to Pavlovian conditioning, previous exposure to stress and pretreatment with opioid agonists and antagonists. As a consequence of Pavlovian conditioning, presentation of an audiovisual signal previously paired with an antigen challenge resulted in a conditioned increase of rat MMC-specific protease RMCPII (MacQueen *et al.*, 1989). Early studies had described the learned release of histamine (Russell *et al.*, 1984). Previous exposure to intermittent inescapable stress had an anti-anaphylactic effect. This can be explained by the stress-induced elevation of corticosteroids and/or by the activation of stress-induced endogenous opioid release, since endorphins and enkephalins alleviate, and pretreatment with naloxone exaggerates anaphylactic shock in the rat. A more extensive review of this area has recently been provided by Djurić & Bienenstock, 1993.

Comparing two genetically related rat strains we demonstrated a strong correlation between different measures of spontaneous activity and susceptibility to immediate hypersensitivity (unpublished observations). This finding indicates that some genetic basis may be responsible for the observed strain-related differences in behaviour and susceptibility to anaphylactic shock and supports some previous observations about the relation between genetic proneness to anxiety and atopic reactions. As a final facet to this field of research the interaction of behaviour and immunology should be considered. Thus, a recent report cites evidence of behaviourly-inhibited children being more susceptible to allergy than non-inhibited age-matched children (controls) (Bell *et al.*, 1990).

Immune cell mediators

Cytokines (monokines, interleukins (ILs)) and growth factors are large glycosylated proteins that were originally identified in macrophages and T cells, but are now known to be synthesised in a variety of resident and recruited immune cells (e.g. MCs (Gordon, Burd & Galli, 1990)) and non-immune cells (e.g. epithelium (Mahida, Ciacci & Podolsky, 1992)). These messenger molecules direct all facets of immune reactions and display both pleiotrophy (multiple roles) and redundancy (multiple cytokines can have similar roles) of function. These attributes confer a great deal of plasticity on the regulation of immune events and are of adaptive value to the host, such that when one cytokine fails to operate then a compensatory mechanism can be employed. The discovery of cytokines has revolutionised the field of immunobiology and the reader is referred to recent reviews on the function of cytokines (Brynskov *et al.*, 1992; Wershil, 1992; Gregory, Magee & Wing, 1991; Jacob, 1989).

An in-depth study of murine T cells, and the cytokines they produce, has revealed that these cells can be classified on the basis of their cytokine profile into TH-1 (IL-2, IFNγ) and TH-2 (IL, 4, 5, 6 and 10) cells (Mosmann, 1992). These cells work antagonistically, with TH-1 cells directing delayed type hypersensitivity reactions and TH-2 cells controlling immediate (allergic) responses. However, a TH-0 cell (ILs 2, 4 and 5, IFNγ) has been identified (Mosmann, 1992) and this may represent a precursor cell whose eventual phenotype may be dictated by microenvironmental cues/switches. For example, fibronectin in the extracellular matrix can evoke TNFα secretion from resting rat CD4+ T cells (Hershkovic *et al.*, 1993). Although less well defined, data have been presented to suggest the existence of a dichotomous T-helper cell system in humans (Romagnani, 1991). More than 20 cytokines/ growth factors have been identified and shown to control: B cell proliferation, T cell maturation, granulocyte growth and development, immunocyte recruitment, antibody synthesis, wound healing and the synthesis and release of cytokines (Mosmann, 1992; Wershil, 1992; Jacob, 1989). Some cytokines are pro-inflammatory, whereas others exert an anti-inflammatory influence. For example, administration of IL-1 or TNFα to rodents results in the development of intestinal features characteristic of IBD, such as necrosis of crypt lining, goblet cell depletion and diarrhoea (Butler *et al.*, 1989). In contrast, interferons (IFNγ and α/β) inhibit the release of histamine from isolated or cultured MCs (Sweiter *et al.*, 1989) and we have shown that IFN-α/β can diminish antigen-induced changes in Isc and therefore reduce water secretion into the gut lumen (Fig. 3.4) (McKay, Bienenstock & Perdue, 1993).

Epithelial function

Cytokines can affect the transport and barrier functions of the gut epithelium. IL-1 can evoke Cl$^-$ secretion from Ussing-chambered rabbit ileum,

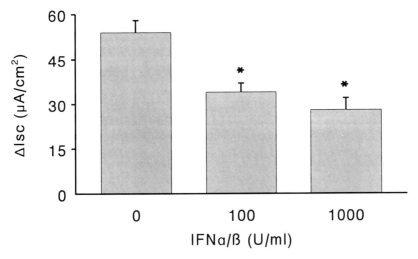

Fig. 3.4. Histogram showing the effect of a 1 h pre-incubation of interferon α/β (IFNα/β, applied to serosal surface) on antigen-induced (egg albumin at 0.1 mg/ml; applied to serosal surface) changes in intestinal short-circuit current (Isc) in jejunal segments from sensitised rats (data are mean ± SEM; $n = 6$–8; *, $p < 0.05$; after McKay, Bienenstock & Perdue, 1993).

however, this effect was indirect being mediated by the release of prosta-glandins from submucosal cells (Chiossone, Simon & Smith, 1990). TNFα and IFNγ have been shown to be cytotoxic to HT-29 cells and IFNγ can increase the permeability of confluent monolayers of the human colonic, 'crypt-like' T84 cells to small molecules (mannitol) (Deem, Shanahan & Targan, 1991; Madara & Stafford, 1989). Moreover, IFNγ treatment increased epithelial expression of MHC II *in vitro* and thus confers an increased capacity of the enterocyte to present antigen to immune cells (McDonald & Spencer, 1988). Similarly, studies with the rat intestinal cell line, IEC-6 have revealed that these cells can express the IL-2 receptor and synthesise IL-6 and transforming growth factor β (TGFβ): paneth cells can also manufacture IL-6 (see Mahida, Ciacci & Podolsky, 1992). In terms of immunomodulation, TGFβ can reduce lymphocyte proliferation, IgG and IgM synthesis and macrophage production of reactive oxygen metabolites. Thus, the epithelial cell must be recognised as a component of the afferent, as well as the efferent limb of mucosal immune events. In this respect, it is now recognised that epithelial cells can manufacture a gamut of cytokines (e.g. IL-1, 6, TNFα, GM-CSF) (Jordana et al., 1992). Furthermore, their 'sentinel' location and the possibility of environmental priming suggests the intriguing scenario where the epithelium may initiate, potentiate and eventually down regulate mucosal inflammatory reactions (Jordana et al., 1992).

Mucus and IgA secretion

Only indirect evidence is available to implicate cytokines in the regulation of mucus secretion. Goblet cell hyperplasia and increased mucus production is characteristic of intestines from rodents that have been infected with *N. brasiliensis*. Early reports suggested that this response was T cell-dependent and could be induced in naive rats by adoptive transfer of thymocytes from infected rats (Miller, Nawa & Parish, 1979). However, the soluble media-tors that control goblet cell activity were not identified. Recently, IL-1 administration to mice resulted in depletion of mucus from colonic goblet cells (Butler *et al.*, 1989). Equivocal data have been presented that cytokines can affect IgA secretion. IgA production in response to a bacterial polysac-charide is preferentially up-regulated following treatment with IL-2 and IFNγ (Murray, Swain & Kagnoff, 1985). In addition, treatment of HT-29 cells with TNFα or IFNγ evoked an increase in the intracellular pool of secretory component and increased expression of this poly-Ig receptor on the membrane (Kvale, Brandtzaeg & Lovhaug, 1988; Phillips *et al.*, 1990).

However, it should be noted that actual immunoglobulin transepithelial transport was not reported.

Cytokine–nerve interaction

To-date most reports have concerned neurone-to-immune cell communication. However, it is becoming apparent that information can be transferred in the opposite direction. Macrophages can remain in the nervous system for long periods as microglial cells and T cells, in conjunction with antigen, can also reside in the central nervous system (Hickey, Hsu & Kimura, 1991). Furthermore, during Crohn's disease immunocytes are frequently observed in the intestinal myenteric plexus (Geboes, Rutgeerts & Desmet, 1991).

Studies with primary cultures of spinal nerve cells have revealed that IL-1 enhances neuronal survival in cultures that were electrically active (Brenneman *et al.*, 1992). Following neuronal injury macrophages are recruited into the site and secrete IL-1, this cytokine in turn promotes the up-regulation of mRNA for NGF and NGF receptor and thus the repair process can proceed (Lindholm *et al.*, 1987). Increases in noradrenaline metabolism in the hypothalamus and the release of pituitary hormones can be elicited by treatment with IL-1 (Dunn, 1988; Bernton *et al.*, 1987). If such findings are applicable to the peripheral nervous system and ENS, this has far reaching implications for the regulation of neuroimmune events. Additionally, the SP content of spinal neurones in mixed culture is increased after two days of culture with IL-1; levels remained elevated until day 5 (end of experiment) (Freidin & Kessler, 1991). However, increased neuronal SP was not evident in cultures of pure neurones and this would imply that, in the former instance, IL-1 was working by release of an unidentified mediator from an intermediate cell type.

This finding is reminiscent of the change in SP-levels in longitudinal muscle-myenteric plexus preparations from rat experimentally infected with the intraepithelial parasitic nematode *Trichinella spiralis* (Swain *et al.*, 1992). Levels of immunoreactive-SP were elevated 24 h after infection and peaked at 6 days post-infection (peak of worm rejection) and were correlated with the degree of inflammation as indicated by elevated levels of myeloperoxidase (neutrophil marker). Also, tissue levels of IL-1 are elevated following infection with this parasite. This model of nematode-induced inflammation in rats has been extensively used by Collins and co-workers to investigate neuroimmunophysiological reactions that may be responsible for some of the pathophysiology associated with human IBD (Collins *et al.*, 1992). This group has shown that the increased SP-levels in this model is T cell dependent and have preliminary data that suggest that IL-1β can elicit increases in SP (Hurst *et al.*, 1992). Furthermore, pretreatment of rat myenteric plexus nerve varicosities (≡synaptosomes) with recombinant human IL-1β (10 ng/ml) for 1 h resulted in a significant reduction in the release of ^{3}H-acetylcholine and ^{3}H-noradrenaline (Hurst & Collins, 1993; Main, Blennerhassett & Collins, 1991). Collectively these *in vitro* studies illustrate that IL-1β may affect intestinal cholinergic, aminergic and peptidergic nerves and suggest an intimate association between IL-1 and SP in the regulation of mucosal nerve function and the control of intestinal inflammation. Furthermore, changes in smooth muscle contractility accompany *T. spiralis* infection and this effect is dependent on the presence of functional T cells, intimating cytokine involvement (Vermillion, Ernst & Collins, 1991).

The few examples sited above are undoubtedly only the 'tip of the iceberg' in relation to cytokine-directed neuroimmune events. Further work in this field will provide a wealth of data, and when intercalated into the present schema of neuroimmune regulation of mucosal defence will provide a more realistic appreciation of the true complexity of the *in situ* situation.

Conclusions

In this chapter we have adopted a panoramic view of mucosal immune events, in an attempt to show the co-operation of multiple cell types, and systems, in the integrated response to antigen (Fig. 3.5). The voluminous amount of data that has accrued pertaining to the regulation of mucosal immunological reactions could easily be the subject of a separate monograph. Thus, we have concentrated on the main concepts of neuroimmunological events and cited examples to illustrate the cell-to-cell signalling and the bi-directional transfer of information within the immuno-neuroendocrine systems. Interactions of neuronal and immune cells/ mediators can be summarised in three categories: 1) change in cell phenotype (e.g. NGF enhancement of MC development from MC precursors); 2) changes in cell expression of receptors, surface molecules or intracellular biochemical pathways (e.g. INFγ induction of neuronal MHC II expression); 3) transient changes in cell proliferation or molecule biosynthesis (e.g. neuropeptide effects on lymphocytes). By emphasising cell cooperation we are not trivialising self-regulation of the immune system, but rather enriching the picture by setting immune events in the context of a multi-system, interactive and dynamic environment: the intestinal mucosa. There can no longer be any doubt that the immune and nervous systems are functionally inter-dependent, and the task with which the neuroimmunophysiologist is now faced, is the unravelling of these intricate regulatory networks. Development of a comprehensive understanding of the neuroimmune system will ultimately allow for extrinsic pharmacological manipu-

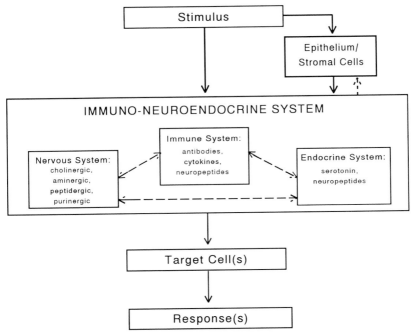

Fig. 3.5. Schematic illustrating the communication pathways within the immuno-neuroendocrine system and how a collective cell effort can be employed to achieve a common goal.

lation of the cells/mediators to counteract pathophysiological reactions and combat disease.

Acknowledgements

Financial support for the studies conducted in our laboratory was provided by The Canadian Medical Research Council, The Crohn's Colitis Foundation of Canada and the National Institutes of Health (NS 29536), and is greatly appreciated.

References

Ader, R. (ed.) (1981). *Psychoneuroimmunology*. New York: Academic Press.
Agro, A., Padol, I. & Stanisz, A. M. (1991). Immunomodulatory activities of the somatostatin analogue BIM 23014c: effects on murine lymphocyte proliferation and natural killer activity. *Regulatory Peptides*, **32**, 129–39.

Arizono, N., Matsuda, S., Hattori, T., Kojima, Y., Meada, T. & Galli, S. J. (1990). Anatomical variation in mast cell nerve associations in the rat small intestine, heart, lung, and skin: similarities of distances between neural processes and mast cells, eosinophils or plasma cells in the jejunal lamina propria. *Laboratory Investigation*, **62**, 626–34.

Augeron, C., Voisin, T., Maoret, J. J., Berthon, B., Laburthe, M. & Laboisse, C. L. (1992). Neurotensin and neuromedin N stimulate mucin output from human goblet cells (Cl.16E) via neurotensin receptors. *American Journal of Physiology*, **262**, G470–6.

Bani-Sacchi, T., Barattini, M., Bianchi, S., Blandina, S., Brunelleschi, S., Fantozzi, R., Mannaioni, P. F. & Masini, E. (1986). The release of histamine by parasympathetic stimulation in guinea pig auricle and rat ileum. *Journal of Physiology*, **371**, 29–43.

Banzhaf, E. J. & Famulener, L. W. (1910). The influence of chloral hydrate on serum anaphylaxis. *Journal of Infectious Diseases*, **7**, 577–86.

Barajas-Lopez, C., Surprenant, A. & North, R. A. (1991). Adenosine A_1 and A_2 receptors mediate presynaptic inhibition and postsynaptic excitation in guinea pig submucosal neurons. *Journal of Pharmacology and Experimental Therapeutics*, **258**, 490–5.

Beagley, K. W. & Elson, C. O. (1992). Cells and cytokines in mucosal immunity and inflammation. *Gastroenterology Clinics of North America*, **21**, 347–66.

Befus, A. D., Johnston, N. & Bienenstock, J. (1979). *Nippostrongylus brasiliensis*: mast cells and histamine levels in tissues of infected and normal rats. *Experimental Parasitology*, **48**, 1–8.

Befus, A. D., Bienenstock, J. & Denburg, J. (eds) (1986). *Mast Cell Differentiation and Heterogeneity*. New York: Raven.

Bell, I. R., Jasnoski, M. L., Kagan, J. & King, D. S. (1990). Is allergic rhinitis more frequent in young adults with extreme shyness? A preliminary review. *Psychosomatic Medicine*, **52**, 517–25.

Bernton, E. W., Beach, J. E., Holaday, J. W., Smallridge, R. C. & Fein, H. G. (1987). Release of multiple hormones by direct action of interleukin-1 on pituitary cells. *Science*, **233**, 652–4.

Bishop, A. E., Polak, J. M., Bryant, M. G., Bloom, S. R. & Hamilton, S. (1980). Abnormalities of vasoactive intestinal polypeptide-containing nerves in Crohn's disease. *Gastroenterology*, **79**, 853–60.

Blennerhassett, M. G., Tomioka, M. & Bienenstock, J. (1991). Formation of contacts between mast cells and sympathetic neurones *in vitro*. *Cell and Tissue Research*, **265**, 121–8.

Brandtzaeg, P., Sollid, L. M., Thrane, P. S. *et al.* (1988). Lymphoepithelial interactions in the mucosal immune system. *Gut*, **29**, 1116–30.

Brenneman, D., Schultz, M., Bartfai, T. & Gozes, I. (1992). Cytokine regulation of neuronal survival. *Journal of Neurochemistry*, **58**, 454–60.

Brynskov, J., Nielsen, O. H., Ahnfelt-Ronne, I. & Bendtzen, K. (1992). Cytokines in inflammatory bowel disease. *Scandinavian Journal of Gastroenterology*, **27**, 897–906.

Butler, L. D., Layman, N. K., Cain, R. I. *et al.* (1989). Interleukin 1-induced pathophysiology: induction of cytokines, development of histopathologic changes and immunopharmacology intervention. *Clinical Immunology and Immunopathology*, **53**, 400–21.

Chelbi-Alix, M. K., Boissard, C., Sripati, C. E., Rosselin, G. & Thang, M. N. (1991). VIP induces HT-29 cell $2'5'$oligoadenylate synthetase and antiviral state via interferon α/β synthesis. *Peptides*, **12**, 1085–93.

Chesa, P. G., Retting, W. J., Thompson, T. M., Old, L. J. & Melamed, M. R. (1988). Immunohistochemical analysis of nerve growth factor receptor expression in normal and malignant human tissues. *Journal of Histochemistry and Cytochemistry*, **36**, 383–9.

Chiossone, D. C., Simon, P. L. & Smith, P. L. (1990). Interleukin-1: effects on rabbit ileal mucosal ion transport *in vitro*. *European Journal of Pharmacology*, **180**, 217–28.

Church, El-Lati, S. & Caulfield, J. P. (1991). Neuropeptide-induced secretion from human skin mast cells. *International Archives of Allergy and Applied Immunology*, **94**, 310–18.

Collins, S. M., Hurst, S. M., Main, C., Stanley, E., Khan, I., Blennerhassett, P. & Swain, M. (1992). Effect of inflammation on enteric nerves: cytokine-induced changes in neurotransmitter content and release. In *Neuro-Immuno-Physiology of the Gastrointestinal Mucosa. Implications for Inflammatory Diseases*. Annals of the New York Academy of Sciences vol. 664, eds. R. H. Stead, M. H. Perdue, H. Cooke, D. W. Powell & K. E. Barrett, pp. 415–24. New York.

Cooke, H. J. (1986). Neurobiology of the intestinal mucosa. *Gastroenterology*, **90**, 1057–81.

Cooke, H. J. (1992). Neuro-modulation of ion-secretion by inflammatory mediators. In *Neuro-Immuno-Physiology of the Gastrointestinal Mucosa. Implications for Inflammatory Diseases*. Annals of the New York Academy of Sciences vol. 664, eds. R. H. Stead, M. H. Perdue, H. Cooke, D. W. Powell & K. E. Barrett, pp. 346–52. New York.

Costa, M. & Furness, J. B. (1989). Structure and neurochemical organisation of the enteric nervous system. In *Handbook of Physiology, The Gastrointestinal System, Neural and Endocrine Biology* (sect. 6), vol. II ed. S. G. Schultz, pp. 97–100. Bethesda, Maryland: American Physiology Society.

Cox, H. M., Cuthbert, A. W., Hakanson, R. & Wahlestedt, C. (1988). The effect of neuropeptide Y and peptide YY on electrogenic ion transport in rat intestinal epithelia. *Journal of Physiology (London)*, **398**, 65–80.

Croitoru, K., Ernst, E. B., Bienenstock, J., Padol, I. & Stanisz, A. M. (1990). Selective modulation of natural killer activity of murine intestinal intraepithelial leucocytes by the neuropeptide substance P. *Immunology*, **71**, 196–201.

Crowe, S. E., Sestini, P. & Perdue, M. H. (1990). Allergic reactions in rat jejunal mucosa. Ion transport responses to luminal antigen and inflammatory mediators. *Gastroenterology*, **99**, 74–82.

Crowe, S. E., Soda, K., Stanisz, A. M. & Perdue, M. H. (1993). Intestinal permeability in allergic rats: abnormalities before and after antigen challenge. *American Journal of Physiology*, **264**, G617–23.

Deem, R. L., Shanahan, F. & Targan, S. R. (1991). Triggered human T cells release tumour necrosis factor-alpha and interferon-gamma which kill human colonic epithelial cells. *Clinical and Experimental Immunology*, **83**, 79–84.

Djurić, V. J. & Bienenstock, J. (1993). Learned sensitivity. *Annals of Allergy*, **71**, 5–15.

Dunn, A. J. (1988). Systemic interleukin-1 administration stimulates hypothalamic norepinephrine metabolism paralleling the increased plasma corticosterone. *Life Science*, **43**, 429–35.

Dvorak, A. M. & Monahan, R. A. (1983). Crohn's disease – mast cell quantification using one micron plastic sections for light microscopic study. *Pathology Annals*, **18**, 181–90.

Elitsur, Y. & Luk, G. D. (1990). Gastrointestinal neuropeptides suppress human colonic lamina propria lymphocyte DNA synthesis. *Peptides*, **11**, 879–84.

Ferri, G-L., Wright, N. A., Soimero, L, Labo, G. & Polak, J. M. (1984). Quantification of the intestinal peptide-containing innervation: length density of nerve fibres and total length of nerve supply to the single villus/crypt unit. *Journal of Histochemistry and Cytochemistry*, **32**, 737–40.

Finch, R., Sreedharan, S. & Goetzl, E. (1989). High affinity receptors for vasoactive intestinal peptide on human myeloma cells. *Journal of Immunology*, **142**, 1977–81.

Freidin, M. & Kessler, J. A. (1991). Cytokine regulation of substance P expression in sympathetic neurons. *Proceedings of the National Academy of Sciences, USA*, **88**, 3200–3.

Freier, S., Eran, M. & Alon, I. (1989). A study of stimuli operative in the release of antibodies in the rat intestine. *Immunological Investigations*, **18**, 431–47.

Freier, S., Eran, M., Alon, Y. & Elath, U. (1991). Verapamil and furosemide prevent cholecystokinin-induced translocation of immunoglobulins in rat intestine. *Digestive Diseases and Sciences*, **36**, 1619–24.

Ganguly, A. K. & Gopinath, P. (1979). Vagus nerves and the gastric histamine concentration in pylorus ligated albino rats. *Quarterly Journal of Experimental Physiology and Cognate Medical Sciences*, **64**, 1–6.

Geboes, K., Rutgeerts, P. & Desmet, V. (1991). Lymphocyte interactions with smooth muscle cells and nerves. In *The Effects of Immune Cells and Inflammation on Smooth Muscle and Enteric Nerves*. ed. W. J. Snape & S. M. Collins, pp. 257–70, Boca Raton, Fl: C.R.C. Press.

Goetzl, E. J., Chernov-Rogan, T., Cooke, M. P., Renda, F. & Payan, D. G. (1985). Endogenous somatostatin-like peptide of rat basophilic leukaemia cells. *Journal of Immunology*, **135**, 2707–12.

Gordon, J. R., Burd, P. R. & Galli, S. J. (1990). Mast cells as a source of multifunctional cytokines. *Immunology Today*, **11**, 458–64.

Greene, L. A. & Shooter, E. M. (1980). Nerve growth factor: biochemistry, synthesis, and mechanism of action. *Annual Reviews of Neuroscience*, **3**, 353–402.

Gregory, S. H., Magee, D. M. & Wing, E. J. (1991). The role of colony-stimulating factors in host defenses. *Proceedings of the Society for Experimental Biology and Medicine*, **197**, 349–60.

Grisham, M. B. & Yamada, T. (1992). Neutrophils, nitrogen oxides, and inflammatory bowel disease. In *Neuro-Immuno-Physiology of the Gastrointestinal Mucosa. Implications for Inflammatory Diseases*. Annals of the New York Academy of Sciences, vol. 664, ed. R. H. Stead, M. H. Perdue, H. Cooke, D. W. Powell & K. E. Barrett, pp. 103–15. New York.

Gudat, F., Laubscher, A., Otten, U. & Pletscher, A. (1981). Shape changes induced by biologically active peptides and nerve growth factor in blood platelets of rabbits. *British Journal of Pharmacology*, **74**, 533–8.

Hafstrom, I. Gyllenhammer, H., Palmblad, J. & Ringertz, B. (1989). Substance P activates and modulates neutrophil oxidative metabolism and aggregation. *Journal of Rheumatology*, **16**, 1033–7.

Hartung, H. P. & Toyka, K. V. (1983). Activation of macrophages by substance P: induction of oxidative burst and thromboxane release. *European Journal of Pharmacology*, **89**, 301–5.

Hershkovic, R., Gilat, D., Miron, S., Mekori, Y. A., Aderka, D., Wallach, D., Vlodavsky, I., Cohen, I. R. & Lider, O. (1993). Extracellular matrix induces tumour necrosis factor-α secretion by an interaction between resting rat CD4+ T cells and macrophages. *Immunology*, **73**, 50–7.

Hickey, W. F., Hsu, B. L. & Kimura, H. (1991). T-lymphocyte entry into the central nervous system. *Journal of Neuroscience Research*, **28**, 254–60.

Hiruma, K., Koike, T., Nakamura, H., Sumida, T., Maeda, T., Tomioka, H., Yoshida, S. & Fujita, T. (1990). Somatostatin receptors on human lymphocytes and leukaemia cells. *Immunology*, **71**, 480–5.

Hogaboam, C. M., Bissonnette, E. Y., Chin, B. C., Befus, A. D. & Wallace, J. L. (1993). Prostaglandins inhibit inflammatory mediator release from rat mast cells. *Gastroenterology*, **104**, 122–9.

Hurst, S. M. & Collins, S. M. (1993). Interleukin-1β modulation of norepinephrine release from rat myenteric nerves. *American Journal of Physiology*, **264**, G30–5.

Hurst, S., Stepien, H., Stanisz, A. (1992). The relationship between pro-inflammatory peptide interleukin-1β and substance P in the inflamed rat intestine (abstract). *Gastroenterology*, **102**, A640.

Jacob, C. O. (1989). Cytokines and anti-cytokines. *Current Opinion in Immunology*, **2**, 249–57.

Jin, G.-F., Guo, Y.-S. & Houston, C. W. (1989). Bombesin: an activator of specific *Aeromonas* antibody secretion in rat intestine. *Digestive Diseases and Sciences*, **34**, 1708–12.

Jordana, M., Clancy, R., Dolovich, J. & Denburg, J. (1992). Effector role of the epithelial compartment in inflammation. In *Neuro-Immuno-Physiology of the Gastrointestinal Mucosa. Implications for Inflammatory Diseases*. Annals of the New York Academy of Sciences vol. 664, ed. R. H. Stead, M. H. Perdue, H. Cooke, D. W. Powell & K. E. Barrett, pp. 181–9. New York.

Kannan, Y., Ushio, H., Koyama, H., Okada, M., Oikawa, M-A, Yoshihara, T., Kaneko, M. & Matsuda, H. (1991). 2.5S nerve growth factor enhances survival, phagocytosis, and superoxide production of murine neutrophils. *Blood*, **77**, 1320–5.

Kock, T. R., Carney, J. A. & Go, V. L. W. (1987). Distribution and quantitation of gut neuropeptides in normal intestine and inflammatory bowel diseases. *Digestive Diseases and Sciences*, **32**, 369–76.

Kvale, D., Brandtzaeg, P. & Lovhaug, D. (1988). Up-regulation of the expression of secretory component and HLA molecules in a human colonic cell line by tumour necrosis factor-α and gamma interferon. *Scandinavian Journal of Immunology*, **28**, 351–7.

Lindholm, D., Heumann, R., Meyer, M. & Thoenen, H. (1987). Interleukin-1 regulates synthesis of nerve growth factor in non-neuronal cells of the rat sciatic nerve. *Nature*, **330**, 658–9.

Lotz, M., Vaughan, J. H. & Carson, D. A. (1988). Effect of neuropeptides on production of inflammatory cytokines by human monocytes. *Science*, **241**, 1218–21.

MacQueen, G., Siegel, S., Marshall, J. S., Perdue, M. H. & Bienenstock, J. (1989). Pavlovian conditioning of rat mucosal mast cells to secrete rat mast cell protease II. *Science*, **243**, 83–5.

Madara, J. L. & Stafford, J. (1989). Interferon-γ affects barrier function of a cultured intestinal epithelial monolayer. *Journal of Clinical Investigation*, **83**, 724–7.

Mahida, Y. R., Ciacci, C. & Podolsky, D. K. (1992). Peptide growth factors: role in epithelial-lamina propria cell interactions. In *Neuro-Immuno-Physiology of the Gastrointestinal Mucosa. Implications for Inflammatory Diseases*. Annals of the New York Academy of Sciences vol. 664, ed. R. H. Stead, M. H. Perdue, H. Cooke, D. W. Powell & K. E. Barrett, pp. 148–56. New York.

Main, C., Blennerhassett, P. & Collins, S. M. (1991). Human recombinant interleukin-1 beta (HrIL-1β) suppresses the release of ^{3}H-acetylcholine (^{3}H-ACh) from rat myenteric plexus (abstract). *Gastroenterology*, **100**, A833.

Manty, P. W., Catton, M. D., Boehmer, C. G., Welton, M. L., Passaro, E. P., Maggio, J. E. & Vigna, S. R. (1989). Receptors for sensory neuropeptides in human inflammatory diseases: implications for the effector role of sensory neurons. *Peptides*, **10**, 627–45.

Marshall, J. S., Stead, R. H., McSharry, C., Nielsen, L. & Bienenstock, J. (1990). The role of mast cell degranulation products in mast cell hyperplasia. I. Mechanism of action of nerve growth factor. *Journal of Immunology*, **144**, 1886–92.

Masson, S. D., Stead, R. H., Agro, A., Stanisz, A. M. & Perdue, M. H. (1990). Increases in substance P containing nerves in altered transport responses during intestinal inflammation in the rat (abstract). *Clinical and Investigative Medicine*, **13**, B27.

Matis, W. L., Lavker, R. M. & Murphy, G. F. (1990). Substance P induces the expression of an endothelial-leukocyte adhesion molecule by microvascular endothelium. *Journal of Investigative Dermatology*, **94**, 492–5.

Matsuda, H., Coughlin, M. D., Bienenstock, J. & Denburg, J. A. (1988). Nerve growth factor promotes hemopoietic colony growth and differentiaton. *Proceedings of the National Academy of Sciences, USA*, **85**, 6508–12.

McDonald, T. T. & Spencer, J. (1988). Evidence that mucosal T cells play a role in the pathogenesis of enteropathy in human small intestine. *Journal of Experimental Medicine,* **167**, 1341–9.

McKay, D. M., Bienenstock, J. & Perdue, M. H. (1993). Inhibition of antigen-induced secretion in jejunum from sensitized rats by interferon α/β. *Regional Immunology,* **5**, 53–9.

McKay, D. M., Halton, D. W., Johnston, C. F., Shaw, C., Fairweather, I. & Buchanan, K. D. (1991). *Hymenolepis diminuta*: changes in the levels of certain intestinal regulatory peptides in infected C57 mice. *Experimental Parasitology,* **73**, 15–26.

McKay, D. M. & Perdue, M. H. (1993). Intestinal epithelial function: the case for immunophysiological regulation – cells and mediators (first of two parts). *Digestive Diseases and Sciences,* **38**, 1377–87.

Miller, H. R. P., Nawa, Y. & Parish, C. R. (1979). Intestinal goblet cell differentiation in *Nippostrongylus*-infected animals rats after transfer of fractionated thoracic duct lymphocytes. *International Archives of Allergy and Applied Immunology,* **59**, 281–5.

Moncada, S., Palmer, R. M. J. & Higgs, E. A. (1991). Nitric oxide; physiology, pathophysiology, and pharmacology. *Pharmacological Reviews,* **43**, 109–42.

Moore, T., Spruck, C. & Said, S. (1988). Depression of lymphocyte traffic in sheep by vasoactive intestinal peptide. *Immunology,* **64**, 475–8.

Mosmann, T. R. (1992). T lymphocytes subsets, cytokines and effector functions. In *Neuro-Immune-Physiology of the Gastrointestinal Mucosa. Implications for Inflammatory Diseases.* Annals of the New York Academy of Sciences vol. 664, ed. R. H. Stead, M. H. Perdue, H. Cooke, D. W. Powell & K. E. Barrett, pp. 89–92. New York.

Murase, K., Murakami, Y., Takayanagi, K., Furukawa, Y. & Hayashi, K. (1992). Human fibroblast cells synthesize and secrete nerve growth factor in culture. *Biochemical and Biophysical Research Communications,* **184**, 373–9.

Murray, P. D., Swain, S. L. & Kagnoff, M. F. (1985). Regulation of the IgM and IgA anti-dextran B1355S response: synergy between IFN-γ, BCGF II, and IL-2. *Journal of Immunology,* **135**, 4015–20.

Neutra, M. R., O'Malley, L. J. & Specian, R. D. (1982). Regulation of goblet cell secretion II. A survey of potential secretagogues. *American Journal of Physiology,* **242**, G380–7.

Nong, Y.-H., Titus, R. G., Ribeiro, J. M. C. & Remold, H. G. (1989). Peptides encoded by the calcitonin gene inhibit macrophage function. *Journal of Immunology,* **143**, 45–9.

O'Dorisio, M. S., O'Dorisio, T. M., Cataland, S. & Balcerzak, S. P. (1980). VIP as a biochemical marker for polymorphonuclear leukocytes. *Journal of Laboratory and Clinical Medicine,* **96**, 666–72.

O'Dorisio, M. S., Shannon, B. T., Fleshman, D. J. & Campolito, L. B. (1989). Identification of high affinity receptors for vasoactive intestinal peptide on human lymphocytes of B cell lineage. *Journal of Immunology,* **142**, 3533–6.

Ottaway, C. A. (1984). *In vitro* alteration of receptors for vasoactive intestinal peptide changes in the *in vivo* localisation of mouse T cells. *Journal of Experimental Medicine,* **160**, 1054–69.

Ottaway, C. A. (1987). Selective effects of vasoactive intestinal peptide on the mitogenic response of murine T cells. *Immunology,* **62**, 291–7.

Ottaway, C. A. (1991). Neuroimmunomodulation in the intestinal mucosa. *Gastroenterology Clinics of North America,* **20**, 511–29.

Ottaway, C. A. & Greenberg, G. R. (1984). Interaction of vasoactive intestinal peptide with mouse lymphocytes: specific binding and the modulation of mitogen responses. *Journal of Immunology,* **132**, 417–23.

Ottaway, C. A., Lay, T. & Greenberg, G. (1990). High affinity specific binding of vasoactive intestinal peptide to human circulating T cells, B cells and large granular lymphocytes. *Journal of Neuroimmunology,* **29**, 149–55.

Pascual, D. W. & Bost, K. L. (1990). Substance P production by macrophage cell lines: a possible autocrine function for this neuropeptide. *Immunology*, **71**, 52–6.

Payan, D. G., Brewster, D. R. & Goetzl, E. J. (1984). Stereospecific receptors for substance P on cultured human IM-9 lymphoblasts. *Journal of Immunology*, **133**, 3269–75.

Payan, D. G., Brewster, D. R., Missirian-Bastian, A. & Goetzl, E. J. (1984). Substance P recognition by a subset of human T lymphocytes. *Journal of Clinical Investigation*, **74**, 1532–9.

Payan, D. G., Hess, C. A. & Goetzl, E. J. (1984). Inhibition by somatostatin of the proliferation of T lymphocytes and Molt-4 lymphoblasts. *Cellular Immunology*, **84**, 433–8.

Pearce, F. L. & Thompson, H. L. (1986). Some characteristics of histamine secretion from peritoneal mast cells stimulated with nerve growth factor. *Journal of Physiology (London)*, **372**, 379–93.

Perdue, M. H., Galbraith, R. & Davison, J. R. (1987). Evidence for substance P as a functional neurotransmitter in guinea pig intestinal mucosa. *Regulatory Peptides*, **18**, 63–74.

Perdue, M. H., Masson, S. D., Wershil, B. K. & Galli, S. J. (1991). Role of mast cells in ion transport abnormalities associated with intestinal anaphylaxis. Correction of the diminished secretory response in genetically mast cell-deficient W/W^v mice by bone marrow transplantation. *Journal of Clinical Investigation*, **87**, 687–93.

Pezzati, P., Stanisz, A. M., Marshall, J. S., Bienenstock, J. & Stead, R. H. (1992). Expression of nerve growth factor-receptor immunoreactivity on follicular dendritic cells from human mucosae associated lymphoid tissues. *Immunology*, **76**, 485–90.

Phillips, T. E. (1992). Both crypt and villus intestinal goblet cells secret mucin in response to cholinergic stimulation. *American Journal of Physiology*, **262**, G327–31.

Phillips, J. O., Everson, M. P., Moldoveanu, Z., Lue, C. & Mestecky, J. (1990). Synergistic effect of Il-4 and IFN-γ on the expression of polymeric Ig receptor (secretory component) and IgA binding by human epithelial cells. *Journal of Immunology*, **145**, 1740–4.

Phillips, T. E., Phillips, T. L. & Neutra, M. R. (1987). Macromolecules can pass through occluding junctions of rat ileal epithelia during cholinergic stimulation. *Cell and Tissue Research*, **247**, 547–54.

Polak, J. M. (1989). Endocrine cells of the gut. In *Handbook of Physiology, The Gastrointestinal System, Neural and Endocrine Biology* (sect. 6), vol. II ed. S. G. Schultz, pp. 79–96. Bethesda, Maryland, American Physiology Society.

Rola-Pleszczynski, M., Bulduc, D. & St. Pierre, A. (1985). The effects of VIP on human NK cell function. *Journal of Immunology*, **135**, 2569–73.

Romagnani, S. (1991). Human T_H1 and T_H2 subsets: doubt no more. *Immunology Today*, **12**, 256–7.

Russell, M., Dark, K. A., Cummins, R. W., Ellman, G., Callaway, E. & Peeke, H. V. S. (1984). Learned histamine release. *Science*, **225**, 733–4.

Sagi-Eisenberg, R., Ben-Neriah, Z., Pecht, I., Terry, S. & Blumberg, S. (1983). Structure activity relationship in the mast cell degranulating capacity of neurotensin fragments. *Neuropharmacology*, **22**, 197–201.

Schultz, S. G. & Zalusky, R. (1964). Ion transport in isolated rabbit ileum. I. Short-circuit current and Na fluxes. *Journal of General Physiology*, **47**: 567–84.

Scicchitano, R., Bienenstock, J. & Stanisz, A. M. (1988). *In vivo* immunomodulation by the neuropeptide substance P. *Immunology*, **63**, 733–5.

Scicchitano, R., Dazin, P., Bienenstock, J., Payan, D. G. & Stanisz, A. M. (1988). The murine IgA-secreting plasmacytoma MOPC-315 expresses somatostatin receptors. *Journal of Immunology*, **141**, 937–41.

Shanahan, F., Denburg, J., Fox, J. & Bienenstock, J. (1985). Mast cell heterogeneity: effects of neuroenteric peptides on histamine release. *Journal of Immunology*, **135**, 1331–7.

Soder, O. & Hellstrom, P. M. (1987). Neutrophil regulation of human thymocyte, guinea pig T lymphocyte and rat B lymphocyte mitogenesis. *International Archives of Allergy and Applied Immunology*, **84**, 205–11.

Stanisz, A. M., Befus, A. D. & Bienenstock, J. (1986). Differential effects of vasoactive intestinal peptide, substance P and somatostatin on immunoglobulin synthesis and proliferation by lymphocytes from Peyer's patches, mesenteric lymph nodes, and spleen. *Journal of Immunology*, **136**, 152–6.

Stanisz, A. M., Scicchitano, R., Dazin, J., Bienenstock, J. & Payan, D. G. (1987). Distribution of substance P receptors on murine spleen and Peyer's patch T and B cells. *Journal of Immunology*, **139**, 749–54.

Stanisz, A. M. (1993). Neural factors (neuropeptides/neurotransmitters, nerve growth factors) acting on cells of the immune system mediating immunity. In *Molecular Basis of Neuroimmune Interactions*. ed. D. G. Payan & M. Hauser, Oxford: Pergamon Press, in press.

Stead, R. H. (1992). Innervation of mucosal immune cells in the gastrointestinal tract. *Regional Immunology*, **4**, 91–9.

Stead, R. H., Tomioka, M., Quinonez, G., Simon, G. T., Felten, S. Y. & Bienenstock, J. (1987). Intestinal mucosal mast cells in normal and nematode-infected rat intestines are in intimate contact with peptidergic fibres. *Proceedings of the National Academy of Sciences, USA*, **84**, 2975–9.

Stead, R. H., Dixon, M. F., Bramwell, N. H., Riddell, R. H. & Bienenstock, J. (1989). Mast cells are closely apposed to nerves in the human gastrointestinal mucosa. *Gastroenterology*, **97**, 575–85.

Stepien, H., Lyson, K., Stanisz, A. M. & Pawlikowski, M. (1991). The effect of nerve growth factor on DNA synthesis, cyclic AMP and cyclic GMP accumulation by mouse spleen lymphocytes. *International Journal of Immunopharmacology*, **13**, 51–6.

Swain, M. G., Agro, A., Blennerhassett, P., Stanisz, A. M. & Collins, S. M. (1992). Increased levels of substance P in the myenteric plexus of *Trichinella*-infected rats. *Gastroenterology*, **102**, 1913–19.

Sweiter, M., Ghali, W. A., Rimmer, C. & Befus, A. D. (1989). Interferon-α/β inhibits IgE-dependent histamine release from rat mast cells. *Immunology*, **66**, 606–10.

Tainsh, K. R. & Pearce, F. L. (1992). Mast cell heterogeneity: evidence that mast cells isolated from various connective tissue locations in the rat display markedly graded phenotypes. *International Archives of Allergy and Applied Immunology*, **98**, 26–34.

Thorpe, L. W., Werbach-Perez, K. & Perez-Polo, J. R. (1987). Effect of nerve growth factor on the expression of interleukin-2 receptors on cultured human lymphocytes. *Annals of the New York Academy of Sciences*, **496**, 310–11.

Vermillion, D. L., Ernst, P. B. & Collins, S. M. (1991). T-lymphocyte modulation of intestinal muscle function in the *Trichinella*-infected rat. *Gastroenterology*, **101**, 31–8.

Waldman, D. B., Gardner, J. D., Zfass, A. M. & Makhlouf, G. M. (1977). Effects of vasoactive intestinal peptide on colonic transport and adenylate cyclase activity. *Gastroenterology*, **73**, 518–25.

Weinstock, J. V., Blum, A., Walder, J. & Walder, R. (1988). Eosinophils from granulomas in murine *Schistosomiasis mansoni* produce substance P. *Journal of Immunology*, **141**, 961–6.

Wershil, B. K. (1992). Immune mediators and cytokines in gastrointestinal inflammation. *Current Opinion in Gastroenterology*, **8**, 975–82.

Whitehead, W. E. (1992). Behavioral medicine approaches to gastrointestinal disorders. *Journal of Consulting and Clinical Psychology*, **60**, 605–12.

Wiik, P., Haugen, A. H., Lvhaug, D., Byum, A. & Opstad, P. K. (1989). Effect of VIP on the respiratory burst in human monocytes *ex vivo* during prolonged strain and energy deficiency. *Peptides*, **10**, 819–23.

Yonei, Y., Oda, M., Nakamura, M. *et al.*, (1985) Evidence for direct interaction between the cholinergic nerve and mast cells in rat colonic mucosa. An electron microscopic cytochemical and autoradiographic study. *Journal of Clinical Electron Microscopy*, **18**, 560–7.

Zimmerman, B. J., Anderson, D. C. & Granger, D. N. (1992). Neuropeptides promote neutrophil adherence to endothelial cell monolayers. *American Journal of Physiology*, **263**, G678–82.

–4–
Gastritis

R. V. HEATLEY

Introduction

Normal gastric mucosa contains few, if any, inflammatory cells. Gastritis represents the inflammatory response within the gastric mucosa resulting from injury, whatsoever the nature. The diagnosis is essentially histological since naked eye appearances are known to be unreliable. The advent of fibre-optic endoscopy and biopsy has considerably increased our knowledge about this condition and its natural history (Heatley & Wyatt, 1994). On a worldwide basis, gastritis is extremely common. Various classifications of gastric inflammation have developed based upon current knowledge at the time but, more recently, existing systems have been swept aside by the current terminology based upon known pathogenic mechanisms (Misiewicz, 1991). Most cases of gastritis are now known to be caused by infection with *Helicobacter pylori*. Other causes, including auto-immune gastritis, probably represent less than 10% of all cases of gastritis in most populations (Heatley & Wyatt, 1994).

Acute gastritis

The histological changes observed are usually simply those associated with acute inflammation, namely hyperaemia, infiltration with polymorphonuclear cells and oedema, together with a variable loss of surface epithelium. Macroscopically, oedema, small superficial haemorrhages and erosions or small ulcers may be visible (Heatley & Wyatt, 1994). A range of external influences have been shown to produce these changes but amongst the most important are alcohol excess, some spices, non-steroidal anti-inflammatory drugs (NSAIDs) including aspirin and metabolic disturbances associated with acute illnesses, in particular uraemia. Salicylate ingestion is one of the most studied models of acute injury. Most believe that aspirin ingestion produces disruption of the postulated superficial epithelial barrier, allowing diffusion of luminal acid to the underlying gastric mucosa and subsequent acute inflammation, as a result possibly of mast cell disruption. It is also now well recognised that acute *H. pylori* infection can occur. The histological changes described include marked neutrophil polymorphonuclear infiltration of the mucosa with surface exudation, in contrast with the acute haemorrhagic gastritis typically occurring with NSAIDs (Rathbone & Heatley, 1986). Acute *H. pylori* gastritis may either spontaneously resolve or progress to chronic gastritis. In association with acute *H. pylori* infection, local production of IgA and IgM by gastric mucosa occurs early but later circulating IgG and IgM become apparent (Sobala *et al.*, 1991a).

Chronic gastritis

Infiltration with chronic inflammatory cells, including lymphocytes and plasma cells, is the hallmark of chronic gastritis. Most cases of chronic gastritis are due to *H. pylori* infection but others, including autoimmune gastritis, also occur. Whatever the cause, in the long-term, atrophy of the mucosa may eventually ensue, which can affect gastric physiology, especially acid secretion (Heatley & Wyatt, 1994). Gastric atrophy and replacement with intestinal-type epithelium may also be relevant in the pathogenesis of gastric carcinoma, but this sequence of events has yet to be clearly understood.

Autoimmune chronic gastritis

Autoimmune gastritis (AIG) is essentially a histological diagnosis since endoscopic abnormalities are unusual, except in cases of extreme atrophy (Heatley & Wyatt, 1994). Pernicious anaemia (PA) can be a complication if chronic atrophic gastritis leads to a markedly reduced intrinsic factor secretion, which can subsequently result in vitamin B12 deficiency and hence a megaloblastic anaemia (Strickland, 1991).

   In autoimmune gastritis, circulating antibodies to gastric intrinsic factor (intrinsic factor antibodies – IFA) exist. Two types have been described – Type 1, blocking type present in 70% and Type 2, binding antibody in 30% of patients (Garrido-Pinson *et al.*, 1966; Samloff *et al.*, 1968). Furthermore, gastric parietal cell antibodies (PCA) have been detected in around 80–90% of sera (Taylor *et al.*, 1962). Parietal cell antibodies occur in auto-immune gastritis at any stage and PCA-positive gastritis is prevalent in relatives of patients with PA. IFA, however, tend to be associated with more advanced forms of gastritis associated with PA (Fisher *et al.*, 1967; TeVelde *et al.*, 1966; Wright *et al.*, 1966). Parietal cell antibodies have been further characterised into those reacting to the surface of parietal cells (PCSA) and a distinct microsomal (cytoplasmic) type (PCMA) (Masala *et al.*, 1980; De Aizpurua, Toh & Ungar, 1983). Some investigators have also suggested that gastrin-receptor auto-antibodies also exist, although these findings have not been generally confirmed (De Aizpurua, Ungar & Toh, 1985; Smith *et al.*,

Table 4.1. *Comparison of human and experimental murine auto-immune gastritis (AIG)* (adapted from Strickland, 1991)

	Human AIG	Mouse AIG
Morphology		
Body gastritis	+	± up to 50% Hypertrophic foveolar cell hyperplasia
Parietal cells destroyed	+	+
Lymphoid infiltrate	T & B cells	T cells <3 months B cells >3 months
Physiology		
Acid secretion	↓	↓
Impaired B12 absorption	↓	↑↓
Assoc. endocrine diseases	+	+
Immune associations		
Genetic predisposition	+	+
PCA	+	+
Parietal cell antigen	Membrane H+K+−ATP-ase	Microsomal, tubo-vesicular membrane protein
IFA	+	Not known

1989). It is now thought, however, that canalicular membrane H^+K^+ATP-ase, the gastric parietal cell proton pump, is the major parietal cell microsomal antigen (Burman *et al.*, 1989; Karlsson *et al.*, 1988). Other studies have also shown reactivity in PA sera to pepsinogen, which may explain concurrent destruction of a different cell type – the chief cell (Mardh & Song, 1989).

The early stages in the development of human auto-immune gastritis (AIG) are not well documented since the condition remains clinically silent until a late stage. The development phases have been studied in an animal model, an inbred, neonatally thymectomised mouse which has also been treated neonatally with cyclosporin (Kojima *et al.*, 1976; Kojima, Taguchi & Nishizuka, 1980; Sakaguchi & Sakaguchi, 1989). These animals develop a variety of organ-specific auto-antibodies, including gastric, and have inflammatory disease of the stomach. The gastritis developing in this model is very similar to human AIG (Table 4.1). Marked mucosal lymphoid infiltration occurs, including T and B cells. Parietal cell microsomal antibodies also develop and similarities are apparent between the microsomal antigen in the mouse model and the human disease. Interestingly, in the murine model, adoptive transfer of the disease can be accomplished by T cells but not serum. The T cell would therefore appear central to disease initiation in the mouse. In human AIG, T cell involvement is much less apparent (Taguchi & Nishizuka, 1987; Elson, 1990).

AIG is not a frequent cause of chronic gastritis. Nevertheless, auto-antibodies to parietal cells occur in up to 5–10% of adult populations of developed countries and the incidence increases with age (Strickland & Hooper, 1972). The major complication of AIG is pernicious anaemia and that itself is associated with the subsequent development of gastric cancer (Heatley & Wyatt, 1994). However, fortunately, only a minority of patients with AIG (usually less than a quarter) will eventually develop PA. The only clear risk factor for this progression is the development of auto-antibody to gastric intrinsic factor. AIG varies in prevalence, being commonest in Caucasians. Family studies suggest inheritance is as an autosomal recessive trait. Some studies have shown associations with HLA A3, B7 and B8 and some HLA DR antigens (Thomsen et al., 1981; Ungar et al., 1981). PA is not infrequently associated with other disorders also having organ-specific auto-antibodies, including thyroid disease, Addison's disease, diabetes mellitus, vitiligo and hypoparathyroidism (Heatley & Wyatt, 1994).

Eosinophilic gastritis (see Fig. 4.1)

This is an unusual condition, in which an eosinophilic infiltration of the gut occurs, particularly in the stomach and is often associated with a peripheral blood eosinophilia (Waldmann et al., 1967). The disorder is probably related to other hypereosinophilic syndromes, including polyarteritis nodosa and eosinophilic leukaemias (Ureles et al., 1961; Robert, Omura & Durant, 1977; Churg & Strauss, 1951; Nicks & Hughes, 1975). The cause is unknown, but some patients have allergic conditions affecting other organs. Treatment with steroids, elimination diets and oral sodium cromoglycate has been reported (Leinbach & Rubin, 1970; Heatley, Harris & Atkinson, 1980).

Lymphocytic gastritis (see Fig. 4.2)

This is another unusual condition, characterised by large numbers of intra-epithelial T lymphocytes in the surface and foveolar epithelium (Heatley & Wyatt, 1994). Some patients also appear to suffer from coeliac disease. In the endoscopic counterpart of this condition, 'varioliform gastritis', increased numbers of IgE-containing cells have been identified in the gastric

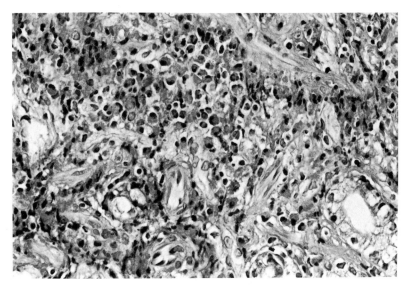

Fig. 4.1. Eosinophilic gastritis. Large numbers of eosinophils are present in the inflammatory infiltrate.

mucosa in some patients. Once again, steroids and sodium cromoglycate have been reported effective in some cases of varioliform gastritis (Haot et al., 1985; Dixon et al., 1988; Wolber et al., 1990).

H. pylori Chronic gastritis

In the majority of patients, chronic gastritis is a microbial disease associated with H. pylori infection, resulting in a gastric mucosal inflammatory response. This disorder is essentially a chronic inflammatory process, often with a polymorph infiltrate indicative of active inflammation, together with associated architectural change to the mucosa (Heatley & Wyatt, 1994). There are usually also marked local mucosal and systemic humoral and mucosal cellular responses. Specific IgA and IgM antibody is produced by cultures of gastric mucosa and mucosal plasma cells and T cell numbers increase in association with local cytokine production. H. pylori gastritis is a chronic infection which persists for many years, despite the presence of an apparently active and intact immune response by the gastric mucosa (Rathbone & Heatley, 1989). The disease is not only persistent but also often progressive, so that mucosal gastric atrophy develops in many affected individuals. The disorder is usually a pangastritis but it predominates largely in the antrum. Prevalence of H. pylori gastritis tends to increase with age. In most developed countries, 50% of the population will be affected by the fifth or sixth decade of life although, in populations with lower socioeconomic

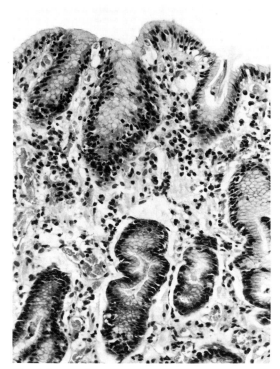

Fig. 4.2. A patient with lymphocytic gastritis. Although the serology for
H. pylori was positive, no organisms could be seen on histological
examination.

status in the developing world, the onset may be at a much lower age.
Progression of *H. pylori* chronic gastritis can profoundly affect gastric
physiology, with reductions occurring in stimulated acid secretion, pepsinogen secretion, output of intrinsic factor, together with a rise in gastrin
secretion (Table 4.2) (Heatley & Wyatt, 1994). Chronic *H. pylori* gastritis
does appear to be associated with an increased risk of peptic ulceration
developing, as well as an increased risk of gastric carcinoma, usually of the
intestinal type.

Transmission

It is not at all clear how *H. pylori* infection is transmitted from one individual
to another. Epidemiological studies show a strong relation between infection rates and low socio-economic conditions, particularly in childhood. The
assumption is that spread is probably by the faecal–oral route, perhaps
through contaminated water in underdeveloped countries.

There have been well-documented cases of transmission, two of which were deliberate, self-infection studies (Morris & Nicholson, 1992). After ingestion of the organism, non-specific symptoms occurred. The histological, physiological and immunological changes of acute infection have been documented in these circumstances and in some incidents in which accidental infection occurred (Heatley & Wyatt, 1994).

Although in some instances self-cure spontaneously occurred, in others changes of chronic gastritis ensued. It is by no means clear what factors are important in developing immunity to this infection or why some of those infected progress to chronic gastritis or subsequently perhaps peptic ulceration or even gastric cancer.

Local humoral immune response

Titres of *H. pylori*-specific IgA and IgM antibodies are measurable by ELISA in gastric juice in approximately one-third of subjects with *H. pylori* gastritis (Rathbone *et al.*, 1986). The lack of IgG could be expected because of degradation in gastric juice. Short-term biopsy cultures have confirmed local production of *H. pylori* specific IgG, IgA and IgM. The presence of both IgG and IgA antibodies correlates well with the initial plasma cell densities in the gastric mucosa. The data therefore confirm that a proportion of the plasma cell infiltrate that characterises chronic gastritis is involved in the local humoral response to *H. pylori* infection. Many of the micro-organisms lining the epithelial surface of affected patients also show a coating with immunoglobulin, using an immunoperoxidase technique (Wyatt, Rathbone & Heatley, 1987). IgG, IgA and IgM coating has been demonstrated but, as expected, IgA coating was the most consistent (see Fig. 4.6). Surprisingly, few organisms appeared coated deep in the gastric pits, an observation which is currently unexplained.

The functional effects of this response remain ill defined. Although the relevance of complement-mediated responses at mucosal surfaces is unclear, *H. pylori* has been demonstrated *in vitro* to be sensitive to antibody-dependent complement-mediated, bactericidal activity of serum. In the presence of serum opsonin, *H. pylori* organisms are phagocytosed and killed by neutrophils. Complement activation may also occur in the presence of lipid A, the lipid moiety of lipopolysaccharide (LPS) which has been shown to be present in *H. pylori*. (Pruul *et al.*, 1987).

Local cellular immune responses

In *H. pylori* gastritis (see Fig. 4.7), submucosal accumulations of lymphocytes and plasma cells frequently occur as lymphoid follicles. T cell numbers are usually increased, both in the epithelial compartment and lamina

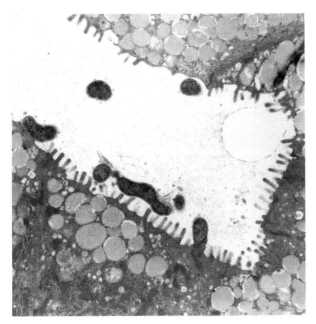

Fig. 4.3. Thin section of *H. pylori* adjacent to epithelial cell surface (magnification ×11 000).

propria, although reports of T cell subsets have given conflicting results (Papadimitriou *et al.*, 1988). In one study, T helper cells from gastritis patients showed increased CD7 expression, a T cell stimulation marker (Rathbone *et al.*, 1988). In *H. pylori* gastritis, inflamed mucosa unlike the normal stomach, becomes HLA-DR positive, suggesting that gastric epithelial cells may be capable of antigen recognition and presentation (Papadimitriou *et al.*, 1988; Engstrand *et al.*, 1988). Macrophage numbers are also usually increased in chronic active gastritis. Tumour necrosis factor α (TNF-α), a cytokine produced chiefly by activated macrophages and monocytes, has a variety of modulatory effects on immune activation. TNF-α secretion is greatly enhanced in antral biopsies from *H. pylori*-positive individuals, in particular those with evidence of activity of the gastritis (Crabtree *et al.*, 1991*a*; Karttunen, 1991). Active gastritis is particularly associated with the presence of neutrophil polymorphs, which appear principally between epithelial cells, especially in the deeper portions of the gastric pits (Craig *et al.*, 1992). It has been suggested that *H. pylori* secretes a chemotactic factor responsible for attracting the neutrophilic infiltrate (Craig *et al.*, 1992). The cytokine interleukin (IL) 8 is a known, potent attractant of neutrophils and may well be important in the gastric mucosa in *H. pylori* infection (Gupta *et al.*, 1991). Mucosal levels of IL6 are also elevated in active *H. pylori*

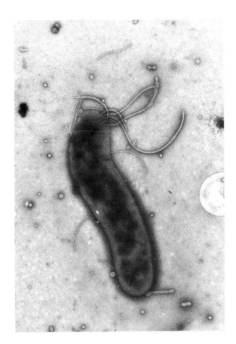

Fig. 4.4. Negatively stained preparation of cultured *H. pylori* (magnification ×25 000).

infection and this may influence neutrophils by augmenting oxidative burst responses and increasing lysozyme and lactoferrin secretion (Crabtree *et al.*, 1991*a*). *H. pylori* organisms have been seen in neutrophil phagocytic vacuoles (Shousha, Bull & Parkins, 1984; Tricottet *et al.*, 1986).

Systemic immune responses

A variety of techniques has been developed to identify circulating antibodies against *H. pylori*, but most would now use an ELISA which has been well validated and is also available commercially (Crabtree *et al.*, 1991*b*). In *H. pylori*-associated gastritis, both circulating IgG and IgA levels are usually elevated, although the most consistent and predictive values are obtained with the IgG titres. Subclass analysis has shown increases in IgG1, IgG2 and IgG4, but not IgG3 (Newell, Hawtin & Steer, 1988). In acute infection, an IgM response is first observed, followed subsequently after about two months by IgG and IgA seroconversion, by which time the IgM

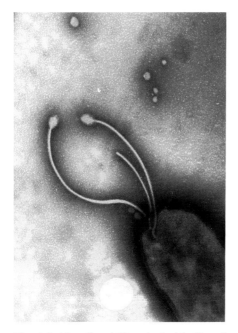

Fig. 4.5. Flagella of *H. pylori* with dilated terminations (magnification ×60 000).

response has declined (Morris & Nicholson, 1992; Sobala *et al.*, 1991*a*). The systemic response is longstanding if colonisation of the gastric mucosa continues. However, a decline in antibody levels accompanies successful eradication of the organism.

H. pylori antigens.   Most investigations have been carried out using the Western immunoblot method. However, significant differences in the molecular weights of the major protein antigens have been reported (Newell, 1987*a*; Newell 1987*b*; Dunn, Perez-Perez & Blaser, 1989; Kist, Apel & Jacobs, 1988; von Wulffen *et al.*, 1988). Most positive individuals produce antibodies that react against 61 and 28 Kd polypeptides, which appear specific for *H. pylori*, and are probably components of the urease enzyme. Other frequently reported antigens have been a 110–120 kD protein, a more recently described CagA antigen and a further urease-associated 56 kD polypeptide. A 54 kD polypeptide, which is flagellin, and 56 kD polypeptide (flagella-associated proteins) are generally consistent findings. The antibody response to *H. pylori* infection is, therefore, highly complex and variable in the experience of most observers (Rathbone & Heatley, 1989).

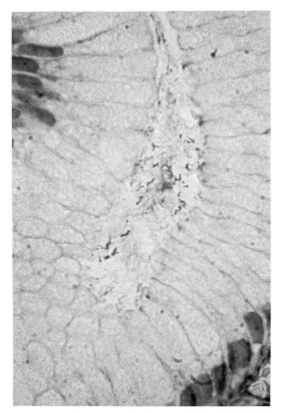

Fig. 4.6. IgA staining of antral mucosa. *H. pylori* strongly positive for IgA are present on the surface, although those deep in the gastric pit are not so strongly positive (magnification ×320). (Reproduced with permission *J. Clin. Path.*).

Practical uses of H. pylori serology

Serology is now a well-established, non-invasive method of diagnosing *H. pylori* infection (Newell & Stacey, 1992). It has to compete with other non-invasive techniques, in particular urea breath testing and invasive procedures including endoscopic biopsy and subsequent histological identification, bacterial culture or indirect identification by urease tests on gastric biopsy material (Heatley & Wyatt, 1994).

Serological studies have to date been used to demonstrate the marked increase of *H. pylori* infection with age in various populations, and also the geographic variation in infection rates throughout different population groups. Further epidemiological studies, using serological techniques, have

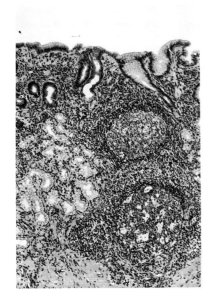

Fig. 4.7. *H. pylori* gastritis with prominent lymphoid follicles.

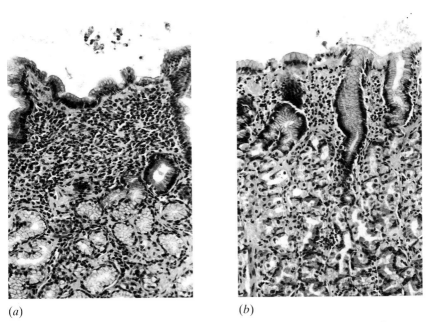

(a)   (b)

Fig. 4.8. Duodenal ulcer patient with antral predominant *H. pylori* gastritis (a) antrum (b) corpus.

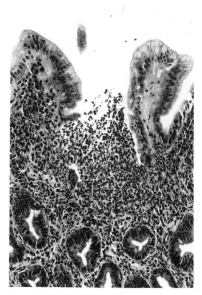

Fig. 4.9. Early duodenal ulcer associated with peptic duodenitis and areas of gastric metaplasia.

found differing infection risks in relation to occupations, concurrent medical conditions and home circumstances. Serological methods of identifying the mode of spread of infection and its sources are most likely to be of great relevance in the future (Heatley & Wyatt, 1994).

   H. pylori serology has also been used as a screening technique in patients presenting with dyspepsia, in view of the close relationship between *H. pylori* infection and many conditions associated with dyspepsia (Sobala *et al.*, 1991*b*). Immunoblotting has also been used to identify particular characteristics of organisms associated with peptic ulcer disease and active gastritis, especially the 120 kD antigen (Crabtree *et al.*, 1991*c*).

Pathogenetic mechanisms in H. pylori *gastritis*

It is by no means clear how *H. pylori* infection of gastric mucosa induces gastric inflammation. The organism has been shown to develop adhesion pedestals to gastric epithelium in a similar manner to enteropathic *E. coli* in the intestine. Furthermore, the organism has a wide range of enzymes capable of causing damage to gastric epithelium, either directly or indirectly. Urease is the one that has received most attention, although there are doubts about whether this is likely to be damaging. Some strains of organism have also been claimed to have pathogenic features, although data are limited and varied. Gastric mucus synthesis is believed to be an

Table 4.2. *Comparison of human autoimmune (AIG) and* H. pylori (H.p)
gastritis

	AIG	H.p
Morphology		
Gastritis	Corpus	Predominantly antral
Progression	Leads eventually to gastric atrophy	Can lead to gastric atrophy
Cellular infiltrate	Mainly B cells (some T cells)	Probably T and B cells increased Neutrophils ↑ in active disease
Physiology		
Acid secretion	↓	May be short-lived ↓ early or when atrophy ensues
Impaired B12 absorption	↓	No specific effects
Immune associations		
Associated immune diseases	+	None known
Genetic predisposition	+	None known
Systemic antibodies	PCA	IgM early in acute infection
	IFA	IgG + IgA in chronic disease
Antigens	Parietal cell Microsomal and cell surface antigens	To variety of *H.p* surface antigens

important means of epithelial defence. Some evidence suggests *H. pylori*
infection can affect gastric mucus glycoprotein secretion (Rathbone &
Heatley, 1992).

There are a number of ways in which *H. pylori* infection could compromise the normal gastric mucosal barrier. If indeed this is the case, then
subsequent exposure to potentially aggressive luminal factors, including
acid, pepsin, bile and some drugs, may trigger the pathways which could
lead to the development of mucosal inflammation.

Treatment prospects

Unfortunately, once established as a chronic infection, *H. pylori* gastritis is difficult to treat. None of the currently available regimens is entirely successful, but best reported results have been obtained with a combination of a bismuth salt with at least two anti-bacterials, such as tetracycline or amoxycillin, together with metronidazole. Other combinations include acid suppressants such as omeprazole or ranitidine, with amoxycillin or clarithromycin, but results with all these different combinations have been extremely variable. One of the principal obstacles to eradication appears to be antibiotic resistance, mainly to metronidazole (Heatley, 1992).

Presumably in the future, immunisation against *H. pylori* is a possibility, in particular as a means of preventing primary infection. Although little progress has been made against human infection, a related organism (*H. felis*), infecting mice, has been used as a model to study immunological responses and possible means of developing immunotherapy against human *H. pylori*-related disease (Lee, 1992).

Conclusions

Gastritis has long been recognised as a clinical entity. Interest in the immunology of chronic gastritis began with the recognition of an auto-immune variant, although the precise stages of development remain poorly understood. An enormous explosion of interest in the immunology and pathogenesis of chronic gastritis has occurred as a result of our recognition of the importance of *H. pylori* in this condition. In the short time we have known about the *H. pylori* organism and its role in chronic gastritis, we are little further forward in understanding how this bacterium promotes gastric inflammation. From what we do know about the immunological response of the host to infection, one would assume this would probably lead to expulsion of the organism. Yet, *H. pylori* gastritis remains probably the most prevalent and widely spread of all chronic human infections. Parallel animal infections may help us to solve this riddle yet, unfortunately, we do not have any entirely suitable animal model of *H. pylori* infection. Probably the most fascinating aspect of this organism is as a means of studying microbiological infection within the human gastrointestinal tract. There can be few, if any, other infectious processes at a mucosal surface which persist for so long and apparently do so little overall harm to the host. Further study of this relationship is likely to be greatly revealing in our endeavours to understand the full repertoire of the gut mucosal immune system.

Acknowledgements

EM photomicrographs, courtesy of Dr Alan Curry and histology Dr J. Wyatt.

References

Burman, P., Mardh, S., Norberg, L. *et al.* (1989). Parietal cell antibodies in pernicious anaemia inhibit H^+, K^+-adenosine triphosphatase, the proton pump of the stomach. *Gastroenterology*, **96**, 1434–8.

Churg, J. & Strauss, L. (1951). Allergic granulomatosis, allergic angiitis and periarteritis nodosa. *American Journal of Pathology*, **27**, 277–301.

Crabtree, J. E., Shallcross, T. M., Heatley, R. V. & Wyatt, J. I. (1991*a*). Mucosal tumour necrosis factor alpha and interleukin-6 in patients with *Helicobacter pylori*-associated gastritis. *Gut*, **44**, 768–71.

Crabtree, J. E., Shallcross, T. M., Heatley, R. V. & Wyatt, J. I. (1991*b*). Evaluation of a commercial ELISA for serodiagnosis of *H. pylori* infection. *Journal of Clinical Pathology*, **44**, 326–8.

Crabtree, J. E., Taylor, J. D., Wyatt, J. I. *et al.* (1991*c*). Mucosal IgA recognition of *Helicobacter pylori* 120 kDa protein, peptic ulceration and gastric pathology. *Lancet*, **338**, 332–35.

Craig, P. M., Territo, M. C., Karnes, W. E. & Walsh, J. H. (1992). *Helicobacter pylori* secretes a chemotactic factor for monocytes and neutrophils. *Gut*, **33**, 1020–3.

De Aizpurua, H. J., Toh, B. & Ungar, B. (1983). Parietal cell surface reactive autoantibody in pernicious anemia demonstrated by indirect membrane immunofluorescence. *Clinical and Experimental Immunology*, **52**, 341–9.

De Aizpurua, H. J., Ungar, B. & Toh, B. (1985). Autoantibody to the gastrin receptor in pernicious anemia. *New England Journal of Medicine*, **313**, 479–83.

Dixon, M. F., Wyatt, J. I., Burke, D. A. *et al.* (1988). Lymphocytic gastritis – relationship to *Campylobacter pylori* infection. *Journal of Pathology*, **154**, 125–32.

Dunn, B. E., Perez-Perez, G. I. & Blaser, M. J. (1989). Two-dimensional gel electrophoresis and immunoblotting of *Campylobacter pylori* proteins. *Infectious Immunology*, **57**, 1825–33.

Elson, C. O. (1990). Do organ-specific suppressor T cells prevent autoimmune gastritis? *Gastroenterology*, **98**, 226–9.

Engstrand, L., Scheynius, A., Grimelius, L. *et al.* (1988). Induced expression of class II transplantation antigens on gastric epithelial cells in patients with *Campylobacter pylori*-positive gastric biopsies. *Gastroenterology*, **94**, A115.

Fisher, J. M., MacKay, I. R., Taylor, K. B. *et al.* (1967). An immunologic study of categories of gastritis. *Lancet*, **i**, 176–80.

Garrido-Pinson, G. C., Turner, M. D., Crookston, J. H. *et al.* (1966). Studies of human intrinsic factor autoantibodies. *Journal of Immunology*, **97**, 897–912.

Gupta, R., Moss, S., Thomas, D. M., Abbott, F., Rees, A., Calam, J. (1991). *Helicobacter pylori* increases release of interleukin 8: a potent attractant of neutrophils. *Gut*, **32**, A1206.

Haot, J., Wallez, A., Jouret-Mourin, A. & Hardy, N. (1985). La gastrite 'a lymphocytes'. Une nouvelle entite? *Acta Endoscopica*, **15**, 187–8.

Heatley, R. V. & Wyatt, J. I. (1994). Gastritis and Duodenitis. In *Bockus Gastroenterology*, 5th edn, ed. W. Haubrich & F. Schaffner. Philadelphia and London: W. B. Saunders Co. (in press).

Heatley, R. V., Harris, A. & Atkinson, M. (1980). Treatment of a patient with clinical features of both eosinophilic gastroenteritis and polyarteritis nodosa with oral sodium cromoglycate. *Digestive Diseases and Sciences*, **25**, 470–2.

Heatley, R. V. (1992). Review article: the treatment of *Helicobacter pylori* infection. *Alimentary Pharmacology and Therapeutics*, **6**, 291–303.

Karlsson, F. A., Burman, P., Loof, L. *et al.* (1988). Major parietal cell antigen in autoimmune gastritis with pernicious anemia is the acid-producing H^+, K^+-adenosine triphosphatase of the stomach. *Journal of Clinical Investigation*, **81**, 475–9.

Karttunen, R. (1991). Blood lymphocyte proliferation, cytokine secretion and appearance of T cells with activation surface markers in cultures with *Helicobacter pylori*. Comparison of the responses of subjects with and without antibodies to *H. pylori*. *Clinical and Experimental Immunology*, **83**, 396–400.

Kist, M., Apel, I. & Jacobs, E. (1988). Protein antigens of *Campylobacter pylori*: the problem of species specificity. In *Campylobacter pylori*, ed. H. Menge, M. Gregor, G. J. J. Tytgat *et al.*, pp. 19–26. Berlin: Springer-Verlag.

Kojima, A., Tanaka-Kojima, Y., Sakakura, T. *et al.* (1976). Spontaneous development of autoimmune thyroiditis in neonatally thymectomized mice. *Laboratory Investigations*, **34**, 550–7.

Kojima, A., Taguchi, O. & Nishizuka, Y. (1980). Experimental production of possible autoimmune gastritis followed by macrocytic anemia in athymic nude mice. *Laboratory Investigations*, **42**, 387–95.

Lee, A. (1992). Helicobacter pylori and Helicobacter-like organisms in animals: overview of mucus-colonizing organisms. In *Helicobacter pylori and Gastroduodenal Disease*, ed. B. J. Rathbone & R. V. Heatley, pp. 259–275. Oxford: Blackwell Scientific Publications.

Leinbach, G. E. & Rubin, C. E. (1970). Eosinophilic gastroenteritis: a simple reaction to food allergens? *Gastroenterology*, **59**, 874–89.

Mardh, S. & Song, Y-H. (1989). Characterization of antigenic structures in autoimmune atrophic gastritis with pernicious anemia. The parietal cell H, K-ATPase and the chief cell pepsinogen are the two major antigens. *Acta Physiologica Scandinavica*, **136**, 581–7.

Masala, C., Smurra, G., De Prima, M. A. *et al.* (1980). Gastric parietal cell antibodies. Demonstration by immunofluorescence of their reactivity with the surface of the gastric parietal cells. *Clinical and Experimental Immunology*, **41**, 271–80.

Misiewicz, J. J. (1991). The Sydney System: a new classification of gastritis. Working Party Report to the World Congresses of Gastroenterology, Sydney 1990. *Journal of Gastroenterology and Hepatology*, **6**, 207–8.

Morris, A. & Nicholson, G. (1992). Helicobacter pylori: human ingestion studies. In *Helicobacter pylori and Gastroduodenal Disease, Campylobacter pylori*, ed. B. J. Rathbone, R. V. Heatley, pp. 209–216. Oxford: Blackwell Scientific Publications.

Newell, D. G., Hawtin, P. R. & Steer, H. W. (1988). Human serum immunoglobulin class and subclass responses to *Campylobacter pylori* acid extract antigens. In *Campylobacter*, IV, ed. B. Kaijser & E. Falsen, pp. 192–93. Göteburg, Sweden: University Göteburg.

Newell, D. G. (1987*a*). Identification of the outer membrane proteins of *Campylobacter pyloridis* and antigenic cross-reactivity between *C. pyloridis* and *C. jejuni*. *Journal of General Microbiology*, **133**, 163–70.

Newell, D. G. (1987*b*). Human antibody responses to the surface protein antigens of *Campylobacter pyloridis*. *Seriodiagnosis Immunotherapy*, **1**, 209–17.

Newell, D. G. & Stacey, A. R. (1992). The Serology of H. pylori Infections. In *Helicobacter pylori and Gastroduodenal Disease*, ed. B. J. Rathbone & R. V. Heatley, pp. 64–73. Oxford: Blackwell Scientific Publications.

Nicks, A. J. & Hughes, F. (1975). Polyarteritis nodosa 'mimicking' eosinophilic gastroenteritis. *Radiology*, **116**, 53–4.

Papadimitriou, C. S., Ioachim-Velogianni, E. E., Tsianos, E. B. *et al.* (1988). Epithelial HLA-DR expression and lymphocyte subsets in gastric mucosa in type B chronic gastritis. *Virchow's Archiv A*, **413**, 197–204.

Pruul, H., Lee, P. C., Goodwin, C. S. *et al.* (1987). Interaction of *Campylobacter pyloridis* with human immune defence mechanisms. *Journal of Medical Microbiology*, **23**, 233–8.

Rathbone, B. J., Wyatt, J. I., Worsley, B. W. *et al.* (1986). Systemic and local antibody responses to gastric *Campylobacter pyloridis* in non-ulcer dyspepsia. *Gut*, **27**, 642–7.

Rathbone, B. J. & Heatley, R. V. (1986). Gastritis. In *Gut Defences in Clinical Practice*, ed. M. S. Losowsky & R. V. Heatley, pp. 228–42. Edinburgh, London, Melbourne & New York: Churchill Livingstone.

Rathbone, B. J., Wyatt, J. I., Trejdosiewicz, L. K. *et al.* (1988). Mucosal T cell subsets in normal gastric antrum and *C. pylori* associated chronic gastritis. *Gut*, **29**, A1438.

Rathbone, B. J. & Heatley, R. V. (1989). Immunology of *C. pylori* infection. In *Campylobacter pylori in Gastritis and Peptic Ulcer Disease*, ed. Martin J. Blaser, pp. 135–45. New York & Tokyo: Igaku-Shoin.

Rathbone, B. J. & Heatley, R. V. (1992). Possible pathogenic mechanisms in *Helicobacter pylori* infection. In *Helicobacter pylori and Gastroduodenal Disease*, ed. B. J. Rathbone & R. V. Heatley, pp. 217–23. Oxford: Blackwell Scientific Publications.

Robert, F., Omura, E. & Durant, J. R. (1977). Mucosal eosinophilic gastroenteritis with systemic involvement. *American Journal of Medicine*, **62**, 139–43.

Sakaguchi, S. & Sakaguchi, N. (1989). Organ-specific autoimmune disease induced by elimination of T cell subset. V. Neonatal administration of cyclosporin A causes autoimmune disease. *Journal of Immunology*, **142**, 471–80.

Samloff, I. M., Kleinman, M. S., Turner, M. D. *et al.* (1968). Blocking and binding antibody to intrinsic factor and parietal cell antibody in pernicious anemia. *Gastroenterology*, **55**, 575–83.

Shousha, S., Bull, T. B. & Parkins, R. A. (1984). Gastric spiral bacteria. *Lancet*, **ii**, 101.

Smith, J. T. L., Garner, A., Hampson, S. E. *et al.* (1989). Absence of gastrin inhibitory activity in the IgG fraction of serum from patients with pernicious anemia. *Gut*, **30**, A721.

Sobala, G. M., Crabtree, J. E., Dixon, M. F. *et al.* (1991*a*). Acute *Helicobacter pylori* infection: clinical features, local and systemic immune response, gastric mucosal histology and gastric juice ascorbic acid concentrations. *Gut*, **32**, 1415–18.

Sobala, G. M., Crabtree, J. E., Pentith, J. A. *et al.* (1991*b*). Screening dyspepsia by serology to *Helicobacter pylori*. *Lancet*, **338**, 94–6.

Strickland, R. G. & Hooper, B. (1972). The parietal cell heteroantibody in human sera: prevalence in a normal population and relationship to parietal cell autoantibody. *Pathology*, **4**: 259–63.

Strickland, R. G. (1991). The Sydney System: auto-immune gastritis. *Journal of Gastroenterology and Hepatology*, **6**, 238–43.

Taguchi, O. & Nishizuka, Y. (1987). Self tolerance and localised autoimmunity. Mouse models of autoimmune disease that suggest tissue-specific suppressor T cells are involved in self-tolerance. *Journal of Experimental Medicine*, **165**, 146–56.

Taylor, K. B., Roitt, I. M., Doniach, D. *et al.* (1962). Autoimmune phenomena in pernicious anemia: gastric antibodies. *British Medical Journal*, **2**: 1347–52.

TeVelde, K., Hoedemaeker, P. J., Anders, G. J. P. A. *et al.* (1966). A comparative morphological and functional study of gastritis with and without autoantibodies. *Gastroenterology*, **51**, 135–48.

Thomsen, M., Jorgensen, F., Brandsborg, M. *et al.* (1981). Association of pernicious anemia and intrinsic factor antibody with HLA-D. *Tissue Antigens*, **17**, 97–103.

Tricottet, V., Bruneval, P., Vire, O. & Camilleri, J. P. (1986). *Campylobacter*-like organisms and surface epithelium abnormalities in active, chronic gastritis in humans: an ultrastructural study. *Ultrastructural Pathology*, **10**, 113–22.

Ungar, B., Mathews, J. D., Tait, B. D. *et al.* (1981). HLA-DR patterns in pernicious anemia. *Lancet*, **i**, 768–70.

Ureles, A. L., Alschibaja, L., Louico, D. & Stabins, S. J. (1961). Idiopathic eosinophilic infiltration of the gastrointestinal tract, diffuse and circumscribed. *American Journal of Medicine*, **30**, 899–909.

von Wulffen, H., Grote, H. J., Gaterman, S. *et al.* (1988). Immunoblot analysis of immune response to *Campylobacter pylori* and its clinical associations. *Journal of Clinical Pathology*, **41**, 653–9.

Waldmann, T. A., Wochner, R. D., Laster, L. & Gordon, R. S. (1967). Allergic gastroentero-pathy: a cause of excessive gastrointestinal protein loss. *New England Journal of Medicine*, **276**, 761–9.

Wolber, R., Owen, D., DelBuono, I. *et al.* (1990). Lymphocytic gastritis in patients with coeliac sprue or spruelike intestinal disease. *Gastroenterology*, **98**, 310–15.

Wright, R., Whitehead, R., Wangel, A. G. *et al.* (1966). Autoantibodies and microscopic appearance of gastric mucosa. *Lancet*, **i**, 618–21.

Wyatt, J. I., Rathbone, B. J. & Heatley, R. V. (1987). Local immune response to gastric *Campylobacter* in non-ulcer disease. *Journal of Clinical Pathology*, **39**, 863–70.

–5–
The immunology of coeliac disease

DERMOT KELLEHER and D. G. WEIR

Introduction

Coeliac disease (CD) is a disease of the small intestine characterised by the development of villous atrophy, in response to ingestion of dietary proteins contained in wheat, barley and rye (Kelly *et al.*, 1990). Villous atrophy, in turn, results in malabsorption of essential nutrients with the development of steatorrhea, weight loss and specific deficiency syndromes. Villous atrophy is associated with a cellular infiltrate comprising increased intra-epithelial lymphocytes, increased lamina propria lymphocytes and plasma cells (Anand *et al.*, 1981; Fry *et al.*, 1972; Ferguson, 1987; Lancaster-Smith, Kumar & Dawson, 1975). Coeliac disease is tightly linked genetically to genes encoded in the major histocompatibility complex (MHC). In this respect it is similar to the auto-immune diseases of thyroid, pancreas and joints. However, since the precipitating agent is known, coeliac disease may serve as a useful model for auto-immune disease in the human if the interactions between genetic and environmental factors can be adequately defined. In this respect, an understanding of the genetic basis of coeliac disease is essential for an understanding of the immune hypotheses of the disease.

Genetic studies of coeliac disease

Coeliac disease shows a geographical predeliction, with a particularly high incidence in Northern Europe. There is a clear familial predisposition to the disease (Myllotte *et al.*, 1974), but this does not follow classical Mendelian patterns, suggesting the possibility of multigenic and/or multifactorial aetiopathogenesis. Concordance in monozygotic twins occurs in approximately 75% of cases (Walker-Smith, 1973). However, discordance in 25% of cases suggests that external environmental factors may be important in the pathogenesis of disease. The hypothesis that an external environmental agent such as a virus may be implicated, has been supported by the observations from epidemiological studies that the incidence of childhood

coeliac disease has declined significantly in regions previously known to
have a high incidence (Littlewood, Crollick & Richards, 1980). Relatives of
patients with coeliac disease may show evidence of gliadin sensitivity, with
increased anti-gliadin antibodies and minor histological changes, without
necessarily progressing to coeliac disease (Corazza *et al.*, 1992; MacDonald,
Dobbins & Rubin, 1965; Marsh *et al.*, 1990).

The major histocompatibility complex (MHC) on chromosome 6

Coeliac disease has been tightly linked to the MHC with a particularly strong
association with the HLA Class II genes. The MHC located on chromosome
6 is a region of considerable interest from an immunological point of view.
Three major families of genes have been identified in this region. Class I,
Class II and Class III (Fig. 5.1). The Class III genes are mainly complement
genes, although the genes coding for tumour necrosis factor (TNF) and for a
heat shock protein also lie within this region. The Class I genes code for the
HLA A, B, and C molecules, all of which are highly polymorphic. The Class
II genes include DR, DQ, DX and DP and DM (Trowsdale & Powis, 1992).
DM differs from other Class II genes in that there is limited polymorphism in
genes coding for this molecule. Each of these genes has one or more genes
coding for an α chain and a β chain and each of these α and β chain genes may
be divided into a number of segments ($\alpha 1$, $\alpha 2$ etc.). In addition, this region
includes a large group of other genes with important immunoregulatory
functions. These genes include the protein transporter genes known as *tap* 1
and *tap* 2 (Trowsdale & Campbell, 1992), which possess a so-called ABC

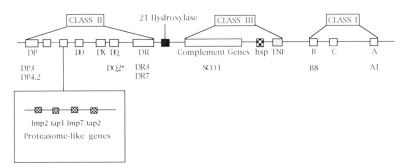

Fig. 5.1. Simplified map of the human major histocompatibility complex
(not to scale). Structural organisation of human MHC genes with
classification into Class I, II and III genes. The coeliac disease associated
haplotype is illustrated underneath. The DQ haplotype associated with
the disease is now designated DQA1*0501 DQB1*0201 at a genetic
level.

cassette typical of other transporter proteins, such as the protein encoded by the multi-drug resistance gene. These genes appear to be of major importance in the processing of antigen for presentation to CD8 T-cells, i.e. cells of the suppressor/cytotoxic phenotype (Kleijmeer et al., 1992; Kelly et al., 1992). In addition, genes within this region code for proteasomes and proteases (Trowsdale & Campbell, 1992). Many of the genes within this region are inducible by γ-interferon (Trowsdale & Powis, 1992). A large number of additional genes within the Class III region remain to be defined. Hence, this is a region of the genome of major immunological dominance containing genes essential for the processing and presentation of antigen to T cells.

Linkage of coeliac disease to HLA genes

DR and DQ

Initial studies linked coeliac disease to HLA Class I gene products, HLA A1 and B8. Subsequently it was noted that HLA DR3 and DR7 and complement haplotypes were also associated with coeliac disease in the majority of cases (Alper et al., 1987). Further studies demonstrated that both HLA DR3 and DR7 were in linkage disequilibrium with HLA DQ2 and that DQ2 (Tosi, Vismara & Tanigaki, 1983), present in over 90% of cases and was the most strongly linked of the HLA haplotypes to coeliac disease. The genetic association of coeliac disease with HLA DQ has been studied in further detail. A number of individuals with coeliac disease do not have either HLA DR3 or 7 but do have the HLA DR5, 7 phenotype. However, the HLA DR5 associated DQ7 AI gene is identical to the HLA DQ2 AI gene in linkage disequilibrium with HLA DR3. Furthermore, the DR7 associated DQ B1 is identical to the DR3 associated DQ B1 gene. Thus, the combination of DQA1*0501 and DQB1*0201 is found in 99% of coeliac patients (Sollid et al., 1989). However, HLA DQ alleles from both normal individuals and from patients with coeliac disease were sequenced and found to be identical (Kagnoff et al., 1989). transComplementation, i.e. the association of the α chain of one HLA allele with the β chain of another would suggest that identical HLA DQ structures could be generated from several specificities. Thus, individuals possessing the HLA types DR3, 3 and DR5, 7 could potentially generate an identical DQ molecule for antigen-presentation to CD4 cells. However, siblings sharing HLA haplotypes with the propositus have only a 30% incidence of disease emphasising the fact that HLA DQ is a disease susceptibility gene, which does not specifically confer disease (Tosi et al., 1983). Furthermore, a recent study of Ashkenazi Jews has demonstrated that up to 20% of individuals with coeliac disease do not possess the

HLA DQ2 haplotype (Tighe *et al.*, 1993). Patients negative for DQ2 appear to possess a DQ β chain negative for Asp on position 57 (Mantovani *et al.*, 1993). Similar data can be inferred from a Californian study in which up to 25% of coeliac patients did not possess the HLA DR3 or 7 haplotype (Kagnoff *et al.*, 1983).

HLA DP

Using oligonucleotide allele specific probes, Erlich demonstrated that two HLA DP haplotypes, 3 and 4.2 are associated with coeliac disease in Italian patients (Bugawan *et al.*, 1989). It was of particular note in this study that polymorphic residues at positions 69, 56 and 57 on the molecule, which may be predicted to interact with the antigen binding groove, are of critical importance in determining this susceptibility. Prior studies had demonstrated restriction fragment length polymorphisms (RFLPs) in DP associated with coeliac disease (Caffrey *et al.*, 1990; Howell *et al.*, 1986, 1988). The question of whether these are in linkage disequilibrium with HLA DQ2 has not been resolved and much of these data are conflicting. Family linkage studies are required to definitively confirm whether HLA DP and DQ polymorphisms are in linkage disequilibrium.

Functional significance of HLA association with coeliac disease

HLA Class II molecules are involved in the presentation of endogenously processed antigen to antigen specific T cells. Foreign antigen undergoes processing in the endosomic compartment of the antigen presenting cell and then binds tightly to an antigen binding groove on the molecule (Strominger, 1986). This complex of antigen and Class II is recognised by the T cell receptor (Davis & Bjorkman, 1988). Specific residues flanking this groove have been noted to be of major importance in the genetics of diabetes mellitus (Todd, Bell & McDevitt, 1987), rheumatoid arthritis (Nepom, Hansen & Nepom, 1987) and pemphigus vulgaris. Since Class II molecules present antigens to CD4 positive T cells, this appears to be the major mechanism of activation of antigen specific help including the production of cytokines, such as interleukins 2 and 4 and γ-interferon (Fig. 5.2). Hence, the tight association of coeliac disease with this haplotype has led to the suggestion that coeliac disease is mediated by some immunological perturbation of this complex. However, the complexity of this region and the presence of multiple non-HLA genes suggests some caution in this interpretation. Other, as yet uncharacterised, genes in this region might also be linked to coeliac disease. The *tap* 2 peptide transporter gene is located between HLA DP and DQ (Powis *et al.*, 1992). The product has a role in the

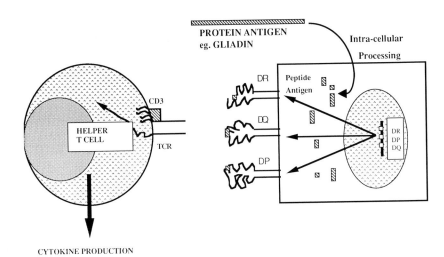

Fig. 5.2. Function of MHC encoded molecules. Antigen processing in accessory cells results in small peptides 7–11 amino-acids long which bind to the antigen binding groove on Class II molecules. The Class II molecules present processed antigen on the surface of accessory cells to T cells. Class II molecules in association with antigen preferentially activate CD4+ T cells.

transport of peptides for presentation by HLA Class I molecules. While this particular gene has been sequenced and found to be normal in coeliac patients, this is obviously a region of major importance in the regulation of antigen presentation and many of the genes in this region are as yet uncharacterised.

A mutation in the promoter region of the TNF-α gene has been found to be in linkage disequilibrium with HLA A1, B8, DR3 (Wilson *et al.*, 1993). Such a mutation would be predicted to have functional properties. In fact it has been reported that TNF microsatellite polymorphisms are associated with differences in lymphocyte TNF production (Pociot *et al.*, 1991). TNF microsatellite polymorphisms have been found to be tightly associated with coeliac disease in one study (McManus *et al.*, 1993).

Immunoglobulin genes and coeliac disease

Genes coding for the MHC and immunoglobulin genes both dictate the nature of the antibody response to wheat proteins in mice (Kagnoff, 1982). Some studies have shown that particular immunoglobulin allotypes defined by Gm haplotypes may be associated with coeliac disease in HLA B8 and DR3 negative individuals (Kagnoff *et al.*, 1983), but this has not been confirmed in other studies. Like the HLA system the Gm allotype system has been further explored using molecular techniques. These techniques have yet to be utilised in this area in coeliac disease. However, coeliac disease may occur in the setting of hypogammaglobulinemia (Webster *et al.*, 1981).

Gliadin chemistry and immunology

The evolutionary genetics of cereals are illustrated in Fig. 5.3. As can be seen, grains known to induce coeliac disease are separated in evolution from non-toxic cereals. Wheat, rye and barley are known to induce villous atrophy in patients with coeliac disease. The toxic component of the wheat protein is contained within the alcohol soluble fraction, the gliadins in the case of wheat. Gliadins are closely related to secalin in rye and to hordeins in barley. Electrophoretic mobility separates gliadins into four major families α, β, γ and ω gliadins. Early studies suggested that α-gliadin was more highly toxic than other components (Ciclitira *et al.*, 1984; O'Farrelly *et al.*, 1982). However, it now appears that all four components are capable of inducing coeliac disease (Cornell, Wieser & Belitz, 1992; Davidson & Bridges, 1987). Toxicity testing of peptides derived from the α-gliadin, A-gliadin has been performed in organ culture studies. These studies depend on the alterations in enterocyte height seen on exposure of jejunal explants to gliadin and it is uncertain whether this truly reflects coeliac disease. However, a number of sequences including residues Pro–Ser–Gln–Gln and Gln–Gln–Gln–Pro have been identified as common to toxic sequences (De Ritis *et al.*, 1988). It is also of note that sequences from A-gliadin have sequence homology to Adenovirus 12 viral protein (Kagnoff *et al.*, 1984) and peptides containing these sequences were found to be toxic in an organ culture system (De Ritis *et al.*, 1988). However, while antibodies to Adenovirus 12 have been

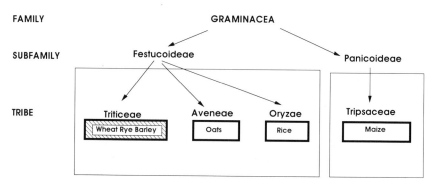

Fig. 5.3. Simplified taxonomy of graminacea (grain) family. The grains known to exacerbate coeliac disease are shown in the hatched box.

detected in some patients (Kagnoff *et al.*, 1987), Adenovirus 12 DNA has not been detected at increased frequency in the coeliac duodenum (Vesy *et al.*, 1993).

Morphology of the coeliac lesion and the lesion of dermatitis herpetiformis (DH)

Dermatitis herpetiformis has provided a useful model to examine varying degrees of gluten sensitivity (O'Mahoney, Vestey & Ferguson, 1990; Scott & Losowsky, 1975; Scott *et al.*, 1976). Total villous atrophy develops in a sizeable minority of patients with dermatitis herpetiformis. Patients with DH may exhibit a continuum of epithelial changes ranging from a (i) simple infiltrative lesion involving an intra-epithelial lymphocyte (IEL) infiltrate to (ii) the hyperplastic lesion characterised by crypt hyperplasia without villous atrophy and (iii) finally a destructive enteropathy characterised by crypt hyperplasia and villous atrophy (Marsh *et al.*, 1990). In fact, Marsh has now documented that this sequence does indeed occur in treated coeliac patients challenged with a gluten-containing diet. This is an important study which utilised a dynamic observation of the consequences of gluten challenge in a dose–response fashion (Marsh *et al.*, 1992). The initial event observed is an increase in the intra-epithelial lymphocyte count which is most marked in the coeliac crypts.

The second phase of coeliac disease is characterised by an influx of lamina propria lymphocytes, followed by crypt hyperplasia. Notably, crypt hyperplasia preceded the development of villous atrophy (Marsh, 1992). Crypt hyperplasia is by no means unique to coeliac disease and is a characteristic feature of graft-versus-host disease of the intestine (Mowat, Borland & Parrott, 1986; Mowat & Ferguson, 1982) and nematode infection (Miller, 1987). These findings suggest that crypt hyperplasia and villous atrophy may be induced by the action of T-cells, possibly by means of cytokines. The time-course of development of these features suggests that the influx of CD4 cells into the lamina propria may be the key factor in the induction of the destructive lesion (Marsh, 1992).

Aetiology of crypt hyperplasia

A number of experimental models have provided clues as to the aetiology of crypt hyperplasia. Firstly, in experimental models of graft-versus-host disease, crypt hyperplasia may be blocked by treatment with cyclosporine, suggesting a T cell aetiology to this condition (Guy-Grand & Vassalli, 1986; Mowat, Borland & Parrott, 1986). Secondly, in one experimental model, antibodies to γ-interferon blocked the development of crypt hyperplasia, suggesting a role for cytokines in the pathogenesis (Mowat, 1989). However, it is notable that increased γ interferon is not detected in infiltrating lymphocytes in the CD mucosa, suggesting that this is not a specific factor in coeliac pathogenesis (Al-Dawoud et al., 1992). In organ culture experiments, using foetal intestine, activation of resident T cells with mitogen or anti-CD3 was found to induce villous atrophy and crypt hyperplasia, suggesting that pure T-cell activation could result in villous atrophy (MacDonald, 1990; MacDonald & Spencer, 1988; Da Cunha Ferreira et al., 1990). Further evidence for T-cell involvement in the pathogenesis of crypt hyperplasia comes from studies involving patients infected with HIV. Patients with AIDS enteropathy who develop gastrointestinal infection frequently have a lymphocyte infiltrate with crypt hyperplasia (Ullrich, Zeitz & Riecken, 1992; Ullrich et al., 1992). However, in the absence of an infiltrate, villous atrophy occurs without crypt hyperplasia. These data taken together strongly suggest that crypt hyperplasia is T cell mediated.

Intra-epithelial lymphocyte compartment

This highly specialised, but poorly understood lymphocyte population, intercalates between epithelial cells of the gastro-intestinal tract. In normal individuals, these cells are predominantly TCR $\alpha\beta$ positive with generally less than 10% expressing the $\gamma\delta$ receptor (Brandtzaeg et al., 1989a; Halstensen, Scott & Brandtzaeg, 1989; Brandtzaeg et al., 1989b; Brandtzaeg, Sollid & Thrane, 1988; Jarry et al., 1990). In coeliac disease, the T-cell $\gamma\delta$ receptor is detected in up to 30% of IEL with dominant expression of the $V\gamma1\delta1$ phenotype (Spencer et al., 1989). However, the proportion of $\gamma\delta$ IEL appears to be fixed and does not reduce when the mucosal lesion is treated by a gluten-free diet (Viney, MacDonald & Spencer, 1990; Kutlu et al., 1993). It has been demonstrated that IEL have the capacity to differentiate in the gastrointestinal tract and it may be that the percentages of $\alpha\beta$ and $\gamma\delta$ lymphocytes are developmentally regulated. It is notable that an increase in the IEL count is the earliest morphological feature of the coeliac lesion (Marsh, 1992). In addition, relatives of coeliac patients have an increased number of IEL (Holm, 1993; Marsh et al., 1990). As the disease progresses, IEL appear to be replicating in situ (Halstensen & Brandtzaeg, 1993). However, the functional understanding of the role of these lymphocytes in coeliac disease is hampered by our lack of understanding of the functional role of normal IEL. While these cells appear to have inducible cytotoxic functions in mice, cytotoxicity is weak in human systems (Cerf-Bensussan, Guy-Grand & Griscelli, 1985). These cells can secrete cytokines including interferon (Yamamoto et al., 1993), TNF and interleukin 5 (Fujihashi et al., 1992) and it has been suggested that they play a role in the development and maintenance of oral tolerance. However, there is a reduction in the percentage of IEL producing interferon in the coeliac lesion (Al-Dawoud *et al.*, 1992). The poor proliferation observed in these cells *in vitro* has hampered the development of our understanding of their function.

Lamina propria lymphocyte (LPL) response

The lymphocyte infiltrate in the coeliac lamina propria is predominantly composed of CD4+ cells (Griffiths *et al.*, 1988; Kelly *et al.*, 1987). These cells appear to have a memory phenotype (CD45R0) (Schieferdecker *et al.*, 1992) and may express the interleukin 2 receptor (Pentilla *et al.*, 1990). Specific antigenic responses have, however, been difficult to detect. Expression of interleukin 2 receptor increases on these cells following exposure to gliadin, suggesting that specific sensitisation does occur (Pentilla *et al.*, 1990). CD4+ gliadin-specific T cells have now been cloned from duodenal biopsies of coeliac patients following gluten challenge (Lundin *et al.*, 1993). Interestingly, the majority of such clones are HLA DQ restricted. Individual clones use different T cell receptors and may respond to different peptides, suggesting a polyclonal response to gliadin. The role of such clones in the pathogenesis of coeliac disease is clearly of major interest, particularly if they secrete cytokines which may potentially affect the enterocytes.

Other inflammatory cells

Macrophages in the lamina propria appear to be activated and express the interleukin 2 receptor. There is also increasing evidence of an intense eosinophil infiltrate (Colombell *et al.*, 1992) with considerable degranulation of eosinophil products (Talley *et al.*, 1992). Studies performed during gluten challenge with an indwelling duodenal tube have indicated that there is a considerable release of eosinophil degranulation products rapidly into the intestinal lumen (Hallgren *et al.*, 1989). Eosinophil degranulation may be of particular relevance to tissue damage, as it is known that factors produced by eosinophils such as major basic protein (MBP), eosinophil derived neurotoxin (EDN) and eosinophil cationic protein (ECP) are neurotoxic. Chemical interference with intestinal innervation with tetrodotoxin has been shown to result in failure of healing of experimentally induced villous atrophy (Moore, Carlson & Madara, 1989). The eosinophil infiltrate could be secondary to T-cell cytokines, as it has been shown that IL-5 in particular is an eosinophil differentiation factor (Denburg, Dolovich & Harnish, 1989). Notably, the intra-epithelial lymphocytes have been shown to secrete IL-5 in murine studies (Yamamoto *et al.*, 1993). The histological features following gluten challenge would support the hypothesis that the eosinophil infiltrate is a late response in the development of the characteristic appearances of disease, occurring after the lamina propria infiltrate (Marsh & Hinde, 1985). This would be consistent with the hypothesis that T-cell derived cytokines are responsible for the generation of the eosinophil response. In addition, eosinophil degranulation is triggered by IgG and IgA (Abu-Ghazaleh *et al.*, 1989) and could potentially be triggered by antibodies to dietary proteins. Specifically, eosinophils are frequently detected in close proximity to IgA plasma cells in the coeliac duodenum (Marsh & Hinde, 1985). Mast cell and neutrophil activity may also be affected by exposure to dietary gliadin (Horvath *et al.*, 1989). In particular, a rapid mast cell involvement is characteristic of changes occurring following rectal challenge with gliadin in coeliac patients (Loft *et al.*, 1989).

Soluble factors

Eosinophil and mast cell degranulation products have been detected in the gut lumen following gluten challenge, suggesting that this is a rapid and immediate response to gluten ingestion (Griffiths *et al.*, 1988). In addition, products of eicosanoid metabolism including 15-HETE (Krillis *et al.*, 1986) and prostaglandin E_2, are detected following stimulation of the duodenum with gliadin (Lavo *et al.*, 1990). These data do suggest that the coeliac small bowel is capable of responding rapidly to gluten and that specific responses to wheat proteins occur far in advance of villous atrophy. Circulating interleukin-2 receptor has also been detected in advance of villous atrophy (Crabtree *et al.*, 1989).

Class II expression

HLA Class II expression is normally limited to the villus tips. In particular, limited DR and DP expression are detected at the villus tip (Kelly, Weir & Feighery, 1988). DQ is not detected in significant quantities and it has been demonstrated that DR and DP may be independently regulated from DQ. In the coeliac patient, HLA DR and DP expression are located throughout the villus and in the crypts. Intra-epithelial lymphocytes have been shown to modulate Class II expression by enterocytes (Cerf-Bensussan *et al.*, 1984). Furthermore, gliadin administration *in vitro* has been shown to stimulate increased enterocyte Class II expression (Ciclitira *et al.*, 1986*a*). Epithelial cells have the capability to present antigen in experimental systems (Bland & Warren, 1986). Hence, induction of Class II expression could potentially induce antigen-specific responses. Aberrant Class II expression has been suggested as a factor in auto-immune thyroid disease (Botazzo *et al.*, 1983).

Complement

Activated complement has been detected at the villus tip in the sub-epithelial layer (Halstensen *et al.*, 1992) and adjacent to Brunner's glands in the duodenum of patients with coeliac disease (Gallagher *et al.*, 1989). It has been suggested that gluten stimulates IgG and IgM mediated sub-epithelial complement activation and that this may interfere with the binding of enterocytes to the basement layer. In addition, complement products may generate an inflammatory response through vasodilation, smooth muscle contraction and leukocyte activation.

Antibodies in coeliac disease

Antibodies to wheat protein have been found in the majority of patients with coeliac disease (Ciclitira *et al.*, 1986*b*; Dias, Unsworth & Walker-Smith, 1987; O'Farrelly *et al.*, 1983). Current data suggest that the IgA antibodies to gliadin have the highest specificity for coeliac disease (Gorczi, Skerritt & Mitchell, 1992; Hallstrom, 1989). However, antibodies to wheat proteins have been found in conditions as diverse as sarcoidosis (McCormack *et al.*, 1988), rheumatoid arthritis (Parke *et al.*, 1984), recurrent oral ulceration (O'Farrelly *et al.*, 1991) and even in normal individuals with high IEL counts (O'Farrelly *et al.*, 1987). While these data could suggest that wheat protein sensitivity is more widespread than previously perceived, it is also possible that these antibodies are low affinity antibodies with a broad specificity.

Anti-endomysial antibodies are identified using monkey oesophagus for detection. These antibodies have been reported to have a high degree of specificity for coeliac disease, with up to 100% specificity reported in certain studies (Chorzelski *et al.*, 1984; Ferreira *et al.*, 1992). However, their general use has been limited by the availability of monkey oesophagus. Recently, the proteins recognised by these antibodies have been characterised (Maki, Hallstrom & Marttinen, 1991). If genes coding for these proteins are cloned, it should be possible to generate recombinant product for enzyme-linked immunosorbent assays.

Pathogenic mechanisms in coeliac disease

Coeliac disease is a HLA-linked disease and as such many of the theories of pathogenesis revolve around its association with HLA Class II genes. Other Class II diseases such as diabetes and rheumatoid arthritis appear to be linked to the presence or absence of specific residues flanking the antigen-binding groove, rather than a particular HLA type. It has been suggested that diabetes is polygenic requiring up to three genes for disease expression (Todd *et al.*, 1991). It is not known whether coeliac disease is linked to genes outside the MHC. However, it is possible that coeliac disease is polygenic, requiring the expression of multiple genes *within* the MHC. Such a hypothesis is difficult to test, however.

The initial event in coeliac disease is an influx of CD8+ T-lymphocytes into the IEL compartment. This influx could be in response to specific antigen, in which case it should be regulated by MHC Class I molecules or alternatively this influx could simply be regulated by adhesion molecule expression. An influx of lymphocytes into the epithelial layer could release cytokines, such as γ-interferon, capable of disrupting the epithelial tight junction integrity (Madara & Stafford, 1988). However, γ-interferon is not increased in coeliac IEL (Al-Dawoud et al., 1992). The existence of a large population of $\gamma\delta$ IEL in the coeliac duodenum which is unchanged by disease activity would suggest a fundamental developmental difference in IEL maturation in the coeliac patient. It has been suggested that the gut is a site of extra-thymic T-cell maturation (Mosley, Styre & Klein, 1990). The antigens recognised by $\gamma\delta$ IEL and their restriction is little understood (Strominger, 1989; Haas, Kaufman & Martinez, 1990), although they may recognise class Ib molecules in mice or CD1 in humans (Strominger, 1989). However, their existence is thought to provide a primitive line of defence against gut pathogens. It has been suggested that $\gamma\delta$ cells may play a role in oral tolerance (Fujihashi et al., 1992). Any unifying hypothesis of coeliac disease pathogenesis would have to incorporate this increased proportion of $\gamma\delta$ IEL, the initial rapid IEL response and in particular the concept that these lymphocytes are CD8+ and not predicted to be regulated by Class II gene products.

In traditional terms, the involvement of lamina propria lymphocytes is more easily rationalised as a Class II mediated phenomenon. CD4 cells in the intestine recognise gliadin in the context of HLA DQ (Lundin et al., 1993). Furthermore, cytokines produced by CD4+ cells could potentially induce crypt hyperplasia (Monk et al., 1988; MacDonald & Spencer, 1988). This might involve over-production of a specific cytokine for example tumour necrosis factor or γ-interferon. In fact DR3+ cells have been shown to produce higher levels of TNF-α than other DR types and this is felt to be due to linkage with TNF polymorphisms (Pociot et al., 1991). How might the LPL infiltrate contribute to villous atrophy? Villous atrophy does not appear to be related to epithelial cell death. The maintenance of the villous structure is poorly understood but it undoubtedly involves the production of a basement membrane, epithelial cell adherence to a basement membrane, a vascular supply and innervation. Interference with any or all of these factors might contribute to villous atrophy. Cytokines produced by LPL could induce alterations in tight junctions (Madara & Stafford, 1988), epithelial proliferation (MacDonald & Spencer, 1988) and potentially enterocyte death (McDevitt et al., 1993). Production of prostaglandins (Lavo et al., 1990) and procoagulants (Deverey et al., 1990) could contribute to ischaemic damage. The eosinophil infiltration could contribute damage to innervation owing to the production of neurotoxins (Hallgren et al., 1989). Significantly, eosinophil behaviour is regulated by T-cell derived cytokines.

However, which of these factors is dominant in the induction of villous atrophy is currently poorly understood.

References

Abu-Ghazaleh, R. I., Fujisawa, T., Mestecky, J., Kyle, R. A. & Gleich, G. J. (1989). IgA induced eosinophil degranulation. *Journal of Immunology*, **142**(7), 2393–400.

Al-Dawoud, A., Nakshabendi, I., Foulis, A. & Mowat, A. M. (1992). Immunohistochemical analysis of mucosal gamma-interferon production in coeliac disease. *Gut*, **33**(11), 1482–6.

Alper, C. A., Fleischnick, E., Awdeh, Z. *et al.* (1987). Extended major histocompatibility complex haplotypes in patients with gluten-sensitive enteropathy. *Journal of Clinical Investigation*, **79**, 251–6.

Anand, B. S., Piris, J., Jerrome, D. W., Offord, R. E. & Truelove, S. C. (1981). The timing of histological damage following a single challenge with gluten in treated coeliac disease. *Quarterly Journal of Medicine*, **197**, 83–94.

Bland, P. W. & Warren, L. G. (1986). Antigen presentation by epithelial cells of the rat small intestine. I. Kinetics, antigen specificity and blocking by Ia antisera. *Immunology*, **58**, 1–7.

Botazzo, G. F., Pujol-Borrell, R., Hanafusa, T. & Feldman, M. (1983). Role of aberrant HLA-DR expression and antigen presentation in induction of endocrine autoimmunity. *Lancet*, **ii**, 1115–18.

Brandtzaeg, P., Bosnes, V., Halstensen, T. S., Scott, H., Sollid, L. M. & Valnes, T. (1989*a*). T lymphocytes in human gut epithelium preferentially express the α/β antigen receptor and are often CD45/UCHL1 positive. *Scandinavian Journal of Immunology*, **30**, 123–8.

Brandtzaeg, P., Halstensen, T. S., Kett, K., Krajci, P., Kvale, D., Rognum, T., Scott, H. & Sollid, L. (1989*b*). Immunobiology and immunopathology of human gut mucosa: humoral immunity and intraepithelial lymphocytes. *Gastroenterology*, **97**, 1562–84.

Brandtzaeg, P., Sollid, L. M., Thrane, P. S. *et al.* (1988). Lympho-epithelial interactions in the mucosal immune system. *Gut*, **29**, 1116–30.

Bugawan, T. L., Angelini, G., Larrick, J., Auricchio, S., Ferrara, G. B. & Erlich, H. A. (1989). A combination of a particular HLA-DP beta allele and an HLA DQ heterodimer confers susceptibility to coeliac disease. *Nature*, **339**, 470–3.

Caffrey, C., Hitman, G. A., Niven, M. J. *et al.* (1990). HLA-DP and coeliac disease: family and population studies. *Gut*, **31**, 663–7.

Cerf-Bensussan, N., Guy-Grand, D., Griscelli, C. (1985). Intraepithelial lymphocytes of human gut: isolation, characterisation and study of natural killer activity. *Gut*, **26**, 81–8.

Cerf-Bensussan, N., Quaroni, A., Kurnick, J. T. & Bhan, A. K. (1984). Intra-epithelial lymphocytes modulate Ia expression by intestinal epithelial cells. *Journal of Immunology*, **132**, 2244–52.

Chorzelski, T. P., Beutner, E. H., Sulej, J. *et al.* (1984). IgA anti-endomysium antibody. A new immunological marker of dermatitis herpetiformis and coeliac disease. *British Journal of Dermatology*, **111**, 395–402.

Ciclitira, P. J., Nelufer, J. M., Ellis, H. J. & Evans, D. J. (1986*a*). The effect of gluten on HLA-DR in the small intestinal epithelium of patients with coeliac disease. *Clinical Experimental Immunology*, **63**, 101–4.

Ciclitira, P. J., Ellis, H. J., Howdle, P. D. & Losowsky, M. S. (1986*b*). Secretion of gliadin antibody by coeliac jejunal mucosal biopsies cultured *in vitro*. *Clinical Experimental Immunology*, **64**, 119–24.

Ciclitira, P. J., Evans, D. J., Fagg, N. L. K., Lennox, E. S. & Dowling, R. H. (1984). Clinical testing of gliadin fractions in coeliac patients. *Clinical Science*, **66**, 357–64.

Colombell, J. F., Torpier, G., Janin, A., Klein, O., Cortot, A. & Capron, M. (1992). Activated eosinophils in adult coeliac disease: evidence for a local release of major basic protein. *Gut,* **33**(9), 1190–4.

Corazza, G., Valentini, R. A., Frisoni, M., Volta, U., Corrao, G., Bianchi, B. & Gasbarrini, G. (1992). Gliadin immune reactivity is associated with overt and latent enteropathy in relatives of celiac patients. *Gastroenterology,* **103**, 1517–22.

Cornell, H., Weiser, H. & Belitz, H. D. (1992). Characterization of the gliadin-derived peptides which are biologically active in coeliac disease. *Clinica Chimica Acta,* **213** (1–3), 37–50.

Crabtree, J. E., Heatley, R. V., Juby, L. D., Howdle, P. D. & Losowsky, M. S. (1989). Serum interleukin-2 receptor in coeliac disease: response to treatment and gluten challenge. *Clinical Experimental Immunology,* **77**, 345–8.

Da Cunha Ferreira, R., Forsyth, L., Richman, P., Wells, C., Spencer, J. & MacDonald, T. (1990). Changes in the rate of crypt epithelial cell proliferation and mucosal morphology induced by a T cell mediated response in human small intestine. *Gastroenterology,* **98**, 1225–63.

Davidson, A.G.F. & Bridges, M. A. (1987). Coeliac disease: a critical review of aetiology and pathogenesis. *Clinica Chimica Acta,* **163**, 1–40.

Davis, M. M. & Bjorkman, P. J. (1988). T-cell receptor genes and T-cell recognition. *Nature,* **334**, 395–402.

Denburg, J. A., Dolovich, J. & Harnish, D. (1989). Basophil mast cell and eosinophil growth and differentiation factors in human allergic diseases. *Clinical and Experimental Allergy,* **19**, 249–54.

De Ritis, G., Auriochio, S., Jones, H. W., Liew, E. J.-L., Bernardin, J. E. & Kasarda, D. D. (1988). *In vitro* (organ culture) studies of the toxicity of specific A-gliadin peptides in celiac disease. *Gastroenterology,* **94**, 41–9.

Deverey, J. M., Geezy, C. L., Declarle, D., Skerrit, J. & Krillis, S. (1990). Macrophage procoagulant activity as an assay of cellular hypersensitivity to gluten peptides in coeliac disease. *Clinical Experimental Immunology,* **82**, 333–7.

Dias, J., Unsworth, D. J. & Walker-Smith, J. A. (1987). Antigliadin and antireticulin antibodies in screening for coeliac disease. *Lancet,* **ii**, 157–8.

Ferguson, A. (1987). Models of immunologically driven small intestinal damage. In *Immunopathology of the Small Intestine,* ed. M. N. Marsh, pp. 225–252. Chichester: John Wiley & Sons.

Ferreira, M. & Davies, S., Butler, M., Scott, D., Clark, M. & Kumar, P. (1992). Endomysial antibody: is it the best screening test for coeliac disease? *Gut,* **33**(12), 1633–7.

Fry, L., Seah, P. P., McMinn, R. M. & Hoffbrand, A. V. (1972). Lymphocytic infiltration of epithelium in diagnosis of gluten-sensitive enteropathy. *British Medical Journal,* **3**, 371–4.

Fujihashi, K., Taguchi, T., McGhee, J. R., Bluestone, J. A., Eldridge, J. H. & Kiyono, H. (1992). Immunoregulatory functions for murine intra-epithelial lymphocytes: gamma/delta T cell receptor-positive (TCR+) T cells abrogate oral tolerance, while alpha/beta TCR+ cells provide B cell help. *Journal of Experimental Medicine,* **75**(3), 695–707.

Gallagher, R. B., Kelly, C. P., Naville, S., Sheils, O., Weir, D. G. & Feighery, C. F. (1989). Complement activation within the coeliac small intestine is localised to Brunner's glands. *Gut,* **30**(11), 1568–78.

Gorczi, J., Skerritt, J. H. & Mitchell, J. D. (1992). Differentiation of coeliac disease and other malabsorption diseases using specific serum antigliadin IgG subclass profiles and IgA1 levels. *International Archives of Allergy Immunology,* **98**(4), 377–85.

Griffiths, C. E., Barrison, I., Leonard, J., Caun, K., Valdimarsson, M. & Fry, L. (1988). Preferential activation of CD4 T lymphocytes within the lamina propria of gluten-sensitive enteropathy. *Clinical Experimental Immunology,* **72**, 280–3.

Guy-Grand, D. & Vassalli, P. (1986). Gut injury in mouse graft-versus-host reaction. *Journal of Clinical Investigation*, **77**, 1584–95.

Haas, W., Kaufman, S. & Martinez, A. C. (1990). The development and function of γδ T cells. *Immunology Today*, **11**, 340–3.

Hallgren, R., Colombel, J. F., Dahle, R. *et al.* (1989). Neutrophil and eosinophilic involvement of the small bowel in patients with coeliac disease and Crohn's disease: studies on the secretion rate and immunohistochemical localization of granulocyte granule constituents. *American Journal of Medicine*, **86**, 56–64.

Hallstrom, O. (1989). Comparison of IgA-class reticulin and endomysium antibodies in coeliac disease and dermatitis herpetiformis. *Gut*, **30**, 1225–32.

Halstensen, T. S. & Brandtzaeg, P. (1993). Activated T lymphocytes in the celiac lesion: non-proliferative activation (CD25) of CD4+ α/β cells in the lamina propria but proliferation (Ki-67) of α/β and γ/δ cells in the epithelium. *European Journal of Immunology*, **23**, 505–10.

Halstensen, T. S., Hvatum, M., Scott, H., Fausa, O. & Brandtzaeg, P. (1992). Association of subepithelial deposition of activated complement and immunoglobulin G and M response to gluten in coeliac disease. *Gastroenterology*, **102**, 751–9.

Halstensen, T. S., Scott, H. & Brandtzaeg, P. (1989). Intraepithelial T cells of the TCR γ/δ CE8⁻ and Vγ₁/δ1 phenotypes are increased in coeliac disease. *Scandinavian Journal of Immunology*, **30**, 665–72.

Holm, K. H. (1993). Correlation of HLA DR alleles to jejunal mucosal morphology in healthy first-degree relatives of coeliac disease patients. *European Journal of Gastroenterology and Hepatology*, **5**, 35–41.

Horvath, K., Nagy, L., Horn, G., Simon, K., Csiszar, K. & Bodansky, H. (1989). Intestinal mast cell and neutrophil chemotactic activity of serum following a single challenge with gluten in celiac children on a gluten-free diet. *Journal of Pediatric Gastroenterology and Nutrition*, **9**, 276–80.

Howell, M. D., Austin, R. K., Kelleher, D., Nepom, G. T. & Kagnoff, M. P. (1986). An HLA-D region restriction fragment length polymorphism associated with celiac disease. *Journal of Experimental Medicine*, **164**, 333–8.

Howell, M. D., Smith, J. R., Austin, R. K. *et al.* (1988). An extended HLA-D region haplotype associated with celiac disease. *Proceedings of the National Academy of Sciences, USA*, **85**, 222–6.

Jarry, A., Cerf-Bensussan, N., Brousse, N., Selz, F. & Guy-Grand, D. (1990). Subsets of CD3+ (T cell receptor α/β or γ/δ) and CD3⁻ lymphocytes isolated from normal human gut epithelium display phenotypical features different from their counterparts in peripheral blood. *European Journal of Immunology*, **20**, 1097–103.

Kagnoff, M. J. (1982). Two genetic loci control the murine immune response A-gliadin, a wheat protein that activates coeliac sprue. *Nature*, **296**, 158–60.

Kagnoff, M. F., Austin, R. K., Hubert, J. K., Bernardin, J. E. & Kasarda, D. D. (1984). Possible role for a human adenovirus in the pathogenesis of coeliac disease. *Journal of Experimental Medicine*, **160**, 1544–57.

Kagnoff, M. F., Harwood, J. I., Bugawan, T. L. & Erlich, H. A. (1989). Structural analysis of the HLA DR, DQ and DP alleles on the celiac disease associated HLA DR3 (Dw 17) haplotype. *Proceedings of the National Academy of Sciences, USA*, **86**, 6274–8.

Kagnoff, M. F., Paterson, Y. J., Kumar, P. J. *et al.* (1987). Evidence for the role of a human intestinal adenovirus in the pathogenesis of coeliac disease. *Gut*, **28**, 995–9.

Kagnoff, M. F., Weiss, J. B., Brown, R., Lee, T. & Schanfield, M. S. (1983). Immunoglobulin allotype markers in gluten-sensitive enteropathy. *Lancet*, **i**, 952–3.

Kelly, A., Powis, S. H., Kerr, L. A. *et al.* (1992). Assembly and function of the two ABC transporter proteins encoded in the human major histocompatibility complex. *Nature*, **355**(6361), 641–4.

Kelly, C. P., Feighery, C. F., Gallagher, R. B. & Weir, D. G. (1990). Diagnosis and treatment of gluten-sensitive enteropathy. *Advances in Internal Medicine*, **35**, 341–64.

Kelly, J., O'Farrelly, C., O'Mahoney, C., Weir, D. G. & Feighery, C. (1987). Immunoperoxidase demonstration of the cellular composition of the normal and coeliac small bowel. *Clinical Experimental Immunology*, **68**, 177–88.

Kelly, J., Weir, D. G. & Feighery, C. (1988). Differential expression of HLA-D gene products in the normal and coeliac small bowel. *Tissue Antigen*, **29**, 151–60.

Kleijmeer, M. J., Kelly, A., Geuze, H. J., Slot, J. W., Townsend, A. & Trowsdale, J. (1992). Location of MHC-encoded transporters in the endoplasmic reticulum and *cis*-Golgi. *Current Opinions in Genetic Developments*, **357**, 342–4.

Krillis, S., MacPherson, J., De Carle, D. J., Daggard, G., Talley, N. & Chesterman, C. (1986). Small bowel mucosa from celiac patients generates 15-hydroxyeicosatetraenoic acid (15-HETE) after *in vitro* challenge with gluten. *Journal of Immunology*, **137**, 3768–71.

Kutlu, T., Brousse, N., Rambaud, C., Le Deist, F., Schmitz, J. & Cerf-Bensusan, N. (1993). Numbers of T cell receptor (TCR) alpha beta+ but not of TcR gamma delta+ intraepithelial lymphocytes correlate with the grade of villous atrophy in coeliac patients on a long term normal diet. *Gut*, **34**(2), 208–14.

Lancaster-Smith, M., Kumar, P. J. & Dawson, A. M. (1975). The cellular infiltrate of the jejunum in adult coeliac disease and dermatitis herpetiformis following the reintroduction of dietary gluten. *Gut*, **16**, 683–8.

Lavo, B., Knutson, L., Loof, L. & Hallgren, R. (1990). Gliadin challenge-induced jejunal prostaglandin E_2 secretion in coeliac disease. *Gastroenterology*, **99**, 703–7.

Littlewood, J. M., Crollick, A. J., Richards, D. G. (1980). Childhood coeliac disease is disappearing. *Lancet*, **ii**, 1359.

Loft, D. E., Marsh, M. N., Crowe, P. T., Sandle, G., Garner, V. & Gordon, D. (1989). Studies of intestinal lymphoid tissue. XII – Epithelial lymphocyte and mucosal response to rectal gluten challenge in celiac sprue. *Gastroenterology*, **97**, 29–37.

Lundin, K. E. A., Scott, H., Hansen, T. *et al.* (1993). Gliadin-specific HLA DQ (α_1*0501, β_1*0201) restricted T cells isolated from the small intestinal mucosa of coeliac disease patients. *Journal of Experimental Medicine*, **178**, 187–96.

McCormack, P. A., Feighery, C., Dolan, C. *et al.* (1988). Altered gastrointestinal immune response in sarcoidosis. *Gut*, **29**, 1628–31.

McDevitt, J., Feighery, C., Martin, G., O'Farrelly, C. & Kelleher, D. (1993). Tumour necrosis factor induced apoplosis of epithelial cells. *Gastroenterology*, **104**, A740.

MacDonald, T. T. (1990). The role of activated T lymphocytes in gastro-intestinal disease. *Clinical Experimental Allergy*, **20**, 247–52.

MacDonald, T. T. & Spencer, J. (1988). Evidence that activated mucosal T cells play a role in the pathogenesis of enteropathy in human intestine. *Journal of Experimental Medicine*, **167**, 1341–9.

MacDonald, W. C., Dobbins, W. O. & Rubin, C. E. (1965). Studies of the familial nature of coeliac sprue using biopsy of the small intestine. *New England Journal of Medicine*, **272**, 448–56.

McManus, R., Moloney, M., Chuan, Y. T., Weir, D. G. & Kelleher, D. (1993). TNF microsatellite polymorphisms in coeliac disease. *Gut*, **34**, S63.

Madara, J. L. & Stafford, J. (1988). Interferon-γ directly affects barrier function of cultured intestinal epithelial monolayers. *Journal of Clinical Investigation*, **83**, 724–7.

Maki, M., Hallstrom, O. & Marttinen, A. (1991). Reaction of human non-collagenous polypeptides with coeliac disease autoantibodies. *Lancet*, **338**(8769), 724–5.

Mantovani, V., Corazza, G. R., Bragliani, M., Frisoni, M., Zaniboni, M. G. & Gasbarrini, G. (1993). Asp 57-negative HLA DQ beta chain and DOA1*0501 allele are essential for the onset of DQw2-positive and DQw2-negative coeliac disease. *Clinical Experimental Immunology*, **91**, 153–6.

Marsh, M. N. (1992). Gluten, major histocompatibility complex, and the small intestine. A molecular and immunobiological approach to the spectrum of gluten sensitivity ('coeliac sprue'). *Gastroenterology*, **102**, 330–54.

Marsh, M. N., Loft, D. E. Garner, V. C. & Gordon, D. (1992). Time/dose response of coeliac mucosae to graded oral challenges with Frazer's fraction III of gliadin. *European Journal of Gastroenterology and Hepatology*, **4**, 667–73.

Marsh, M. N., Bjarnason, I., Shaw, J., Ellis, A., Baker, R. & Peters, T. J. (1990). Studies of intestinal lymphoid tissue. XIV – HLA status, mucosal morphoogy, permeability and epithelial lymphocyte populations in first degree relatives of patients with coeliac disease. *Gut*, **31**, 32–6.

Marsh, M. & Hinde, J. (1985). Inflammatory component of coeliac sprue mucosa. I. Mast cells, basophils and eosinophils. *Gastroenterology*, **89**, 92–101.

Miller, H. R. P. (1987). Immunopathology of nematode infestation and expulsion. In *Immunopathology of the Small Intestine*, ed. M. N. Marsh, pp. 177–208. Chichester: John Wiley & Sons.

Monk, T., Spencer, J., Cerf-Bensussan, N. & MacDonald, T. T. (1988). Stimulation of mucosal T cells *in situ* with anti-CD3 antibody: location of the activated T cells and their distribution with the mucosal micro-environment. *Clinical Experimental Immunology*, **74**, 216–22.

Moore, R., Carlson, S. & Madara, J. L. (1989). Villus contraction aids repair of intestinal epithelium after injury. *American Journal of Physiology*, **257**, (Gastrointest. Liver Physiol. 20) G274–83.

Mosley, R. L., Styre, D. & Klein, J. R. (1990). Differentiation and functional maturation of bone marrow-derived intestinal epithelial T cells expressing membrane T cell receptor in athymic radiation chimeras. *Journal of Immunology*, **145**, 1369–75.

Mowat, A. Mcl. (1989). Antibodies to interferon-gamma prevent immunologically mediated damage in murine graft versus host reaction. *Immunology*, **68**, 18–23.

Mowat, A. Mcl., Borland, A. & Parrott, D. M. V. (1986). Hypersensitivity reactions in the small intestine. VII – Induction of the intestinal phase of murine graft-versus-host reaction by Lyt2⁻ T cells activated by I-A alloantigens. *Transplantation*, **41**, 192–8.

Mowat, A. McI. & Ferguson, A. (1982). Intra-epithelial lymphocyte count and crypt hyperplasia measure the mucosal component of the graft-versus-host reaction in the mouse small intestine. *Gastroenterology*, **83**, 417–23.

Myllotte, M., Egan-Mitchell, B., Fottrell, P. F., McNicol, B. & McCarthy, C. F. (1974). Family studies in coeliac disease. *Quarterly Medical Journal*, **171**, 359–69.

Nepom, G. T., Hansen, J. A. & Nepom, B. S. (1987). The molecular basis for HLA Class II associations with rheumatoid arthritis. *Journal of Clinical Immunology*, **7**, 1–7.

O'Farrelly, C., Feighery, C., Greally, J. F. & Weir, D. G. (1982). Cellular response to alpha-gliadin in untreated coeliac disease. *Gut*, **23**, 83–7.

O'Farrelly, C., Kelly, J., Hekkens, W. *et al.* (1983). Alpha gliadin antibody levels: a serological test for coeliac disease. *British Medical Journal*, **286**, 2007–10.

O'Farrelly, C., Graeme-Cook, F., Hourihane, D. O'B., Feighery, C. & Weir, D. G. (1987). Histological changes associated with a humoral response to wheat protein in the absence of acute enteropathy. *Journal of Clinical Pathology*, **40**, 1228–30.

O'Farrelly, C., O'Mahony, C., Graeme-Cook, F., Feighery, C., McCartan, B. & Weir, D. G. (1991). Gliadin antibodies identify gluten-sensitive oral ulceration in the absence of villous atrophy. *Journal of Oral Medicine and Pathology*, **20**, 476–8.

O'Mahoney, S., Vestey, J. P. & Ferguson, A. (1990). Similarities in intestinal humoral immunity in dermatitis herpetiformis without enteropathy in coeliac disease. *Lancet*, **335**, 1487–90.

Parke, A. L., Fagan, E. A., Chadwick, V. S. & Hughes, G. R. V. (1984). Coeliac disease and rheumatoid arthritis. *Annals of Rheumatic Disorders*, **43**, 378–80.

Pentilla, I. A., Gibson, C. E., Forrest, B. D., Cummins, A. G. & LaBrooy, J. T. (1990). Lymphocyte activation as measured by interleukin-2 receptor expression to gluten fraction III in coeliac disease. *Clinical Experimental Immunology*, **68**, 155–60.

Pociot, F., Molvig, J., Wogensen, L., Worsaae, H., Dalboget, H., Back, L. & Nerup, J. (1991). A tumour necrosis factor beta gene polymorphism in relation to monokine secretion and insulin-dependent diabetes mellitus. *Scandinavian Journal of Immunology*, **33**, 37–42.

Powis, S. H., Mockridge, I., Kelly, A. *et al.* (1992). Polymorphism in a second ABC transporter gene located within the class II region of the human major histocompatibility complex. *Proceedings of the National Academy of Sciences, USA*, **89**(4), 1463–7.

Schieferdecker, H. L., Ullrich, R., Hirseland, H. & Zeitz, M. (1992). T cell differentiation antigens on lymphocytes in the human intestinal lamina propria. *Journal of Immunology*, **149**(8), 2816–22.

Scott, B. B., Losowsky, M. S. (1975). Coeliac disease: a cause of various associated diseases. *Lancet*, **ii**, 956–7.

Scott, B. B., Young, S., Rajah, S., Marks, J. & Losowsky, M. (1976). Coeliac disease and dermatitis herpetiformis: further studies of their relationship. *Gut*, **17**, 759–62.

Sollid, L. M., Markussen, G., Ek, J., Gjerde, H., Vartdal, F. & Thorsby, E. (1989). Evidence for a primary association of coeliac disease to a particular DQ heterodimer. *Journal of Experimental Medicine*, **169**, 345–50.

Spencer, J., MacDonald, T. T., Diss, T. C., Walker-Smith, J. A., Ciclitira, P. & Isaacson, P. (1989). Changes in the intra-epithelial lymphocyte subpopulation in coeliac disease and enteropathy associated T cell lymphoma. *Gut*, **30**, 339–46.

Strominger, J. L. (1986). Biology of the human histocompatibility leucocyte antigen (HLA) system and a hypothesis regarding the generation of autoimmune disease. *Journal of Clinical Investigation*, **77**, 1411–15.

Strominger, J. L. (1989). The $\gamma\delta$ T cell receptor and class 1b major histocompatibility complex-related proteins: enigmatic molecules of immune recognition. *Cell*, **57**, 895–8.

Talley, N. J., Kephart, G. M., McGovern, T. W., Carpenter, H. A. & Gleich, G. J. (1992). Deposition of eosinophil granule major basic protein in eosinophilic gastroenteritis and celiac disease. *Gastroenterology*, **103**, 137–45.

Tighe, M. R., Hall, M. A., Cardi, E., Ashkenazi, A., Siegler, E., Lanchbury, J. S. & Ciclitira, P. J. (1993). Coeliac disease among Ashkenazi Jews and the associations with polymorphisms of the HLA Class II genes. *Gut*, **34**, Suppl. 1, S34.

Todd, J. A., Aitman, T. J., Cornall, R. J. *et al.* (1991). Genetic analysis of autoimmune type 1 diabetes mellitus in mice. *Nature*, **351**(6327), 542–7.

Todd, J. A., Bell, J. I. & McDevitt, O. (1987). DQ beta gene contributes to susceptibility and resistance to insulin dependent diabetes mellitus. *Nature*, **329**, 599–604.

Tosi, R., Vismara, D. & Tanigaki, N. (1983). Evidence that coeliac disease is primarily associated with a DC locus allelic specificity. *Clinical Immunology and Immunopathology*, **28**, 395–404.

Trowsdale, J. & Campbell, R. D. (1992). Complexity in the major histocompatibility complex. *European Journal of Immunogenetics*, **19**(1–2), 45–55.

Trowsdale, J. & Powis, S. H. (1992). The MHC: relationship between linkage and function. *Current Opinions in Genetic Developments*, **2**(3), 492–7.

Ullrich, R., Heise, W., Bergs, C., L'age, M., Riecken, E. O. and Zeitz, M. (1992). Effects of zidovudine treatment on the small intestinal mucosa in patients infected with the human immunodeficiency virus. *Gastroenterology*, **102**(5), 1483–92.

Ullrich, R., Zeitz, M. & Riecken, E. O. (1992). Enteric immunologic abnormalities in human immunodeficiency virus infection. *Seminars in Liver Diseases*, **12**(2), 167–74.

Vesy, C. J., Greenson, J. K., Papp, A. C., Snyder, P. J., Qualman, S. J. & Prior, T. W. (1993). Evaluation of celiac disease biopsies for Adenovirus 12 DNA using a multiplex polymerase chain reaction. *Modern Pathology*, **6**, 61–4.

Viney, J., MacDonald, T. T. & Spencer, J. (1990). Gamma/delta T cells in the gut epithelium. *Gut*, **31**, 841–4.

Walker-Smith, J. A. (1973). Discordance for childhood coeliac disease in monozygotic twins. *Gut*, **14**, 374–5.

Webster, A. D. B., Slavin, G., Shiner, M., Platts-Mills, T. A. E. & Asherson, G. L. (1981). Coeliac disease with severe hypogammaglobulinaemia. *Gut*, **22**, 153–7.

Wilson, A. G., de-Vries, N., Pociot, F., de-Giovine, F. S., van-der-Putte, L. B., Duff, G. W. (1993). An allelic polymorphism within the human tumour necrosis factor alpha promoter region is strongly associated with HLA A1, B8 and DR3 alleles. *Journal of Experimental Medicine*, **177**(2), 557–60.

Yamamoto, M., Fujihashi, K., Beagley, K. W., McGhee, J. R. & Kiyono, H. (1993). Cytokine synthesis by intestinal intraepithelial lymphocytes. Both gamma/delta T cell receptor-positive and alpha/beta T cell receptor-positive T cells in the GI phase of cell cycle produce IFN-gamma and IL-5. *Journal of Immunology*, **150**(1), 106–14.

Young, R. A. & Elliott, T. J. (1989). Stress proteins, infection and immune surveillance. *Cell*, **59**, 5–8.

–6–
Inflammatory bowel disease

H. R. DALTON and R. V. HEATLEY

Introduction

The cause of inflammatory bowel disease (IBD) remains unknown. Over the years there have been many hypotheses regarding the aetiopathogenesis of both ulcerative colitis (UC) and Crohn's disease, none of which has been proven. However, it seems probable that a combination of genetic and environmental factors is involved. As with any chronic disease of unknown cause, there may be an initiating factor which triggers the disease, ultimately allowing a series of secondary effector mechanisms to induce chronic intestinal inflammation. Quite separate factors may be responsible for causing a relapse.

This chapter will consider, from an immunological perspective, the role of genetic factors, infective agents and other environmental factors in the aetiology of IBD. In addition, the role of humoral and cellular immunity will be discussed in more general terms.

Genetic factors

Genetic factors are of considerable importance in the aetiology of both UC and Crohn's disease. The bulk of evidence to support this suggestion comes from prevalence studies within families and ethnic groups.

First-degree relatives of patients with Crohn's disease or UC have a ten-fold risk of developing the same disease (Orholm et al., 1991). Another study showed that, compared with a control population, the prevalence of UC was 15 times higher and Crohn's disease 3.5 times higher in first-degree relatives of patients with UC (Monsen et al., 1987). Inflammatory bowel disease has an increased concordance in twins (Tysk et al., 1988). This is particularly so in monozygotic twins (compared with dizygotic twins) and for Crohn's disease (compared with UC).

In contrast, there is a low prevalence of IBD amongst the spouses of patients with IBD (Pena, 1990). Taken together with the data on the familial aggregation of IBD, this represents indirect evidence to support the concept that a genetic predisposition is required for the development of this disease in a given environment.

Data from the USA and South Africa indicate that the incidence and prevalence of IBD is higher in Jews than non-Jews (Monk *et al.*, 1969; Wright *et al.*, 1986). Inflammatory bowel disease appears to be more common in American-born Jews and Jewish women compared with other Jewish populations (Odes, Fraser & Krawiec, 1989).

In terms of histocompatability antigen (HLA) markers, no consistently clear-cut relationship to IBD has been found. However, there is some evidence from Japan of an increased incidence of HLA DR2 and HLA DQ1w1 in patients with UC (Kobayashi *et al.*, 1990). In Crohn's disease, there is an association with HLA B44 (Purrman *et al.*, 1990). When Crohn's disease and ankylosing spondylitis occur concomitantly, there is a particularly strong association with the HLA B27, B44 phenotype (Purrman *et al.*, 1988). Although the prevalence of HLA B8 and DR3 is not increased in patients with UC, a patient with UC unfortunate enough to possess this phenotype has a ten-fold increase in the relative risk of developing primary sclerosing cholangitis (Chapman *et al.*, 1983; Schrumpf *et al.*, 1982). There is a particularly strong relationship between primary sclerosing cholangitis and the HLA DRw 52a antigen, which is situated on the DR3 β chain (Prochazka *et al.*, 1990).

Studies using genetic segregation analysis have, as expected, failed to show that simple Mendelian segregation is operative in IBD (Monsen *et al.*, 1989; Küster *et al.*, 1988). The results are far from clear-cut, but are in keeping with the widely held belief that the hereditary aspects of IBD are multifactorial (Monsen *et al.*, 1987; Begleiter & Harris, 1985).

Infective agents

Ever since Crohn's disease and UC were recognised as disease entities, there has been interest in various micro-organisms as possible causative agents. To date, there is no conclusive evidence to support a primary pathophysiological role of any infective agent in either of these disorders (Heatley *et al.*, 1975). Most of the current interest centres around the role of atypical mycobacteria in Crohn's disease.

Mycobacteria

Interest has focused on *M. paratuberculosis* which causes a granulomatous ileocolitis in ruminants. This disease is called Johne's disease and has many similarities to human Crohn's disease (Patterson & Allen, 1972). It has been hypothesised that Crohn's disease and Johne's disease could be caused by the same organism.

Mycobacteria are fastidious organisms, and successful culture of some strains often takes many months. However, acid-fast organisms can be cultured from up to 50% of patients with Crohn's disease, UC and also from controls (Stanford *et al.*, 1988; Graham, Markesich & Yoshimura, 1987). *Mycobacterium paratuberculosis* has been isolated from a few patients with Crohn's disease by prolonged culture of affected tissue. The organism has not been isolated from control or UC specimens (Blaauwgeers *et al.*, 1990). Routine acid-fast staining of Crohn's disease tissue has been uniformly unsuccessful. Immunohistochemical studies have also failed to demonstrate mycobacteria in Crohn's tissue (Whorwell *et al.*, 1978; Haga, 1986; Van Kruiningen *et al.*, 1988; Kobayashi, Blaser & Brown, 1989).

More recently, molecular biological techniques employing DNA probes specific for *M. paratuberculosis* and the polymerase chain reaction have been used. The results so far are discordant, with one group unable to detect any DNA from *M. paratuberculosis* (Rosenberg, Bell & Jewell, 1991), whilst another group found *M. paratuberculosis* DNA in up to 65% of patients with Crohn's disease and only 14% of controls (Sanderson *et al.*, 1992).

Studies of mycobacterial antibodies in Crohn's disease have been inconclusive. Some studies have found no difference between Crohn's and controls (Tanaka *et al.*, 1991; Stainsby *et al.*, 1993; Markesich *et al.*, 1991; Cho *et al.*, 1986). Other studies have reported increased titres of antibody to mycobacteria in Crohn's disease (Chiodini *et al.*, 1984; Jiwa *et al.*, 1988; Haagsma *et al.*, 1988; Elsaghier *et al.*, 1992). However, raised titres can be found in control and UC patients (Jiwa *et al.*, 1988; Haagsma *et al.*, 1988). It seems more likely that the constant exposure to environmental mycobacterial antigens in the gut of normal subjects is responsible for this lack of specific difference (Cho *et al.*, 1986). A wide variety of mycobacteria can be isolated from the stools of normal volunteers (Portaels, Larsson & Smeets, 1988).

Much less is known about cell-mediated responses to mycobacteria in Crohn's disease. Intestinal T cells from normal subjects proliferate poorly to antigens. Lamina propria T cells from patients with active Crohn's disease have heightened proliferative responses to a range of antigens, including *M. paratuberculosis* (Pirzer *et al.*, 1991). Macrophages from patients with Crohn's disease have been reported to inhibit growth of mycobacteria when compared with controls (Markesich, Graham & Yoshimura, 1988). Other studies have found no alterations in cell-mediated responses to mycobacteria in Crohn's disease (Ibbotson *et al.*, 1992; Seldenrijk *et al.*, 1990). Ebert *et al.* (1991) reported that there are increased *M. paratuberculosis* specific suppressor cells in Crohn's disease. In contrast, Dalton, Hoang & Jewell (1992) reported that antigen-induced suppression to a range of mycobacterial and non-mycobacterial antigens was reduced both in patients with Crohn's disease and UC.

Other infective agents

E. coli (Ljungh *et al.*, 1988), *bacteroides sp.* (Dragsteadt, Dack & Kirsner, 1941), *C. difficile* (Greenfield *et al.*, 1983), *Yersinia enterocolitica* (Ibbotson *et al.*, 1992), *Salmonellae* (Taylor-Robinson *et al.*, 1989), cell wall-deficient bacteria (Parent & Mitchell, 1976; Belsheim *et al.*, 1983), viruses (Thayer, 1987), parasites (Fradkin, 1937) and fungi (McKenzie *et al.*, 1990) have all created interest at different times for one reason or another. From an immunological viewpoint, antibodies to many commensal and pathogenic organisms have been found in IBD (Tabaqchalit, O'Donoghue & Bettleheim, 1978; Persson & Danielsson, 1979; Matthews *et al.*, 1980; Weinsink, Van de Merwe & Mayberry, 1983; Blaser *et al.*, 1984). The conclusion from these studies is that these elevated immunoglobulin titres probably represent increased bowel wall permeability to luminal micro-organisms rather than any primary pathogenic mechanism (Blaser *et al.*, 1984).

Kunin antigen

One bacterial antigen which has aroused particular interest is the enterobacterial common antigen (Kunin antigen), which is a surface antigen common to the enterobacteriacae. *Escherichia coli* strains rich in content of Kunin antigen have been found in the stools under normal circumstances. Patients with IBD have high titres of circulating antibodies to Kunin antigen which cross-react with antigens found in colonic epithelial cells (Lagercrantz *et al.*, 1968; Cooke, Philipe & Dawson, 1968). Patients with infectious colitis also have antibodies to Kunin antigen, although in much lower titre than found in IBD (Thayer *et al.*, 1969), suggesting that these findings may be just an epiphenomenon. However, using an immune complex model of colitis in rabbits, Mee *et al.* (1979) showed that a chronic colitis developed in animals who had been immunised with Kunin antigen. Augmented T cell responses to Kunin antigen have also been found in IBD (Bartnik, Swarbrick & Williams, 1974). In addition, sera from patients with IBD can induce normal lymphocytes to become cytotoxic to human colonic epithelial cells and Kunin antigen can also induce cytotoxicity against colonic targets (Shorter, Huizenga & Spencer, 1972).

These data led Shorter *et al.* (1972) to suggest the following sequence of events as a possible aetiological mechanism of IBD. A non-specific colonic injury results in increased antigen exposure to gut-associated lymphoid tissue. Continued absorption of gut contents (including Kunin antigen), might then lead to the local secretion of Kunin-specific antibodies, which cross-react with colonic epithelial cell antigens, leading to the development of local cell-mediated responses and further epithelial cell damage. This is an elegant hypothesis and remains to be disproved.

In summary, although infective agents can occasionally cause a relapse of disease, there is no convincing evidence for a primary role for a micro-organism in the aetiopathogenesis of IBD. Interest in this area has waxed and waned over the years, but until Koch's postulates can be fulfilled to prove the pathogenicity of any putative organism, the role of micro-organisms must remain speculative. It is much more likely that micro-organisms play a secondary role once the mucosa is damaged. Evidence for this comes from carrageenan-induced colitis in guinea pigs (an animal model of UC). Normal animals fed carregeenan develop chronic ulceration of the large intestine. This affect is not seen in germ-free animals (Onderdonk, Franklin & Cisneros, 1981). Furthermore, the results of treatment of IBD with antibiotics, including anti-tuberculous therapy in Crohn's disease, has been disappointing (Chapman, Selby & Jewell, 1986; Afdhal et al., 1991; Shaffer et al., 1984). Although metronidazole can be effective in IBD, its effect may be immunological (by suppressing cell-mediated responses), rather than antibacterial (Grove, Mahmoud & Warren, 1977).

Other environmental factors in IBD

Epidemiological studies have suggested that many environmental factors are associated with IBD (see Tables 6.1(a), 6.1(b)). The strength of association between many of these factors and IBD is questionable, but the association between smoking and IBD seems the most consistent. The relation between cigarette smoking and intestinal defences is of interest (Cope & Heatley, 1992). Smoking has been shown to influence colonic mucus production, rectal mucosal blood flow, colonic mucosal immuno-globulin production and colonic mucosal eicosanoid levels (Cope & Heatley, 1992). The exact role of these environmental factors with regard to the aetiology of IBD is not clear. It is also not known what effects (if any) these factors have on the mucosal immunological effector mechanisms which are operative in this disorder.

Nutrition also has profound effects on immune parameters in patients with Crohn's disease (Harries, Danis & Heatley, 1984; Animashaun et al., 1990). It has been clearly shown that elemental diets and parenteral nutrition can be useful adjuncts in the management of Crohn's disease (Harries et al., 1983; Driscoll & Rosenberg, 1978; O'Morain, Segal & Levi, 1984; Ostro, Greenberg & Jeejeebhoy, 1985). The therapeutic efficacy of dietary exclusion in this situation is probably a result of a generalized reduction in luminal antigenic load, rather than the exclusion of a specific single antigen. However, interestingly, treatment of Crohn's disease with an

Table 6.1a. *Other environmental factors in ulcerative colitis*

Factor	Effect	Comments	References
Diet	Response to milk-free diet in some (1) Some patients are lactase-deficient (3,4)	↑ antibody titre to milk protein (2) ? secondary to ↑ mucosal permeability	(1) Truelove (1961) (2) Taylor & Truelove (1961) (3) Struthers, Singleton & Kern (1965) (4) Pena & Truelove (1973)
	Fibre ⎤ No effect Refined sugar ⎦		
Breast feeding	Incidence of UC ↑ in people never breast-fed (5)	? real effect	(5) Acheson & Truelove (1961)
Smoking	↑ incidence in non-smokers Risk inversely proportional to consumption ↑ risk after stopping smoking (6,7)		(6) Heatley *et al.* (1982) (7) Benoni & Nilsson (1984)
Oral contraceptive	—		
Other drugs	?		
Place of residence	No effect		
Occupation	No effect		
Season	No effect		
Stress	? no effect		

Table 6.1b. *Other environmental factors in Crohn's disease*

Factor	Effect	Comments	References
Diet	Milk: no effect	Studies show variable results	(9) Martini & Brandes (1976)
	↑ Refined sugar intake (9)	Large prospective study of low sugar,	(10) Panza *et al.* (1987)
	↓ Fruit and veg intake (10)	high fruit and veg diet as adjunctive therapy in Crohn's showed no effect (11)	(11) Ritchie *et al.* (1987)
Breast feeding	? ↑ Incidence of Crohn's in people never breast-fed (12,13)	? real effect	(12) Koletzko *et al.* (1989) (13) Bergstrand & Hellers (1983)
Smoking	↑ Incidence of Crohn's disease in smokers (14)		(14) Somerville *et al.* (1984)
Oral contraceptive	Weak association with colonic disease (15)		(15) Vessey *et al.* (1986)
Other drugs	?		
Place of residence	? Urban dwellers		
Occupation	No effect		
Season	No effect		
Stress	? No effect		

elemental diet reduces evidence of immune activation (Duane *et al.*, 1991). This view is indirectly supported by the fact that, in patients with IBD, there is an increased prevalence of circulating antibodies to a range of dietary antigens, including wheat, maize and milk. A considerable body of evidence has accumulated to support the existence of an immediate type hypersensitivity reaction in the intestinal mucosa, with increased incidence of atopy in patients, local tissue and peripheral blood eosinophilia, basophilia and colonic mast cell degranulation with increased IgE plasma cells in the rectal mucosa (Heatley, Smart & Danis, 1986). Furthermore, basophils degranulate following antigen challenge in patients with IBD (Smart, Danis & Heatley, 1986). In other inflammatory conditions of the bowel, such as coeliac disease, there are also raised immunoglobulin titres to a range of dietary constituents, including cows' milk and yeast (Gaiffer, Clark & Holdsworth, 1992).

In contrast, in an elegant study of twins with IBD, it has been suggested that baker's yeast (*Saccharomyces cerevisiae*) may have an aetiopathological role in Crohn's disease. This is based on the finding that antibodies to *S. cerevisiae* and yeast cell wall mannan were found in significantly higher titres than in the subjects with UC or controls. This appears to be a specific finding, as antibodies to gliadin, ovalbumin and beta lactoglobulin were not raised compared with the control group (Lindberg *et al.*, 1992).

Humoral immunity in IBD

IgG

Immunohistochemistry shows that there is a large increase in immunoglobulin-containing cells in the lamina propria in both UC and Crohn's disease. All classes of immunoglobulin-containing cells are increased, but the proportional increase in IgG is greatest (Heatley, Smart & Danis, 1986; Brandtzaeg *et al.*, 1990). The relative preponderance of IgG production in IBD is also seen in populations of mucosal lymphocytes isolated from areas of inflammation (Wu *et al.*, 1989). What is fascinating is that in UC the IgG_1-subclass predominate, whereas in Crohn's disease there is an increase in IgG_2 (Scott *et al.*, 1986; Kett, Rognum & Brandtzaeg, 1987; MacDermott *et al.*, 1989). This finding is one of the few consistent differences in immunological response between Crohn's disease and UC, and has created considerable interest.

IgG_1 is normally produced in response to soluble protein antigens and has more complement-activating properties than IgG_2. In contrast, IgG_2 is synthesised predominantly in response to carbohydrates and bacterial antigens. It is conceivable, therefore, that the putative primary insult in UC is mediated by a protein antigen, and in Crohn's disease by a carbohydrate or bacterial antigen. Another explanation for the differing IgG sub-class responses is that they may be determined genetically. A recent study has provided evidence that an IgG_1 response in UC may be genetically determined (Helgeland *et al.*, 1992). However, other provisional data (Quaderi & Jewell, 1991) suggest that patients with Crohn's disease and UC mount normal IgG sub-class responses when challenged with protein or carbohydrate antigens, which mitigates against the genetically determined theory.

IgA

Immunohistochemical techniques have shown that in both UC and Crohn's disease there is a striking shift towards IgA_1 production by B-cells of the intestinal mucosa (Brandtzaeg *et al.*, 1990). The significance of this finding is uncertain, although mucosal IgA secretion overall may be defective (Badr-El Din, Trejdosiewicz & Heatley, 1988). It is not known whether the shift towards IgA_1-production represents a primary phenomenon or is secondary to a massive exposure to luminal antigens and mitogens through the diseased mucosa. Moreover, it is questionable whether such alterations in local IgA production actually compromise secretory immunity. However, it is interesting to note that a recent study (Marteau *et al.*, 1990) showed that, compared with controls, histologically uninvolved jejunum secreted significantly less polymeric IgA in Crohn's disease compared with UC. The implication is that this defect in gut humoral defence could allow increased entry of antigens into the mucosa, subsequently causing immune activation. These findings require confirmation.

Auto-antibodies

Circulating auto-antibody directed against the mucopolysaccharide of goblet cells of the small and large intestine in UC was first described in 1959 (Broberger & Perlmann, 1959). It was subsequently discovered that this antibody was also present in the sera of a large proportion of patients with Crohn's disease. This auto-antibody is not related to disease activity, does not bind complement and is also found following gastroenteritis in otherwise normal subjects.

Another circulating auto-antibody in IBD was described by Roche and co-workers in 1983 (Aronson, Cook & Roche, 1983). This antibody is directed against a water-soluble fraction of intestinal epithelium known as ECAC (epithelial cell associated component). It is also found in some healthy relatives of patients with IBD and it has the ability to fix complement.

More recently, Das (Das, 1991) described a colonic mucosal antibody directed against the colonic epithelial cell in UC but not in Crohn's disease. This is an IgG auto-antibody directed against a 40 kD epithelial cell membrane protein expressed by skin, gallbladder and colon. It is not found in normal subjects, but it is found in the systemic circulation of patients with UC. Its discovery was an exciting development, and its existence could help to explain some of the extraintestinal manifestations such as primary sclerosing cholangitis and pyoderma gangrenosum. However, other workers have been unable to detect any tissue-bound auto-antibody in UC (Snook *et al.*, 1991).

Auto-antibodies directed against neutrophils (pANCA) are found in 70–90% of patients with UC (Snook *et al.*, 1989; Chapman, Selby & Jewell, 1986; Duerr *et al.*, 1991; Seibold *et al.*, 1992; Cambridge *et al.*, 1992). They are much less common in patients with Crohn's disease and even less so in control subjects. In contrast to the cytoplasmic staining seen in vasculitic

Table 6.2. *Major auto-antibodies in inflammatory bowel disease*

Target	Origin	Prevalence UC	Prevalence Crohn's	Comments
Goblet cell	Serum	++	+	Cannot fix complement
ECAC	Serum	++	+	Fixes complement Found in relatives of IBD patients
Epithelial cell	Mucosa and serum	++	−	40 kD protein
Neutrophil	Serum	++	+	Found in relatives of IBD patients Strong association with primary sclerosing cholangitis

disorders, this antibody gives a perinuclear pattern. The target antigen is not known, but one possibility is that it is directed against cathepsin G, which is a 26 kD chymotrypsin-like protease, contained in azurophilic granules of neutrophils and monocytes (Halbwachs-Mecarelli *et al.*, 1992).

The significance of anti-neutrophil antibodies is not known. It is interesting to note that they are particularly prevalent in patients with primary sclerosing cholangitis (which is usually associated with a total colitis) and are rarely found in patients with disease restricted to the rectum (Seibold *et al.*, 1992; Cambridge *et al.*, 1992). It is unlikely that they are merely an epiphenomenon, as their presence is unrelated to disease activity (Oudkerk Pool *et al.*, 1993; Cambridge *et al.*, 1992). Whatever their significance, anti-neutrophil antibodies are found in a significant proportion of probands and unaffected family members of patients with UC (Shanahan *et al.*, 1992). Furthermore, relatives of pANCA-positive probands have a higher prevalence of antibodies compared with relatives of pANCA-negative probands. These findings suggest that anti-neutrophil antibodies represent a potential marker for genetic susceptibility to UC and also give weight to the view that genetic heterogeneity is important in UC (Shanahan *et al.*, 1992).

Other, rather more esoteric, auto-antibodies have also been reported in IBD. These include antibodies directed against lymphocyte cell membranes and a Crohn's-related antibody. These antibodies are not specific for patients with IBD.

In summary, there is a range of auto-antibodies which have been reported in IBD, particularly in UC (Table 6.2). However, their significance in the aetiopathogenesis of these disorders remains to be established.

Complement

Complement levels are normal or only slightly raised in IBD. However, dynamic studies indicate that there is increased turnover of C_3 and $C1_q$ in active UC and Crohn's disease. The activated complement component C_3b is deposited in association with IgG_1 in areas of inflammation, in the brush border of epithelial cells in UC, but not uninflamed mucosa (Halstensen *et al.*, 1990). Although C_3b is seen in epithelial cells in Crohn's disease, there is no co-localisation of IgG or complement components involved in the classical pathway (Halstensen *et al.*, 1992). The implication of this study is that initiators of the alternative pathway are more important in Crohn's disease than UC.

UC: an auto-immune disorder?

Ulcerative colitis is associated with well-recognised auto-immune disorders, such as auto-immune thyroid disease, haemolytic anaemia, vitiligo, etc. (Snook, de Silva & Jewell, 1989). This contrasts with Crohn's disease, where the incidence of associated auto-immune diseases is no different from that in a control population. This lends weight to the theory that UC is itself an auto-immune disease. However, for a disease to be classified as auto-immune, several additional criteria need to be met:

   (i)   circulating disease-specific auto-antibodies
   (ii)   an association with one or more HLA haplotypes
  (iii)   a prominent lymphocytic infiltration at the site of disease
  (iv)   steroid responsiveness.

Whilst UC fulfils the latter two criteria, there is no consistent association with any particular HLA haplotype. Moreover, although there is a range of auto-antibodies found in UC (and Crohn's disease), none of these can be definitely described as truly disease specific. Therefore, although there is some evidence that UC is an auto-immune disorder, further work is required, particularly to define the specificity of the auto-antibodies found in this condition.

Lymphocytes

Lymphocytes are important in the immunopathogenesis of IBD. Despite normal serum populations (except in active Crohn's disease where lympho-penia is seen), the number of lymphocytes seen in the mucosa of both

Crohn's and UC is vastly increased. It is, therefore, logical to ask whether there is a functional defect in lymphocytes in these conditions. An answer to this question would help us understand whether the immunological events in IBD are a primary or secondary phenomenon.

Phenotype

Lymphocytes can be categorised by immunological markers carried on their surface. These markers, often prefixed with the term 'CD' (cluster differentiation), are usually (but not invariably) correlated with functional capability. Thus, CD4+ lymphocytes are designated 'helper cells' and provide help for other T and B lymphocytes. In contrast, CD8+ lymphocytes usually have suppressor or cytotoxic functions. In many 'auto-immune' disorders there is a relative preponderance of CD4+ helper cells (raised CD4/CD8 ratio). However, the CD4/CD8 ratio is unchanged in IBD, compared with controls, in both peripheral blood mononuclear cells (PBMC) and lamina propria mononuclear cells (LPMC). In the lamina propria, there may be an increase in CD8+ cells, with a decrease in the CD4/CD8 ratio in patients with Crohn's disease, but the differences are not marked and have not been found by all investigators (Selby *et al.*, 1984; Senju *et al.*, 1992).

Mucosal lymphocytes are also important (Smart *et al.*, 1988; Smart, Heatley & Trejdosiewicz, 1989). To complicate matters further, the lamina propria contains an increased proportion of CD45Ro cells (a marker for 'memory' or 'helper-inducer' cells). There are increased numbers of CD4+CD45Ro cells in areas of mucosal inflammation, compared with uninflamed lamina propria (Senju *et al.*, 1992; James *et al.*, 1986). CD45Ro is considered a marker for activated T cells which have been in contact with antigen ('memory cells') and have helper-inducer functions. It appears from these phenotypic studies that the resting tone of the lamina propria is likely to be that of 'help' rather than suppression and that this situation is heightened when the lamina propria is inflamed. However, there is little evidence from functional studies to support this concept.

Another area of interest regarding the phenotype of lymphocytes in IBD is that of the activation markers 4F2, transferrin receptor, HLA-DR and IL2R. Peripheral blood mononuclear cells normally do not carry such markers, but do so when activated. In contrast, normal LPMC do express these markers, although only to a limited extent. This alteration may possibly be due to differences in the micro-environment between PBMC and LPMC; LPMC are constantly exposed to luminal antigens and may, therefore, be in a state of low-grade activation (Trejdosiewicz *et al.*, 1989). Raedler *et al.* (1985) and Fais *et al.* (1985) have both demonstrated that there is increased expression of early activation markers (4F2 and transferrin receptor) in PBMC of patients with IBD. There also appears to be similar

Table 6.3. *Summary of suppressor assays in IBD: PBMC*

	Comments
Reduced suppression in IBD	
Hodgson, Wands & Isselbacher (1978)	Active IBD only
	Allogeneic system
Victorino & Hodgson (1981)	↓ Spontaneous suppression
	Active and inactive IBD
Ginsburg & Falchuk (1982)	Active and inactive IBD
Danis & Heatley (1983)	Autologous system
Doldi *et al.* (1984)	↓ Spontaneous suppression in Crohn's
Auer, Roer & Frölich (1984)	Active IBD only
Kelleher *et al.* (1989)	Active and inactive Crohn's
Dalton, Hoang & Jewell (1992)	Inactive IBD
	Antigen-induced
No difference in suppression IBD vs controls	
Holdstock, Chastenay & Krawitt (1982)	Allogeneic system
Elson *et al.* (1981)	'Covert' suppressor cells in Crohn's
Davidsen & Kristensen (1987)	Inactive or moderately active IBD
Indomethacin-sensitive suppressor cells	
Holdstock, Chastenay & Krawitt (1981)	—
Kelleher *et al.* (1990)	Prostaglandin-secreting monocytes

activation within the mucosa (Pallone *et al.*, 1987). In contrast, the expression of HLA-DR or IL2R, which are late-activation markers, is not markedly raised in either PBMC or LPMC (Senju *et al.*, 1992; Pallone *et al.*, 1987; Trejdosiewicz *et al.*, 1989; Smart *et al.*, 1987).

Function

Immunoregulation

Many studies have attempted to assess immunoregulation by lymphocytes in inflammatory bowel disease as a functional corollary of the phenotypic CD4/CD8 studies. In general, the information generated by these functional studies is crude and the results rather confusing. However, the majority of studies of PBMC have shown that there is a defect in suppressor function in IBD, particularly in active disease. As shown in Table 6.3, there is considerable divergence in the results obtained, depending on the method used, patients studied, etc.

The functional significance of these studies is open to debate. If reduced suppressor function of PBMC in IBD does exist, it has been postulated that this could explain the immune activation seen in IBD. However, it could equally be argued that such an immunoregulatory defect could be secondary to chronic low-grade antigen exposure through a 'leaky' gut. Whatever the correct explanation, there is no doubt that most of these studies used non-specific assays and were probably only capable of detecting a 'global' defect at best. Moreover, *in vivo* antigen(s) will be responsible for the induction of suppression, and none of these studies has addressed this issue. However, recent work has shown that there is a defect in antigen-induced suppression in the PBMC of patients with IBD to a range of antigens (Dalton, Hoang & Jewell, 1992).

As regards immunoregulation in the mucosa, the results are even more discordant than for PBMC. To date, there have been several studies in this area (Shorter, 1981; Elson, Machelski & Weiserbs, 1985; Kanof *et al.*, 1988; Goodacre & Bienenstock, 1982; Fiocchi, Youngman & Farmer, 1983; Dalton, Hoang & Jewell, 1992; Danis, Harries & Heatley, 1984), with some showing reduced suppression, no difference or increased suppression in LPMC of patients with IBD. No consistent theme emerges from these results and the issue of mucosal immunoregulation remains an open one. Mucosal immunoglobulins may be regulated by intestinal lymphocytes (Danis & Heatley, 1987).

Cytotoxicity

Studies of MHC-restricted cytotoxicity in IBD have been beset by methodological problems, and so it is difficult to understand their relevance to pathogenesis. For example, it has been reported that LPMC demonstrate cytotoxicity against autologous gut epithelial cells. However, epithelial cells are known to undergo a high rate of spontaneous lysis following isolation, which makes interpretation of the results difficult.

Natural killer (NK) cells isolated from the gut are normal in IBD, but may be subnormal in active Crohn's disease (Gibson & Jewell, 1986). The significance of this is not known.

Intraepithelial lymphocytes

Intraepithelial lymphocytes (IEL) are found interspersed between the epithelial cells of the gastrointestinal tract, and so have a close spatial relationship to luminal antigens. It is difficult to isolate a pure population of IEL and this is the major reason why, until recently, their function in the human has remained unknown.

IEL are large granular lymphocytes, the majority of which express the CD8+ cytotoxic/suppressor phenotype. This contrasts with lamina propria cells which are predominantly CD4+ (helper) cells. IEL express little HLA-DR, IL2-R or transferrin receptor (conventional markers of activation), although a large proportion express HML-1 which is thought to be a marker of activation. There is no evidence that IEL from patients with IBD express increased markers of activation (Hoang, P., personal communication). However, Class II-bearing epithelial cells do increase the expression of activation markers in IEL (Hoang et al., 1992), a phenomenon which may have considerable relevance to mucosal immunological responses.

Despite IEL being predominantly of the CD8+ cytotoxic/suppressor phenotype, and in contrast to studies in mice, there is little evidence from functional studies that IEL have cytotoxic activity in man (Ebert, 1990). In addition, human IEL do not express H366, which is a phenotypic marker found on most cytotoxic cells.

There is evidence that human IEL have potent suppressive properties. Human colonic IEL suppress non-specific proliferative responses of autologous LPMC and also allogeneic PBMC (Hoang, Dalton & Jewell, 1991). This phenomenon is CD8-dependent, $\gamma\delta$-independent and mediated by a soluble factor. IEL from patients with IBD have no defect in this down-regulatory capacity. Colonic IEL also down-regulate IgA production by autologous LPMC and PBMC (Sachdev et al., 1993; Danis, Harries & Heatley, 1984).

Recent data suggest a defect in IBD and that is IEL's down-regulatory capacity to respond to antigen-primed lymphocytes on recall to several different antigens (Dalton et al., 1993).

The epithelial cell, class II expression and antigen presentation

Normal colonic epithelial cells express negligible or only small amounts of class II products (Mayer et al., 1991). In contrast, in inflammatory bowel disease, there is intense expression of class II molecules (Selby et al., 1983). There is considerable debate as to the functional relevance of class II expression on gut epithelial cells in IBD. Most workers believe it is a 'bystander effect', secondary to γ interferon production by activated mucosal T cells. However, there is some evidence to suggest that this may not be the whole story.

T cells can only recognise antigen in the presence of class II molecules. Bland & Warren were the first to describe that enterocyte class II can function as a restriction molecule, as it does in other cell types (Bland & Warren, 1986a,b). Enterocytes isolated from the rat small intestine were found to present soluble proteins to primed lymph node T cells *in vitro*. This was an antigen-specific effect, and was blocked by anti-class II antibodies. Furthermore, following presentation of antigen the lymph node T cells demonstrated antigen-specific suppressive properties, the antigen-responsive cells being largely of the CD8+ phenotype. Induction of these CD8+ cells was also blocked by anti-class II antibody.

Using similar methodology, Mayer & Shlien reported similar (although antigen non-specific) findings using isolated normal human gut epithelial cells, (Mayer & Shlien, 1987). However, in patients with IBD, Mayer observed that Class II-bearing epithelial cells presented antigen to CD4+, rather than CD8+, T cells (Mayer & Eisenhardt, 1990). This effect was seen in non-inflamed, as well as inflamed, areas of bowel mucosa from patients with ulcerative colitis and Crohn's disease.

The mechanism by which gut epithelial cells alter the immunological 'tone' of the underlying lamina propria is not known. Recent evidence suggests that intra-epithelial lymphocytes (IEL) may be important in this process. Epithelial cells bearing class II molecules are capable of activating IEL *in vitro* (Hoang *et al.*, 1992), and normally IEL down-regulate proliferative responses of lamina propria lymphocytes (Hoang, Dalton & Jewell, 1991). However, under certain circumstances, IEL from patients with IBD can up-regulate lymphocyte responses to antigen (Dalton *et al.*, 1993) (see Fig. 6.1).

The implications of these studies are that, under normal circumstances, the epithelium exerts a down-regulatory influence on mucosal immune responses to antigens. However, in IBD (but not in non-IBD-inflamed controls, e.g. ischaemic colitis, diverticulitis) this changes to up-regulation. This may explain several previous findings in the mucosa in IBD. For example, the increase in spontaneous secretion of IgG by lamina propria lymphocytes in IBD (Scott *et al.*, 1986) may be due to the presence of activated CD4+ T cells. As epithelial cells in non-inflamed mucosa from patients with IBD also present antigen in this 'aberrant' manner, it has been proposed that the primary defect in IBD lies in the epithelial cell and the way in which it processes and presents antigen (Mayer & Eisenhardt, 1990). This is an elegant hypothesis, but requires confirmation.

Macrophages and monocytes

In active IBD there are increased numbers of macrophages found in the lamina propria, particularly in Crohn's disease where they form an integral part of the granuloma. Intestinal macrophages are both phenotypically and functionally activated in Crohn's disease and UC (see Table 6.4) and have an important role in mediating and regulating the immune response in the

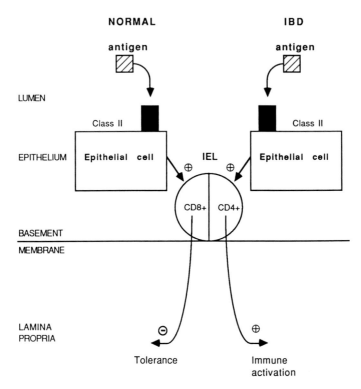

Fig. 6.1. Hypothesis to explain the role of the gut epithelium in mucosal immune events.

Table 6.4. *Phenotypic and functional activation of macrophages/monocytes in inflammatory bowel disease*

Phenotype	↑ IL2R
Function	↑ Release of acid hydrolases
	↑ Respiratory burst activity
	↑ Secretion of IL1α, IL1β, TNF
	↑ Antigen presentation

After Mahida, 1990.

mucosa (Mahida, 1990). Of interest is a recent report that suggests peripheral blood monocytes from patients with Crohn's disease produce significantly greater amounts of TNFα and ILβ, than patients with UC or controls (Mazlam & Hodgson, 1992). There is no evidence to suggest that intestinal macrophages have a primary role in the aetiopathogenesis of IBD. It is more likely that they are merely responding appropriately to an increased antigen load.

Cytokines

Interleukin-1 (IL1)

IL1 is a pro-inflammatory cytokine and is capable of causing release of prostaglandins, thromboxane and platelet activating factor from inflammatory cells. In the gut IL1 is derived predominantly from intestinal macrophages and there is now overwhelming evidence that IL1 production is up-regulated in IBD (see Table 6.5). Furthermore, 5-aminosalicylic acid (5ASA) and corticosteroids reduce the amount of IL1 produced in the mucosa (Mahida *et al.*, 1991; Pullman *et al.*, 1992; Rachmilewitz *et al.*, 1992). This may explain, at least in part, their efficacy in IBD. Of interest for the future is the work of Cominelli *et al.* (1990). Using an immune-complex model of colitis in rabbits, they have demonstrated enhanced mucosal IL1 production. What is fascinating is that tissue damage was inhibited by an IL1 receptor antagonist (IL1ra). This has now been cloned and sequenced and offers a novel approach to the treatment of immunologically mediated inflammation, such as that seen in the gastrointestinal mucosa in IBD.

Interleukin-2 (IL2)

Interleukin-2 (IL2) is a cytokine secreted by T cells, which plays a pivotal role in the immune response by inducing activation and differentiation of lymphoid cells. Under normal circumstances, IL2 is not detectable in the peripheral blood, but is found in inflammatory conditions such as rheumatoid arthritis.

There is considerable controversy regarding the role of IL2 and IBD. Divergent results have been obtained in several studies (see Table 6.6), which probably represent methodological differences (isolated cells vs biopsy specimens; cytokine protein assays vs mRNA assays). What is clear, however, is that soluble IL2-receptors (IL2R) can be detected in serum and mucosa and the levels appear to be related to the activity of the disease. This is not specific for IBD as it is found in other inflammatory conditions, such as rheumatoid arthritis and systemic lupus erythematosus (Crabtree *et al.*, 1990).

Table 6.5. *IL1 in inflammatory bowel disease*

Study	Isolated cells		Biopsy		Conclusion
	P	M	P	M	
Brynskov et al., 1992			√		↑ IL1β in CD and UC ∝ severity
Isaacs et al., 1992				√	↑ IL1 in active UC No difference in IL1 active vs inactive CD ↓ IL1ra in CD
Nakamura et al., 1992	PBMC				↑ In active UC and CD
Pullman et al., 1992	LPMC	LPMC			↑ In IBD. Hydrocortisone and 5ASA → ↓ IL1 production
Capello et al., 1992				√	*in-situ* technique ↑ IL1 in IBD
Mahida et al., 1989			√		↑ IL1 in IBD IL1 production reduced by 5ASA
Mahida et al., 1991	LPMC				↑ IL1 in UC and CD
Youngman et al., 1993	LPMC	LPMC			↑ In UC and CD Gut epithelial cells do not express IL1 mRNA
Stevens et al., 1992				√	↑ Active UC
Rachmilewitz et al., 1992			√		Rat model 5ASA → ↓ IL1 release

Key: M = assay for mRNA.
P = immunobiological assay for cytokine protein.

Interleukin-6 (IL6)

IL6 can be produced in a variety of cells, including macrophages, T cells, B cells, endothelial cells and fibroblasts. Its biological functions include B cell differentiation and growth induction of acute-phase protein synthesis by hepatocytes and T cell activation and differentiation.

Several studies have shown that IL6 production is up-regulated in UC and CD (see Table 6.7). Interestingly, serum IL6 in patients with IBD does not seem to relate to disease activity (Gross *et al.*, 1992).

Table 6.6. *IL2 and IL2R in inflammatory bowel disease*

Study	Isolated cells		Biopsy		Conclusion
	P	M	P	M	
Brynskov et al., 1992			√		↑ IL2 and sIL2R in UC and CD ∝ to activity
Mullin et al., 1992		PBMC			IL2 mRNA in PBMC low in UC, CD and controls
				√	↑ IL2 mRNA in Bx in active CD only
Nakamura et al., 1992	PBMC				↑ in active UC only CD=controls
Schreiber et al., 1992	LPMC				↑ sol IL2R from CD but not UC or controls
Matsura et al., 1993	LPMC	LPMC			↑ IL2R mRNA in UC and CD
	PBMC	PBMC			↓ IL2 mRNA in UC and CD
					↑ IL2, IL2R in LPMC vs PBMC
Crabtree et al., 1990					Serum IL2R assayed ↑ IL2R in CD ∝ to disease activity

Key: M = assay for mRNA.
P = immunobiological assay for cytokine protein.

Interleukin-8 (IL8)

IL8 is a peptide which can be produced by a variety of cell types, but monocytes and macrophages are probably the major source. Its biological activities affect mainly the neutrophils, for which it is a very potent chemo-attractant. IL8 also induces expression of adhesion molecules and causes release of stored enzymes. Chemotactic activity for T cells has also been demonstrated.

In view of the predominant neutrophil infiltration of the mucosa in active ulcerative colitis, production of this cytokine in IBD has been studied. As expected, IL8 production is up-regulated in active UC, but not CD (Mahida et al., 1992a; Isaacs, Balfour, Sartour & Haskill, 1992). Anti-IL8 antibodies are also found in UC, presumably as a defence mechanism to the toxic effects of IL8 in the systemic circulation.

Table 6.7. *IL6 in inflammatory bowel disease*

Study	Isolated cells		Biopsy		Conclusion
	Source of cytokine				
	P	M	P	M	
Isaacs *et al.*, 1992				√	↑ IL6 active UC No difference in IL6 active vs inactive CD
Gross *et al.*, 1992					Serum IL6 assayed IL6 ↑ in IBD CD>UC No correlation to disease activity
Jones *et al.*, 1993			√		↑ In active UC and CD ↑ In inactive UC also
Stevens *et al.*, 1992				√	↑ In active UC and CD

Key: M = assay for mRNA.
P = immunobiological assay for cytokine protein.

γ-Interferon

γ-Interferon (γIFN) is a cytokine produced by T cells. γIFN enhances several functions of phagocytes and lymphocytes and also plays a crucial role in the induction and modulation of major histocompatibility complex Class II antigens on several cell types, including gut epithelial cells. Leiberman *et al.* (1988) reported that polyclonally activated LPMC from patients with IBD produced less γIFN after 72 hours culture *in vitro*, compared with control LPMC. However, a recent in-depth assessment of γIFN production in Crohn's disease came to different conclusions. Fais *et al.* (1991) showed that LPMC from patients with Crohn's disease spontaneously release γIFN, a feature not shared by normal LPMC. Moreover, following polyclonal stimulation of LPMC, the kinetics of γIFN production are also different. In patients with Crohn's disease the production of γIFN peaks at 24 hours, compared with 72 hours for control LPMC.

The implications of this work are that γIFN may have an important role in the maintenance of immune activation in the mucosa in Crohn's disease, possibly by induction of Class II molecules on the adjacent epithelial cells. It is interesting to note that corticosteroids reduce γIFN production, and cyclosporin A and 5-amino salicylic acid reduce Class II expression on epithelial cells. These drugs have been found to be of use in the treatment of IBD.

Table 6.8. *TNFα in inflammatory bowel disease*

Study	Isolated cells		Biopsy		Conclusion
	P	M	P	M	
Isaacs *et al.*, 1992				√	No difference controls/IBD
Capello *et al.*, 1992				√	In situ technique ↑ in IBD
Jones *et al.*, 1993			√		↑ in active UC and CD UC > CD
MacDonald *et al.*, 1990			√		Spot-ELISA technique ↑ TNFα in UC and CD in children
Stevens *et al.*, 1992				√	No difference controls/IBD
Mahida *et al.*, 1992(*b*)	√				No difference controls/IBD

Key: M = assay for mRNA.
P = immunobiological assay for cytokine protein.

Tumour necrosis factor-α

Tumour necrosis factor-α (TNF-α) is produced by macrophages and, in common with other cytokines, has a diverse range of actions. As its name suggests, TNF-α was initially found to have the ability to kill certain tumour cells. TNF-α has subsequently been shown to be an important mediator of endotoxic shock and of cachexia in chronic inflammation. In addition, TNF-α is known to cause acute injury to the gastrointestinal mucosa.

High levels of this cytokine have been reported in the serum and stools of children with active UC and Crohn's disease (Murch *et al.*, 1991; Braegger *et al.*, 1992). It has been suggested that TNF-α may be partially responsible for the growth retardation seen in these subjects. However, studies of TNF-α production at mucosal level in IBD have yielded conflicting results (see Table 6.8), which again is probably a reflection of methodological differences.

In summary, there is mounting evidence that cytokines are involved in the development and amplification of the immune/inflammatory response in the mucosa in IBD. Cytokines have a range of functions, including T and B cell activation (IL1, IL2, γIFN), pro-inflammatory mediation (IL1), enhanced

Table 6.9. *Cytokines in inflammatory
bowel disease: summary*

Up-regulated	Conflicting data
IL1	IL2
IL6	TNFα
IL8	γIFN

Class II expression (γIFN) and direct toxicity to the gastrointestinal mucosa
(TNF-α). It comes as no surprise that secretion of most, if not all, of these
cytokines is up-regulated in the mucosa in IBD.

There is now a solid body of evidence to support the roles of IL1, IL6 and
IL8 in the inflammatory process in IBD. The roles of αIFN, IL2 and TNF-α
are rather less clear-cut at present (Table 6.9).

Summary and conclusions

The cause of UC and Crohn's disease is not known. Despite this, immunological studies, particularly over the last ten years and more, have begun to
shed some light on mucosal immune responses both in normal subjects and
patients with IBD. Furthermore, some interesting immunological differences are beginning to emerge between UC and Crohn's disease, such as the
IgG$_1$/IgG$_2$ responses, anti-neutrophil antibodies, and cytokine production
profiles. Further work in these areas may shed some light on the elusive
initiating event.

Whatever this is, it is clear that immunological effector mechanisms are
important in the aetiopathogenesis of IBD. This hypothesis is supported by
the observation that there are increased numbers of immune cells in the
lamina propria, many of which are in a state of activation. Moreover, some
patients with severe IBD show a clinical response to immunosuppressive
agents (including cyclosporin A) and lymphocyte depletion. This under-
scores the importance of lymphocyte-mediated reactions in the aetiopathogenesis of IBD.

References

Acheson, E. D. & Truelove, S. C. (1961). Early weaning in the aetiology of ulcerative colitis.
British Medical Journal, **2**, 929–33.
Afdhal, N. H., Long, A., Lennon, J., Crowe, J. & O'Donoghue, D. P. (1991). Controlled trial
of antimycobacterial therapy in Crohn's disease. *Digestive Diseases and Science*, **36**, 449–53.

Animashaun, A., Kelleher, J., Heatley, R. V., Trejdosiewicz, L. K. & Losowsky, M. S. (1990). The effect of zinc and Vitamin C supplementation on the immune status of patients with Crohn's disease. *Clinical Nutrition*, **9**, 137–46.

Aronson, R. A., Cook, S. L. & Roche, J. K. (1983). Sensitisation to epithelial antigens in chronic mucosal inflammatory disease. *Journal of Immunology*, **131**, 2796–804.

Auer, I. O., Roder, A. & Frölich, J. (1984). Immune status in Crohn's disease. VI Immuno-regulation evaluated by multiple, distinct T-suppressor cell assays of lymphocyte prolifer-ation, and by enumeration of immunoregulatory T-lymphocyte subsets. *Gastroenterology*, **86**, 1531–43.

Badr-el Din, S., Trejdosiewicz, L. K. & Heatley, R. V. (1988). Local immunity in ulcerative colitis. Evidence for defective secretory IgA production. *Gut*, **29**, 1070–5.

Bartnik, W., Swarbrick, E. T. & Williams, C. (1974). A study of peripheral leucocyte migration in agarose medium in inflammatory bowel disease. *Gut*, **15**, 294–300.

Begleiter, M. L. & Harris, D. J. (1985). Familial incidence of Crohn's disease. *Gastroenter-ology*, **88**, 221.

Belsheim, M. R., Darwish, R. Z., Watson, W. C. & Shieven, B. (1983). Bacterial L-form isolation from inflammatory bowel disease patients. *Gastroenterology*, **85**, 364–9.

Benoni, C. & Nilsson, A. (1984). Smoking habits in patients with inflammatory bowel disease. *Scandinavian Journal of Gastroenterology*, **19**, 824–30.

Bergstrand, O. & Hellers, G. (1983). Breast feeding during infancy in patients who later develop Crohn's disease. *Scandinavian Journal of Gastroenterology*, **18**, 903–6.

Blaauwgeers, H. J. L., Mullder, C. J. J., Das, P. K., Haagsma, J. & Tytgat, G. N. J. (1990). Crohn's disease, a mycobacterial aetiology? *European Journal of Gastroenterology*, **2**, 237–40.

Bland, P. W. & Warren, L. G. (1986a). Antigen presentation by epithelial cells of the rat small intestine. I. Kinetics, antigen specificity and blocking by Ia anti-sera. *Immunology*, **58**, 1–7.

Bland, P. W. & Warren, L. G. (1986b). Antigen presentation by epithelial cells of the rat small intestine. II. Selective induction of suppressor T cells. *Immunology*, **58**, 9–14.

Blaser, M. J., Miller, R. A., Lacher, J. & Singleton, J. W. (1984). Patients with active Crohn's disease have elevated serum antibodies to antigens of seven enteric bacterial pathogens. *Gastroenterology*, **87**, 888–94.

Braegger, C. P., Nicholls, S., Murch, S. H., Stephens, S. & MacDonald, T. T. (1992). Tumour necrosis factor alpha in stool as a marker of intestinal inflammation. *Lancet*, **339**, 89–91.

Brandtzaeg, P., Kett, K., Halstensen, T. S. & Helgeland, L. (1990). Pathogenesis of ulcerative colitis and Crohn's disease: humoral mechanisms. *European Journal of Gastroenterology and Hepatology*, **2**, 256–66.

Broberger, O. & Perlmann, P. (1959). Autoantibodies in human ulcerative colitis. *Journal of Experimental Medicine*, **110**, 657–74.

Brynskov, T., Tvede, N., Andersen, C. B. & Vilien, M. (1992). Increased concentrations of interleukin 1β, IL2, and soluble interleukin-2 receptors in endoscopic mucosal biopsy specimens with active inflammatory bowel disease. *Gut*, **33**, 55–8.

Cambridge, G., Rampton, D. S., Stevens, T. R. J. *et al.* (1992). Anti-neutrophil antibodies in inflammatory bowel disease: prevalence and diagnostic role. *Gut*, **33**, 668–74.

Capello, M., Keshav, S., Prince, C., Jewell, D. P. & Gordon, S. (1992). Detection of mRNAs for macrophage products in inflammatory bowel disease by *in situ* hybridisation. *Gut*, **33**, 1214–19.

Chapman, R. W., Varghese, Z., Gaul, R., Patel, G., Kikinon, N. & Sherlock, S. (1983). Association of primary sclerosing cholangitis with HLA-B8. *Gut*, **24**, 38–41.

Chapman, R. W., Selby, W. S. & Jewell, D. P. (1986). Controlled trial of intravenous metronidazole as an adjunct to corticosteroids in severe ulcerative colitis. *Gut*, **17**, 1210–12.

Chiodini, R. J., Van Kruiningen, H. J., Merkal, R. S., Thayer, W. R. & Coutu, J. A. (1984). Characteristics of an unclassified mycobacterium species isolated from patients with Crohn's disease. *Journal of Clinical Microbiology*, **20**, 966–71.

Cho, S. N., Brenna, P. J., Yoshimura, H. H., Korelitz, B. H. & Graham, D. Y. (1986). Mycobacterial aetiology of Crohn's disease: serologic study using common mycobacterial antigens and a species-specific glycolipid antigen from myobacterium paratuberculosis. *Gut*, **27**, 1353–6.

Cominelli, F., Nast, C. C., Llerena, R., Dinarello, C. A., Zipser, R. D. (1990). Interleukin-1 gene expression, synthesis and effect of specific IL-1 receptor blockade in rabbit immune complex colitis. *Journal of Clinical Investigation*, **86**, 972–80.

Cooke, E. M., Philippe, M. I. & Dawson, I. M. P. (1968). The production of colonic autoantibodies in rabbits by immunisation with *Escherichia coli*. *Journal of Pathology Bacteriology*, **96**, 125–30.

Cope, G. F. & Heatley, R. V. (1992). Cigarette smoking and intestinal defences. *Gut*, **33**, 721–3.

Crabtree, J., Juby, L. D., Heatley, R. V. *et al.* (1990). Soluble IL2R in Crohn's disease: relation of serum concentrations to disease activity. *Gut*, **31**, 1033–6.

Dalton, H. R., Hoang, P. & Jewell, D. P. (1992). Antigen-induced suppression in peripheral blood and lamina propria lymphocytes in inflammatory bowel disease. *Gut*, **33**, 324–30.

Dalton, H. R., DiPaolo, M. C., Sachdev, G. K., Hoang, P. & Jewell, D. P. (1993). Human colonic intraepithelial lymphocytes down-regulate proliferative responses of primed allogenic peripheral blood lymphocytes after re-challenge with antigen in control subjects but not inflammatory bowel disease. *Clinical and Experimental Immunology*, **93**, 97–102.

Danis, V. A. & Heatley, R. V. (1983). Pokeweed mitogen stimulated immunoglobulin production by peripheral blood lymphocytes *in vitro*: evidence for disordered immunoregulation in patients with colitis and Crohn's disease. *Clinical and Experimental Immunology*, **54**, 739–46.

Danis, V. A., Harries, A. D. & Heatley, R. V. (1984). *In vitro* immunoglobulin tissues, and alterations in patients with inflammatory bowel disease. *Clinical and Experimental Immunology*, **56**, 159–66.

Danis, V. A. & Heatley, R. V. (1987). Evidence for regulation of human colonic mucosal immunoglobulin secretion by intestinal lymphoid cells. *Journal of Clinical Laboratory Immunology*, **22**, 7–11.

Das, K. M. (1991). Some current perspectives on the aetiology and pathogenesis of ulcerative colitis. In *Ulcerative Colitis*, ed. C. O'Morain, pp. 47–54. Bora Raton, Ann Arbor, Boston: CRC Press.

Davidsen, B. & Kristensen, E. (1987). Lymphocytes subpopulations, lymphoblast transformation activity and Con A induced suppressor activity in patients with ulcerative colitis and Crohn's disease. *Scandinavian Journal of Gastroenterology*, **22**, 785–90.

Doldi, K., Manger, B., Kock, B., Riemann, J., Hermanek, P. & Kalden, J. R. (1984). Spontaneous suppressor cell activity in the peripheral blood of patients with malignant and chronic inflammatory bowel diseases. *Clinical and Experimental Immunology*, **55**, 655–63.

Dragstaedt, L. R., Dack, G. M. & Kirsner, J. B. (1941). Chronic ulcerative colitis: a summary of evidence implicating bacterium necropharum as an etiologic agent. *Annals of Surgery*, **114**, 653–62.

Driscoll, R. H. & Rosenberg, I. H. (1978). Total parenteral nutrition in inflammatory bowel disease. *Medical Clinics of North America*, **62**, 185–201.

Duane, P. D., Taehon, K., Crabtree, J. E. & Levi, A. J. *et al.* (1991). The relationship between nutritional status and serum soluble interleukin-2 receptor concentrations in patients with Crohn's disease treated with elemental diet. *Clinical Nutrition*, **10**, 222–7.

Duerr, R. H., Targan, S. R., Landers, C. J., Sutherland, L. R. & Shanahan, F., (1991). Neutrophil autoantibodies in ulcerative colitis: comparison with other colitides/diarrhoeal diseases. *Gastroenterology*, **100**, 1590–6.

Ebert, E. C. (1990). Intraepithelial lymphocytes: interferon γ-production and suppressor/cytotoxic activities. *Clinical and Experimental Immunology*, **82**, 81–5.

Ebert, E. C., Bhatt, B. D., Liu, S. & Das, K. M. (1991). Induction of suppressor cells by Mycobacterium paratuberculosis antigen in inflammatory bowel disease. *Clinical and Experimental Immunology*, **83**, 320–5.

Elsaghier, A., Prantera, G., Moreno, C. & Ivanyi, J. (1992). Antibodies to Mycobacterium paratuberculosis-specific protein antigens in Crohn's disease. *Clinical and Experimental Immunology*, **90**, 503–8.

Elson, C. O., Graeff, A. S., James, S. P. & Strober, W. (1981). Covert suppressor T cells in Crohn's disease. *Gastroenterology*, **80**, 1513–21.

Elson, C. O., Machelski, E. & Wieserbs, D. B. (1985). T cell–B cell regulation in the intestinal lamina propria in Crohn's disease. *Gastroenterology*, **89**, 321–7.

Fais, S., Capobianchi, M. R., Pallone, F. *et al.* (1991). Spontaneous release of interferon γ by intestinal lamina propria lymphocytes in Crohn's disease. Kinetics of *in vitro* response to interferon γ inducers. *Gut*, **32**, 403–7.

Fais, S., Pallone, F., Squarcia, O., Boirivant, M. & Pozzilli, P. (1985). T cell early activation antigens expressed by peripheral lymphocytes in Crohn's disease. *Journal of Clinical Laboratory Immunology*, **16**, 75–6.

Fiocchi, C., Youngman, K. R. & Farmer, R. G. (1983). Immunoregulatory function of human intestinal mucosa lymphoid cells: evidence for enhanced suppressor cell activity in inflammatory bowel disease. *Gut*, **24**, 692–701.

Fradkin, W. Z. (1937). Ulcerative colitis: bacteriological aspects. *New York Journal of Medicine*, **37**, 249.

Gaiffer, M. H., Clark, A. & Holdsworth, C. D. (1992). Antibodies to *Saccharomyces cerevisiae* in patients with Crohn's disease and their possible pathogenic importance. *Gut*, **33**, 1071–5.

Gibson, P. R. & Jewell, D. P. (1986). Local immune mechanisms in inflammatory bowel disease and colorectal carcinoma. Natural killer cells and their activity. *Gastroenterology*, **90**, 12–19.

Ginsburg, C. H. & Falchuk, Z. M. (1982). Defective autologous mixed-lymphocyte reaction and suppressor cell generation in patients with inflammatory bowel disease. *Gastroenterology*, **83**, 1–9.

Goodacre, R. L. & Bienenstock, J. (1982). Reduced suppressor cell activity in intestinal lymphocytes from patients with Crohn's disease. *Gastroenterology*, **82**, 653–8.

Graham, D. Y., Markesich, D. C. & Yoshimura, H. H. (1987). Mycobacteria and inflammatory bowel disease: results of culture. *Gastroenterology*, **92**, 436–42.

Greenfield, C., Aguilar, Ramirez, Jr., Pounder, R. E. *et al.* (1983). Clostridium difficile and inflammatory bowel disease. *Gut*, **24**, 713–17.

Gross, V., Andus, T., Caesar, I., Roth, M. & Scholmerich, J. (1992). Evidence for continuous stimulation of IL6 production in Crohn's disease. *Gastroenterology*, **102**, 514–19.

Grove, D. I., Mahmoud, A. A. F. & Warren, K. S. (1977). Suppression of cell-mediated immunity by metronidazole. *International Archive of Allergy and Applied Immunology*, **54**, 422–7.

Haagsma, J., Mulder, C. J. J., Eger, A. & Tytgat, G. N. J. (1988). A study of antibodies to Mycobacterium paratuberculosis in IBD. In *IBD. Current Status and Future Approach*, ed. R. P. MacDermott, pp. 539–542. Amsterdam: Elsevier Science Publishing.

Haga, Y. (1986). Mycobacteria in Crohn's disease. Nippon Shokakibyo Gakki Zarshi, **83**, 2325–33.

Halbwachs-Mecarelli, L., Nusbaum, P., Nöel, L. H. *et al.* (1992). Anti-neutrophil cytoplasmic antibodies (ANCA) directed against cathepsin G in ulcerative colitis, Crohn's disease and primary sclerosing cholangitis. *Clinical and Experimental Immunology*, **90**, 79–84.

Halstensen, T. S., Mollnes, T. E., Garred, P., Fausa, O. & Brandtzaeg, P. (1990). Epithelial deposition of immunoglobulin G^1 and activated complement (C^3b and terminal complement complex) in ulcerative colitis. *Gastroenterology*, **98**, 1264–71.

Halstensen, T. S., Mollnes, T. E., Garred, P., Fausa, O. & Brandtzaeg, P. (1992). Surface epithelium related activation of complement differs in Crohn's disease and ulcerative colitis. *Gut*, **33**, 902–8.

Harries, A. D., Danis, V. A. & Heatley, R. V. (1984). Influence of nutritional status on immune function in patients with Crohn's disease. *Gut*, **25**, 465–72.

Harries, A. D., Jones, L. A., Danis, V., Fifield, R., Heatley, R. V., Newcombe, R. G. & Rhodes, J. (1983). Controlled trial of supplemented oral nutrition in Crohn's disease. *Lancet*, **i**, 887–90.

Heatley, R. V., Bolton, P. M., Owen, E., Jones Williams, W. & Hughes, L. E. (1975). A search for a transmissible agent in Crohn's disease. *Gut*, **16**, 528–32.

Heatley, R. V., Smart, C. J. & Danis, V. A. (1986). Inflammatory bowel disease. In *Gut Defences in Clinical Practice*, ed. M. S. Losowsky, R. V. Heatley. London & Edinburgh: Churchill Livingstone.

Heatley, R. V., Thomas, P., Prokipchuk, E. J. *et al.* (1982). Pulmonary function abnormalities in patients with inflammatory bowel disease. *Quarterly Journal Medicine*, **203**, 241–50.

Helgeland, L., Tysk, C., Jänerot, G. *et al.* (1992). IgG subclass distribution in serum and rectal mucosa of monozygotic twins with or without inflammatory bowel disease. *Gut* **33**, 1358–64.

Hoang, P., Dalton, H. R. & Jewell, D. P. (1991). Human colonic intraepithelial lymphocytes are suppressor cells. *Clinical and Experimental Immunology*, **85**, 498–503.

Hoang, P., Crotty, B., Dalton, H. R. & Jewell, D. P. (1992). Epithelial cells bearing Class II molecules stimulate allogeneic intraepithelial lymphocytes. *Gut*, **33**, 1089–93.

Hodgson, H. J. F., Wands, J. R. & Isselbacher, K. J. (1978). Decreased suppressor cell activity in inflammatory bowel disease. *Clinical and Experimental Immunology*, **32**, 451–8.

Holdstock, G., Chastenay, B. F. & Krawitt, E. L. (1981). Increased suppressor cell activity in inflammatory bowel disease. *Gut*, **22**, 1025–30.

Holdstock, G., Chastenay, B. F. & Krawitt, E. L. (1982). Functional suppressor T cell activity in Crohn's disease and the effects of sulphasalazine. *Clinical and Experimental Immunology*, **48**, 619–24.

Ibbotson, J. P., Lowes, J. R., Chahal, H. *et al.* (1992). Mucosal cell-mediated immunity to mycobacterial, enterobacterial and other microbial antigens in inflammatory bowel disease. *Clinical and Experimental Immunology*, **87**, 224–30.

Isaacs, K. L., Balfour Sartor, R. & Haskill, S. (1992). Cytokine messenger RNA profiles in inflammatory bowel disease mucosa detected by polymerase chain reaction amplification. *Gastroenterology*, **103**, 1587–95.

James, S. P., Fiocchi, C., Graeff, A. S. & Strober, W. (1986). Phenotypic analysis of lamina propria lymphocytes. Predominance of helper-inducer and cytolytic T-cell phenotypes in Crohn's disease and control patients. *Gastroenterology*, **91**, 1483–9.

Jiwa, N. M., Mulder, C. J. J., Van den Berg, F. M. *et al.* (1988). Elevated IgG to mycobacterial PPD's in Crohn's disease. In *IBD. Current Status and Future Approach*. ed. R. P. MacDermott, pp. 543–546. Amsterdam: Elsevier Science Publishing.

Jones, S. C., Haidar, A., Hagan, P. *et al.* (1993). Cytokine production in the mucosa of patients with inflammatory bowel disease. *European Journal of Gastroenterology and Hepatology* (in press).

Kyanof, M. E., Strober, W., Fiocchi, C., Zeitz, M. & James, S. P. (1988). CD4-positive Leu-8-negative helper-inducer T cells predominate in the human intestinal lamina propria. *Journal of Immunology*, **141**, 3029–36.

Kelleher, D., Murphy, A., Feighery, C., Weir, D. G., Keeling, P. W. N. (1989). Defective suppression in the autologous mixed lymphocyte reaction in patients with Crohn's disease. *Gut*, **30**, 839–44.

Kelleher, D., Murphy, A., Whelan, C. A., Feighery, C., Weir, D. G., Keeling, P. W. N. (1990). Lymphocyte proliferation in inflammatory bowel disease: effect of monocyte suppressor cell. *European Journal of Gastroenterology and Hepatology*, **2**, 457–61.

Kett, K., Rognum, T. O. & Brandtzaeg, P. (1987). Mucosal subclass distribution of immuno-globulin G-producing cells is different in ulcerative colitis and Crohn's disease of the colon. *Gastroenterology*, **93**, 919–24.

Kobayashi, K., Blaser, M. J. & Brown, W. R. (1989). Immunohistochemical examination for mycobacteria in intestinal tissues from patients with Crohn's disease. *Gastroenterology*, **96**, 1009–15.

Kobayashi, K., Atoh, M., Konoeda, Y. *et al.* (1990). HLA, DR, DQ and T cell antigen receptor constant beta genes in Japanese patients with ulcerative colitis. *Clinical and Experimental Immunology*, **80**, 400–3.

Koletzko, S., Sherman, P., Corey, M., Griffiths, A. & Smith, C. (1989). Role of infant feeding practices in the development of Crohn's disease in childhood. *British Medical Journal*, **289**, 1617–18.

Küster, W., Pascoe, L., Purrmann, J., Funk, S., Majewski, F. (1988). The genetics of Crohn's disease: complex segregation analysis of a family study with 265 patients with Crohn's disease and 5287 relatives. *American Journal of Medical Genetics*, **32**, 105–8.

Lagercrantz, R., Hammarström, S., Perlmann, P. & Gustafsson, B. E. (1968). Immunological studies in ulcerative colitis IV. *Journal of Experimental Medicine*, **128**, 1339–52.

Lieberman, B. Y., Fiocchi, C., Youngmann, K. R., Sapatnekar, W. K. & Proffit, M. R. (1988). Interferon production by human intestinal mucosal mononuclear cells. Decreased levels in inflammatory bowel disease. *Digest of Diseases Science*, **33**, 1297–304.

Lindberg, E., Magnusson, E.-K, Tysk, C. & Jänerot, G. (1992). Antibody (IgG, IgA and IgM) to baker's yeast (*Saccharomyces cerevisiae*), yeast mannan, gliadin, ovalbumin and betalacto-globulin in monozygotic twins with inflammatory bowel disease. *Gut*, **33**, 909–13.

Ljungh, A., Eriksson, M., Eriksson, Ö. *et al.* (1988). Shiga-like toxin production and connective tissue protein binding of *E. coli* isolated from a patient with ulcerative colitis. *Scandinavian Journal of Infectious Diseases*, **20**, 443–6.

MacDermott, R. P., Nash, G. S., Auer, I. O. *et al.* (1989). Alterations in immunoglobulin subclasses in patients with ulcerative colitis and Crohn's disease. *Gastroenterology*, **96**, 764–8.

MacDonald, T. T., Hutchings, P., Choy, M.-Y., Murch, S. & Cooke, A. (1990). Tumour necrosis factor-alpha and interferon-gamma production measured at the single cell level in normal and inflamed human tissue. *Clinical and Experimental Immunology*, **81**, 301–5.

Mahida, Y. R. (1990). Macrophage function in inflammatory bowel disease. *European Journal of Gastroenterology and Hepatology*, **2**, 251–5.

Mahida, Y. R., Lamming, C. E. D., Gallagher, A., Hawthorne, A. B. & Hawkey, C. J. (1991). 5-aminosalicylic acid is a potent inhibitor of interleukin 1β production in organ culture of colonic biopsy specimens from patients with inflammatory bowel disease. *Gut*, **32**, 50–4.

Mahida, Y. R., Ceska, M., Effenberger, R., Lindley, I. & Hawkey, C. J. (1992a). Enhanced synthesis of neutrophil-activating peptide-1/interleukin 8 in active ulcerative colitis. *Clinical Sciences*, **82**, 273–5.

Mahida, Y. R., Scott, E., Kurlak, L., Gallagher, A. & Hawkey, C. J. (1992b). Interleukin 1β, tumour necrosis factor α and interleukin 6 synthesis by circulating mononuclear cells isolated from patients with active ulcerative colitis and Crohn's disease. *European Journal of Gastroenterology and Hepatology*, **4**, 501–7.

Mahida, Y. R., Wu, K. & Jewell, D. P. (1989). Enhanced production of interleukin 1β by mononuclear cells isolated from mucosa with active ulcerative colitis and Crohn's disease. *Gut*, **30**, 835–8.

Markesich, D. C., Graham, D. Y. & Yoshimura, H. H. (1988). Interaction of human monocytes and mycobacteria: studies comparing Crohn's disease to controls. In *IBD. Current Status and Future Approach*, ed. R. P. MacDermott, pp. 553–558. Amsterdam: Elsevier Science Publishing.

Markesich, D. C., Sawai, E. T., Butel, J. S. & Graham, D. Y. (1991). Investigations on etiology of Crohn's disease: humoral immune response to stress (heat shock) proteins. *Digest of Disease Science*, **36**, 454–60.

Marteau, P., Colombel, J. F., Nemeth, J. *et al.* (1990). Immunological study of histologically non-involved jejunum during Crohn's disease: evidence for reduced *in vivo* secretion of secretory IgA. *Clinical and Experimental Immunology*, **80**, 196–201.

Martini, G. A. & Brandes, J. W. (1976). Increased consumption of refined carbohydrates in patients with Crohn's disease. *Klin Wochenschr*, **54**, 367–71.

Matsuura, T., West, G. A., Youngmann, K. R., Klein, J. S. & Fiocchi, C. (1993). Immune activation genes in inflammatory bowel disease. *Gastroenterology*, **104**, 448–58.

Matthews, N., Mayberry, J. F., Rhodes, J. *et al.* (1980). Agglutinins to bacteria in Crohn's disease. *Gut*, **21**, 376–80.

Mayer, L. & Shlien, R. (1987). Evidence for function of Ia molecules on gut epithelial cells in man. *Journal of Experimental Medicine*, **66**, 1471–83.

Mayer, L. & Eisenhardt, D. (1990). Lack of induction of suppressor T cells by intestinal epithelial cells from patients with inflammatory bowel disease. *Journal of Clinical Investigations*, **86**, 1255–60.

Mayer, L., Eisenhardt, D., Salomon, P, Bauer, W., Plous, R. & Piccinini, L. (1991). Expression of class II molecules on intestinal epithelial cells in humans. Differences between normals and inflammatory bowel disease. *Gastroenterology*, **100**, 3–12.

Mazlam, M. Z., Hodgson, H. J. F. (1992). Peripheral blood monocyte cytokine production and acute phase response in inflammatory bowel disease. *Gut*, **33**, 773–8.

McKenzie, H., Main, J., Pennington, C. R. & Parratt, D. (1990). Antibody to selected strains of *Saccharomyces cerevisiae* (baker's and brewer's yeast) and *Candida albicans* in Crohn's disease. *Gut*, **31**, 536–8.

Mee, A. S., McLaughlin, J. E., Hodgson, H. J. F. & Jewell, D. F. (1979). Chronic immune colitis in rabbits. *Gut*, **20**, 1–5.

Monk, M., Mendeloff, A. I., Siegel, C. I. & Lilienfeld, A. (1969). An epidemiological study of ulcerative colitis and regional enteritis among adults in Baltimore. II. Social and demographic factors. *Gastroenterology*, **56**, 847–57.

Monsen, U., Broström , O., Nordenvall, B., Sörstad, J. & Hellers, G. (1987). Prevalence of inflammatory bowel disease among relatives of patients with ulcerative colitis. *Scandinavian Journal of Gastroenterology*, **22**, 214–18.

Monsen, U., Iselius, L., Johansson, C. & Hellers, G. (1989). Evidence for a major additive gene in ulcerative colitis. *Clinical Genetics*, **36**, 411–14.

Mullin, G. E., Lazenby, A. J., Harris, M. L., Bayless, T. M. & James, S. P. (1992). Increased interleukin-2 messenger RNA in the intestinal mucosal lesions of Crohn's disease but not ulcerative colitis. *Gastroenterology*, **102**, 1620–6.

Murch, S. H., Lamkin, V. A., Savage, M. O., Walker-Smith, J. A., MacDonald, T. T. (1991). Serum concentrations of tumour necrosis factor α in childhood chronic inflammatory bowel disease. *Gut*, **32**, 193–7.

Nakamura, M., Saito, H., Kasanuki, J., Tamura, Y. & Yoshida, S. (1992). Cytokine production in patients with inflammatory bowel disease. *Gut*, **33**, 933–7.

Odes, H. S., Fraser, D. & Krawiec, J. (1989). Inflammatory bowel disease in migrant and native Jewish populations of southern Israel. *Scandinavian Journal of Gastroenterology*, **24**, (Suppl. 170), 36–8.

O'Morain, C., Segal, A. W. & Levi, A. J. (1984). Elemental diets as primary therapy of acute Crohn's disease: a controlled trial. *British Medical Journal*, **288**, 1859–62.

Onderdonk, A. B., Franklin, M. L., Cisneros, R. L. (1981). Production of experimental colitis in gnotobiotic guinea pigs with simplified microflora. *Infections and Immunology*, **32**, 225–31.

Orholm, M., Munkholm, P., Langholz, E., Nielsen, O. H., Sorensen, T. I. A. & Binder, V. (1991). Familial occurrence of inflammatory bowel disease. *New England Journal of Medicine*, **324**, 84–8.

Ostro, M. J., Greenberg, G. R. & Jeejeebhoy, K. N. (1985). Total parenteral nutrition and complete bowel rest in the management of Crohn's disease. *Journal of Parent Ent Nutrition*, **9**, 280–7.

Oudkerk Pool, M., Ellerbroek, P. M., Ridwan, Bu. *et al.* (1993). Serum anti-neutrophil cytoplasmic antibodies in inflammatory bowel disease are mainly associated with ulcerative colitis. A correlation study between perinuclear anti-neutrophil cytoplasmic antibodies and clinical parameters, medical and surgical treatment. *Gut*, **34**, 46–50.

Pallone, F., Fais, S., Squarcia, O. *et al.* (1987). Activation of peripheral blood and intestinal lamina propria lymphocytes in Crohn's disease. In vivo state of activation and in vitro response to stimulation as defined by the expression of early activation antigens. *Gut*, **28**, 745–53.

Panza, E., Franceshi, S., LaVecchia, S. *et al.* (1987). Dietary factors in the aetiology of inflammatory bowel disease. *International Journal of Gastroenterology*, **19**, 205–9.

Parent, K. & Mitchell, P. D. (1976). Bacterial variants: aetiological agent in Crohn's disease. *Gastroenterology*, **71**, 365–8.

Patterson, D. S. P. & Allen, W. M. (1972). Chronic mycobacterial enteritis in ruminants as a model of Crohn's disease. *Proceedings of the Royal Society of Medicine*, **65**, 998–1001.

Pena, A. S. & Truelove, S. C. (1973). Hypolactasia and ulcerative colitis. *Gastroenterology*, **64**, 400–4.

Pena, A. S. (1990). Genetics of inflammatory bowel disease. In *Inflammatory Bowel Disease and Coeliac Children*, ed. D. Hadziselimovic, B. Herzog, A. Bürgin-Wolff, pp. 45–58. Kluwer Academic Publ.

Persson, S. & Danielsson, D. (1979). On the occurrence of serum antibodies to *Bacteroides fragilis* and serogroups of *E. coli* in patients with Crohn's disease. *Scandinavian Journal of Infectious Diseases*, **19**, (Suppl.), 61–7.

Pirzer, U., Schönhaar, R., Fleischer, B. Ferman, E. & Meyer zum Buschenfelde, K. H. (1991). Reactivity of infiltrating T lymphocytes with microbial antigens in Crohn's disease. *Lancet*, **338**, 1238–9.

Portaels, F., Larsson, L. & Smeets, P. (1988). Isolation of mycobacteria from healthy persons' stools. *International Journal of Leprosy*, **56**, 468–71.

Prochazka, E. J., Terasaki, P. I., MinSik Park, D. V. M., Goldtein, L. I. & Busuttil, R. W. (1990). Association of primary sclerosing cholangitis with HLA-DRw52a. *New England Journal of Medicine*, **322**, 1842–4.

Pullman, W. E., Elsbury, S., Kobayashi, M., Hapel, A. J. & Doe, W. F. (1992). Enhanced mucosal cytokine production in inflammatory bowel disease. *Gastroenterology*, **102**, 529–37.

Purrmann, J., Zeidler, H., Bertrams, J. *et al.* (1988). HLA antigens in ankylosing spondylitis associated with Crohn's disease. Increased frequency of the HLA phenotype B27, B44. *Journal of Rheumatology*, **15**, 1658–61.

Quaderi, M. A. & Jewell, D. P. (1991). IgG subclasses in inflammatory bowel disease. *Gut*, **32**, A1259.

Rachmilewitz, D., Karmeh, F. Schwartz, L. W. & Simon, P. L. (1992). Effect of aminopherols (5-ASA and 4-ASA) on colonic interleukin-1 generation. *Gut*, **33**, 929–32.

Raedler, A., Frankels, ?., Klose, G. & Thiele, H. G. (1985). Elevated numbers of peripheral T cells in inflammatory bowel disease displaying T9 antigen and Fc-alpha receptors. *Clinical and Experimental Immunology*, **60**, 518–24.

Ritchie, J. K., Wadsworth, J., Lennard Jones, J. E. & Rogers, E. (1987). Controlled multicentre trial of an unrefined carbohydrate, fibre-rich diet in Crohn's disease. *British Medical Journal*, **295**, 517–20.

Rosenberg, W. M. C., Bell, J. I. & Jewell, D. P. (1991). Mycobacterium paratuberculosis cannot be detected in Crohn's disease tissues. *Gastroenterology*, **100**, A611.

Sachdev, G. K., Dalton, H. R., Hoang, P., DiPaolo, M. C., Crotty, B. & Jewell, D. P. (1993). Human colonic intraepithelial lymphocytes suppress in vitro immunoglobulin synthesis by autologous peripheral blood lymphocytes and lamina propria lymphocytes. *Gut*, **34**, 257–63.

Sanderson, J. D., Moss, M. T., Tizard, M. L. V. & Hermon-Taylor, J. (1992). Mycobacterium paratuberculosis DNA in Crohn's disease tissue. *Gut*, **33**, 890–6.

Schreiber, S., Raedler, A., Conn, A. R., Rombeau, J. L. & MacDermott, R. P. (1992). Increased *in vitro* release of soluble interleukin 2 receptor by colonic lamina propria mononuclear cells in inflammatory bowel disease. *Gut*, **33**, 236–41.

Schrumpf, E., Fausa, O., Forre, O. *et al.* (1982). HLA antigens and immunoregulatory T cells in ulcerative colitis associated with hepatobiliary disease. *Scandinavian Journal of Gastroenterology*, **17**, 187–91.

Scott, M. G., Nahm, M. H., Macke, K., Nash, G. S., Bertovich, M. J. & MacDermott, R. P. (1986). Spontaneous secretion of IgG subclasses by intestinal mononuclear cells: differences between ulcerative colitis, Crohn's disease and controls. *Clinical and Experimental Immunology*, **66**, 209–15.

Seibold, F., Weber, P., Klein, R., Berg, P. A. & Wiedmann, K. H. (1992). Clinical significance of antibodies against neutrophils in patients with inflammatory bowel disease and primary sclerosing cholangitis. *Gut*, **33**, 657–62.

Selby, W. S., Janossy, G., Mason, D. Y. & Jewell, D. P. (1983). Expression of HLA-DR antigens by colonic epithelium in inflammatory bowel disease. *Clinical and Experimental Immunology*, **53**, 614–18.

Selby, W. S., Janossy, G., Boffil, M. & Jewell, D. P. (1984). Intestinal subpopulations in inflammatory bowel disease: an analysis by immunohistological and cell isolation techniques. *Gut*, **32**, 779–83.

Seldenrijk, C. A., Drexhage, H. A., Meuwissen, S. G. M. & Meijer, C. J. L. M. (1990). T cell immune reactions (in macrophage inhibition factor assay) against *Mycobacterium paratuberculosis, Mycobacterium kansasii, Mycobacterium tuberculosis, Mycobacterium avium* in patients with chronic inflammatory bowel disease. *Gut*, **31**, 529–35.

Senju, M., Wu, K. C., Mahida, Y. R. & Jewell, D. P. (1992). Two colour immunofluorescence and flow cytometric analysis of lamina propria lymphocyte subsets in ulcerative colitis and Crohn's disease. *Digest of Disease in Science* (in press).

Shaffer, J. L., Hughes, S., Linaker, B. D., Baker, R. D. & Turnberg, L. A. (1984). Controlled trial of rifampicin and ethambutol in Crohn's disease. *Gut*, **25**, 203–5.

Shanahan, F., Duerr, R. H., Rotter, J. I. *et al.* (1992). Neutrophil autoantibodies in ulcerative colitis: familial aggregation and genetic heterogeneity. *Gastroenterology*, **103**, 456–61.

Shorter, R. F., Huizenga, K. A. & Spencer, R. J. (1972). A working hypothesis for the aetiology and pathogenesis of non-specific inflammatory bowel disease. *American Journal of Digestion Diseases*, **17**, 1024.

Shorter, R. G. (1981). Ty cells in non-specific concanavalin A-induced suppressor activity in vitro in colonic inflammatory bowel disease and in colorectal carcinoma. In *Recent Advances in Crohn's Disease,* ed. A. S. Pena, *et al.,* pp. 448–455. The Hague: Martinus Nijhoff.

Smart, C. J., Crabtree, J. E., Heatley, R. V., Trejdosiewicz, L. K. & Losowsky, M. S. (1987). Functional and phenotypic analysis of lymphocytes isolated from human intestinal mucosa. In *Advances in Experimental Biology and Medicine,* ed. J. Mestecky, J. R. McGhee, J. Bienenstock, P. L. Ogra, New York & London: Plenum Press.

Smart, C., Danis, V. A., Heatley, R. V. (1986). *In vitro* IgE production by peripheral blood lymphocytes and rectal mucosal biopsies and antigen-induced basophil degranulation in patients with inflammatory bowel disease. *Journal of Clinical Laboratory Immunology,* **20,** 183–5.

Smart, C. J., Heatley, R. V. & Trejdosiewicz, L. K. (1989). Expression of CD6 and UCHL1-defined CD45 (pl80) antigen by human colonic T lymphocytes. *Immunology,* **66,** 90–5.

Smart, C. J., Trejdosiewicz, L. K., Badr-El Din, S. & Heatley, R. V. (1988). T lymphocytes of the human colonic mucosa: functional and phenotypic analysis. *Clinical and Experimental Immunology,* **73,** 63–9.

Snook, J. A., Chapman, R. W., Fleming, K. & Jewell, D. P. (1989). Anti-neutrophil nuclear antibody in ulcerative colitis, Crohn's disease and primary sclerosing cholangitis. *Clinical and Experimental Immunology,* **76,** 30–3.

Snook, J. A., de Silva, H. J. & Jewell, D. P. (1989). The association of autoimmune disorders with inflammatory bowel disease. *Quarterly Journal of Medicine,* **72,** 835–40.

Snook, J. A., Lowes, J. R., Wu, C. K., Priddle, J. D. & Jewell, D. P. (1991). Serum and tissue autoantibodies to colonic epithelium in ulcerative colitis. *Gut,* **32,** 163–6.

Somerville, K. W., Logan, R. F. A., Edmond, M. & Langman, M. J. G. (1984). Smoking and Crohn's disease. *British Medical Journal,* **288,** 954–6.

Stainsby, K. J., Lowes, J. R., Allan, R. N. & Ibbotson, J. P. (1993). Antibodies to *Mycobacterium paratuberculosis* and nine species of environmental mycobacteria in Crohn's disease and control subjects. *Gut,* **34,** 371–4.

Stanford, J. L., Dourmashkin, R., McIntyre, G. & Visuvanathan, S. (1988). Do mycobacteria exist in alternative physical forms and what part do they play in the aetiology of inflammatory bowel disease. In *Inflammatory Bowel Disease. Current Status and Future Approach.* ed. R. P. MacDermott, pp. 503–508. Amsterdam: Elsevier Science Publishing.

Stevens, C., Walz, G., Singaram, C. *et al.* (1992). Tumour necrosis factor α, interleukin-1β and interleukin 6 expression in inflammatory bowel disease. *Digestive Diseases in Science,* **37,** 818–26.

Struthers, J. E., Singleton, J. W. & Kern, F. (1965). Intestinal lactase deficiency in ulcerative colitis and regional ileitis. *Annals of Internal Medicine,* **63,** 221–8.

Tabaqchalt, S., O'Donoghue, D. P. & Bettleheim, K. A. (1978). *Escherichia coli* antibodies in patients with inflammatory bowel disease. *Gut,* **19,** 108–13.

Tanaka, K., Wilks, M., Coates, P. J. *et al.* (1991). *Mycobacterium paratuberculosis* and Crohn's disease. *Gut,* **32,** 43–5.

Taylor, K. B. & Truelove, S. C. (1961). Circulating antibodies to milk proteins in ulcerative colitis. *British Medical Journal,* **2,** 924–9.

Taylor-Robinson, S., Miles, R., Whitehead, A. & Dickinson, R. J. (1989). Salmonella infection and ulcerative colitis. *Lancet,* **i,** 1145.

Thayer, W. R., Brown, M., Sangree, M. H., Katz, J. & Hersch, T. (1969). *Escherichia coli* and colon haemagglutinating antibodies in inflammatory bowel disease. *Gastroenterology,* **57,** 311–18.

Thayer, W. R. (1987). Infectious agents in inflammatory bowel disease. In *Inflammatory Bowel Disease,* ed. G. Jänerot, pp. 101–108. Raven Press.

Trejdosiewicz, L. K., Badr-El Din, S., Smart, C. J. *et al.* (1989). Colonic mucosal T lymphocytes in ulcerative colitis: expression of the CD7 antigen in relation to MHC Class II (HLA-D) antigens. *Digest Disease Science*, **34**, 1449–56.

Truelove, S. C. (1961). Ulcerative colitis provoked by milk. *British Medical Journal*, **2**, 929–33.

Tysk, C., Linberg, E., Järnerot, G. & Floderus-Myrhed, B. (1988). Ulcerative colitis and Crohn's disease in an unselected population of monozygotic and dizygotic twins. A study of heritability and the influence of smoking. *Gut*, **29**, 990–6.

Van Kruiningen, J. H., Thayer, W. R., Chiodini, R. J., Meuton, D. J. & Couta, J. A. (1988). An immunoperoxidase search for mycobacteria in Crohn's disease. In *Inflammatory Bowel Disease. Current Status and Future Approach*, ed. R. P. MacDermott, pp. 547–552. Amsterdam: Elsevier Science Publishing.

Vessey, M., Jewell, D. P., Smith, A., Yeates, D. & McPherson, K. (1986). Chronic inflammatory bowel disease, cigarette smoking and use of oral contraceptives: findings in a large cohort study of women of childbearing age. *British Medical Journal*, **292**, 1101–3.

Victorino, R. M. M. & Hodgson, H. J. F. (1981). Spontaneous suppressor cell function in inflammatory bowel disease. *Digest of Diseases in Science*, **26**(9), 801–6.

Weinsink, F., van de Merwe, J. P. & Mayberry, J. F. (1983). An international study of agglutinins to *Eubacterium, Peptostreptococcus*, and *Coprococcus* species in Crohn's disease, ulcerative colitis and control subjects. *Digestion*, **27**, 63–9.

Whorwell, P. J., Davison, I. W., Beeken, W. L. & Wright, R. (1978). Search by immunofluorence for antigens of rotavirus, *Pseudomonas maltophilia* and *Mycobacterium kansasii* in Crohn's disease. *Lancet*, **ii**, 697–8.

Wright, J. P., Forggat, J., O'Keefe, E. A. *et al.* (1986). The epidemiology of inflammatory bowel disease in Cape Town 1980–1984. *South African Medicine Journal*, **70**, 10–15.

Wu, K. C., Mahida, Y. R., Priddle, J. D. & Jewell, D. P. (1989). Immunoglobulin production by isolated intestinal mononuclear cells from patients with ulcerative colitis. *Clinical and Experimental Immunology*, **78**, 37–41.

Youngman, K. R., Simon, R. L., West, G. A. *et al.* (1993). Localisation of interleukin 1 activity and protein and gene expression to lamina propria cells. *Gastroenterology*, **104**, 749–58.

–7–
Food intolerance and allergy

STEPHAN STROBEL

Introduction

Adverse, allergic clinical reactions attributable to food intake tend to divide medical practitioners into two groups: those who ascribe a wide range of medical complaints to food allergy in the broadest sense and those who virtually deny the existence of this disorder.

As a consequence of clinical and basic research, only cynics would deny the existence of immunologically mediated adverse clinical reactions to foods. On the other hand, one has to remember that a number of clinical syndromes previously thought to be caused by food could not always be confirmed in objective double-blind food provocation studies.

At the beginning of the discussion it is important to define the terms food allergy and food intolerance (Table 7.1).

Food allergy incorporates all conceivable immunological reactions to foods and not only the 'classic' IgE-mediated responses. Clinical symptoms that disappear after specific dietary elimination procedures and recur on food challenges (preferably in a double-blind fashion) will be termed *food intolerance*. In this way, this definition may include certain non-immunological mechanisms (e.g. histamine-induced migraine) but also

Table 7.1. *Working definition of food allergy, intolerance and aversion*

A   Food allergy (hypersensitivity): involving all known immunological pathogenetic mechanisms to food proteins (IgE mediated and other humoral and cellular immune responses).

B   Food intolerance: non-allergic reactions to food affecting susceptible individuals. The basis for these reactions can be 1) lack of digestive enzymes, 2) metabolic defects or 3) possibly direct, chemically-triggered, reaction, or 4) as yet, undiscovered, non-immunological mechanisms.

C   Food aversion: in subjects with suspected but unconfirmed, non-specific symptoms to foods.

From Strobel (1993), with kind permission of the editor and publisher. Modified after Royal College of Physicians Report, London 1992 (Kay & Lessoff (eds.) 1992).

clinical symptoms which, at a later stage, may well reveal an immunological aetiology. The spectrum of food-induced clinical symptoms will be addressed by focusing on the intestinal tract of cows' milk-induced entero-pathy in childhood as an example and will present evidence for an underly-ing immune aetiology, based on human studies and experimental models.

Food induced symptoms in clinical practice

Food intolerance to virtually all foods has been described. Most common in childhood are intolerance to cows' milk, wheat, soy protein, fruits, eggs and fish. The overall frequency of specific food substances responsible for clinical symptoms varies from country to country depending on the prevail-ing infant feeding practices (Table 7.2).

Natural history and incidence of food sensitivities

The natural history and incidence of adverse reactions to foods were investigated in detail by Bock & Atkins, 1990. They followed 480 children prospectively from birth to the 3rd year of life. 137 parents (28%) thought the clinical symptoms in their infants were caused by foods. In 8% these reactions were reproduced either in a blind (3.4%) or in an open challenge (4.4%). Most of the symptoms affected the gastrointestinal tract, followed by cutaneous, respiratory and behavioural symptoms, although virtually all organ systems can be affected.

Clinical symptoms of cows' milk allergies

Milk sensitive gastrointestinal symptoms

In a recent prospective study by Høst, Husby & Osterballe (1988) investigat-ing the incidence of cows' milk allergy in 1749 Danish infants, 2.2% were identified in a double-blind challenge to have cows' milk induced gastro-intestinal symptoms Bock & Atkins (1990), in a continuation of their earlier study (Bock, 1987), showed a delayed onset of cows' milk sensitivity (>4 hours) in 8 children under 3 years of age (who did not have a positive skin test result), who exclusively exhibited gastrointestinal symptoms. Six had milk and/or combined milk and soy (2/6) protein gastroenteropathy and 1 child had a biopsy proven gluten sensitive gastroenteropathy (coeliac disease).

Table 7.2. *Foods most commonly implicated in food allergic reactions in childhood*

Immediate (IgE) hypersensitivity reactions (n=355) Esteban (1992)		Associated food intolerance in CMPA (n=100) Bishop et al. (1990)		Reactions to foods (atopic disease, n=144) Kjellman et al. (1989)		Reactions to foods (atopic disease, n=185) Bock & Atkins (1990)	
Egg	34	Egg	58	Citrus	17	Egg	26
Fish	30	Soy	47*	Strawberries	14	Peanut	25
Vegetables	26	Orange	35	Chocolate	8	Milk	23
Milk	25	Peanut	34	Tomato	8	Nuts	10
Fruits	21	Casein hydr.	22*	Egg	8	Soy	6
Leguminosae	19	Wheat	16	Fish	6	Fish	3
Other	11			Nuts	6	Wheat	2
				Milk	4	Pea	2
				Others	29	Others	3

*The percentages given for adverse clinical reactions are unusually high and are most likely overestimates of their 'true' prevalence, since some clinical reactions may have been caused by an intolerance to sucrose or an initially high osmolality of the hydrolysate used. The reactions were not confirmed with a challenge protocol.

Values are given as percentages.

CMPA: cows' milk protein allergy.

From Strobel (1993), with kind permission of the editor and publisher.

Clinical diagnosis of cows' milk allergies

The gold standard for the diagnosis of cows' milk allergy is a reproducible double-blind placebo controlled challenge (Bock & Atkins, 1990). Infants with a particularly high degree of hypersensitivity and the risk of an anaphylactic reaction should not be challenged for diagnostic purposes alone. In addition to a good clinical history, a high level of skin test reactivity, associated with increased levels of serum anti-cows' milk antibodies, provides further corroborative evidence.

Onset of clinical symptoms

In the majority of children, the onset of clinical symptoms in cows' milk protein allergy is within the first year of life. A great number of children present before 3 months of age (Bock, 1987; Esteban, 1992; Bishop, Hill & Hosking, 1990; Høst & Halken, 1990), in direct association with cows' milk intake. In a non-prospective study of 383 cases of immediate-type food allergy, 70% presented under 2 years of age, while only approximately 10% of children exhibited their first symptoms between 7 and 14 years of age (Esteban, 1992).

Immediate onset of symptoms

Children in whom there is a close time relationship between ingestion of cows' milk and the onset of clinical symptoms, have a high probability of suffering from cows' milk allergy. Clinical symptoms of anaphylaxis, urticaria, angioedema, vomiting and diarrhoea develop within minutes or hours after ingestion of small amounts of cows' milk (see Table 7.3). These patients can often be identified by positive skin tests and radioallergosorbent test (RAST).

Infantile colic   It was noted in a large cows' milk allergy cohort study that extremely colicky behaviour of infants with cows' milk allergy resolved when cows' milk was excluded from the diet (Lothe & Lindberg, 1989). Despite this observation and other studies, the frequency with which infants with colic respond to cows' milk withdrawal, remains to be established.

Laboratory diagnosis of cows' milk allergy

Predictive accuracy of skin testing (IgE)

Skin tests have been frequently used in confirming a diagnosis of immediate-type food allergy. Whereas its accuracy in (presumably) IgE-mediated

Table 7.3. *Common symptoms in children with (suspected) food allergy*

Skin	Eczema
	Urticaria
	Conjunctivitis
	Contact dermatitis
Respiratory tract	Rhinitis
	Cough
	Dyspnoea
	Wheeze
	Asthma
Gastrointestinal tract	Regurgitation
	Vomiting
	Bloating
	Infantile colic
	Diarrhoea
	Failure to thrive
	Constipation

Other organ systems (for example ENT, central nervous system, urinary tract etc.), can also be a target for food-related clinical symptoms.
From Strobel, 1993, with kind permission of the editor and publisher.

clinical symptoms (Bock & Atkins, 1990; Kjellman *et al.*, 1989), studies have shown that IgE antibody production to common foods is normally encountered during development (Hattevig *et al.*, 1984) and can also occur during breast feeding indicating a possible sensitisation during lactation (Cant, Bailes & Marsden, 1985; Gerrard & Shenassa, 1983). A positive skin test can be an indicator of a developing atopic disease preceding clinical symptoms (Hattevig *et al.*, 1984; Dreborg, 1989). On the other hand, individuals that have lost their clinical sensitivity can still maintain their skin test responsiveness for a variable period. Skin testing for presumably only partially IgE-mediated clinical symptoms, such as food-induced gastro-enteropathies, is unhelpful. The lack of positive skin test, in children with a cows' milk protein enteropathy, has been demonstrated by Bishop *et al.* (1990).

Mucosal morphology in acute onset (?IgE mediated) disease

There is little information concerning the small intestinal mucosa in these immediate-onset syndromes, since children with these disorders are usually not biopsied. Theoretically, deduced from animal studies discussed below, the biopsy could be histologically normal, but its function could be impaired and exhibiting signs of mucosal oedema and eosinophilic infiltration. The pathogenetic role of intestinal eosinophils in acute (or chronic) intestinal reactions is not clear and the relationship of food allergy to the hypereosinophilic syndrome needs clarification (Katz *et al.*, 1984; Walker-Smith, 1988; Wershil & Walker, 1992). A subgroup of infants under one year, with eosinophilic gastroenteritis and diarrhoea associated with atopy and evidence of IgE-mediated hypersensitivity, may respond to dietary elimination therapy (Walker-Smith, 1988; Wershil & Walker, 1992).

A picture of degranulated IgE positive mast cells on conventional histology (Cooper *et al.*, 1992; Bengtsson *et al.*, 1991) may be helpful in making the diagnosis. However, IgE positive mucosal mast cells are also seen in patients with a negative skin test and this histological finding is only of limited usefulness in the individual case (Bengtsson *et al.*, 1991). IgE levels in faeces may be increased during allergic intestinal reactions (Kolmannskog *et al.*, 1986, 1991).

Cows' milk induced enteropathies with delayed onset

Cows' milk allergy with a slow onset, where the clinical symptoms are not in direct relationship with the food intake, often presents with gastrointestinal problems and failure to thrive to the paediatrician. In these cases there is often no clear history and the diagnosis may be difficult and appropriate diagnostic procedures include investigation of the gastrointestinal structure, assessment of gastrointestinal function and of mucosal immunity. Cows' milk-induced enteropathies often present as chronic diarrhoeal syndromes, with failure to thrive, with or without associated atopic features and can mimic inflammatory bowel diseases.

There is no single and simple laboratory test for routine screening of children with slow-onset intestinal symptoms. In children, these problems often overlap with intestinal infections and a full microbiological study (including electron microscopy for viruses) is needed to distinguish between food allergy and infection.

Small intestinal mucosal morphology

The characteristic feature of a food-sensitive gastroenteropathy, is a small intestinal mucosal damage of varying extent and severity. The mucosa is often thin, the lesion may be patchy and within one biopsy there may be a range of morphological appearances, from a normal mucosa to severe villus atrophy. The changes are often described as non-specific although their presence in children with a typical clinical presentation, is highly suggestive, once infectious causes have been excluded. The typical lesion is crypt hyperplasia and villus atrophy of variable severity, but often less severe than in coeliac disease. The intraepithelial lymphocyte (IEL) count is often within the normal range, although all cows' milk sensitive enteropathies on a milk elimination diet, respond with a significant rise of their IEL counts during a milk challenge (Walker-Smith, 1988; Walker-Smith et al., 1978). An increase of IEL with the γ,δ T cell phenotype, originally thought to be pathognomonic for coeliac disease, has also been reported in children with cows' milk allergy, post-enteritis syndrome (Walker-Smith, 1992). A major difference is that γ,δ positive IEL numbers, return to normal in cows' milk allergy, whereas they stay elevated in coeliac disease, indicating that the increase in cows' milk allergy is transient and most likely a secondary phenomenon.

The immunological basis of food-sensitive enteropathies

Before entering into the discussion on the presumed (immune) aetiology of food-sensitive enteropathies, it is important to remember that a great number of immunological and non-specific factors are likely to affect antigen handling at mucosal surfaces and the subsequent immune response. The factors and their hypothetical effects on gastrointestinal immune regulation are summarised in Table 7.4.

Macromolecular antigen uptake

Minor proportions of most protein antigens that have been investigated, reach the circulation undegraded. Circulating immunoreactive antigen levels vary between 10^{-2} to 10^{-4} of the administered dose in rodents and humans. Achlorhydria has been found to increase macromolecular absorption of bovine serum albumin (BSA) in adults. In an animal model of intestinal anaphylaxis, neutralisation of gastric pH retarded digestion and in this way increased macromolecular absorption from the intestinal tract. This process may play a role in the neonate where gastric output and possibly also proteolytic activity is reduced, compared to older children. Investigations into macromolecular (protein) uptake and the permeability of sugar molecules in premature and term infants, have shown that increased permeability is correlated with reduced gestational age, returning to 'normal' (postnatal) levels at about the 36th or 38th gestational week.

The role of the mucosal barrier during development

The role of the mucosal barrier in antigen handling has been extensively investigated (Walker, 1981, 1987; Sanderson & Walker, 1993). Macromolecules are more adherent to the surface of immature cells than mature cells.

Table 7.4. *Factors controlling antigen handling and immune regulation at mucosal sites*

Gut lumen
  Bacterial/viral colonisation
  Digestion
  Secretion
  Peristalsis

Mucosal surface (non-specific and immunological factors)
  Barrier function
  Antigen:
    Binding, Processing (?), Uptake
    Presentation to gut associated lymphoid tissue (GALT) (?)
    Interaction with intraepithelial lymphocytes (?)
  Local immune defences
    Secretory IgA, IgM
    Cell-mediated immunity
    Other Immunoglobulin (Ig) isotypes

Lamina propria and GALT
  Antigen presentation
  Induction of secretory immunity
  Induction of oral tolerance:
  Suppression of humoral immunity
  Suppression of cell-mediated immunity
  Clonal anergy
  Generation of memory

These increased binding patterns of antigens to (epithelial) microvillus membrane preparations were demonstrated in neonatal rats and in other studies correlated to maturational changes of the phospholipid composition of microvillus membranes and changes in the intestinal mucous.

The specialised role of the M-cells overlaying the Peyer's patch has been the subject of intensive studies. M-cells are known to transport luminal antigen from the gut to the underlying tissue. The immune response of underlying T-lymphocytes to luminal antigens may be enhanced, owing to their close proximity to the surface (Sanderson & Walker, 1993). The exact role of enhanced macromolecular absorption is still not resolved, but is clearly important in the maintenance of a homeostatic balance in the gut-associated lymphoid tissue (GALT). Disruption of the barrier function, e.g. during virus infection, has been linked to development of intestinal sensitisations. An increase of macromolecular permeability may contribute to the continuation of clinical symptoms after sensitisation. A study in our hospital of eczematous children without gastrointestinal symptoms, has identified a subgroup of children with atopy under 6 years of age, with an increased lactulose/rhamnose urinary excretion ratio, possibly indicating an overall increased gastrointestinal permeability (Pike *et al.*, 1986). It remains unresolved whether the observed increased permeability indicates an atopic state (primary phenomenon) or was secondarily caused by the disease, through a constant low grade intestinal antigen challenge. Nor is it known whether such changes are correlated with altered protein uptake.

Uptake of dietary protein antigen in man

Over the past decade there have been several studies measuring dietary antigen uptake in healthy adults, using mainly ovalbumin and β-lactoglobulin as probes. Generally, the results with the egg protein (ovalbumin) are in broad agreement, those obtained using β-lactoglobulin are more controversial.

Husby and colleagues have extensively investigated patterns of antigen uptake *between* individuals and *within* one individual at different times (Husby, 1988; Husby, Høst & Hansen, 1991). It was found that, after a test meal, peak levels (mg/ml) of ovalbumin were reached at times ranging from 120 to 240 minutes, but there was no evidence that low molecular weight fragments of ovalbumin were present. In some individuals, circulating antigen could be detected for up to 48 hours after the test meal.

As mentioned previously, gut closure in man is generally regarded as *in utero* event. One group, however, found evidence of increased intestinal permeability to lactulose during the neonatal period and it (closure) certainly may not have occurred in preterm infants by the time of delivery. More recently Axelsson *et al.* (1989) have confirmed these observations, using α-lactalbumin as a molecular weight marker.

Macromolecular uptake in cows' milk protein intolerance

Using different sized polyethylene glycol (PEG) polymers to assess gut permeability, Fälth-Magnusson *et al.* (1986) reported significant changes in the excretion of PEG, following challenge with cows' milk and similar observations have been made by other groups using sugar probes.

The group mentioned above and others, have recently made a detailed study of macromolecular absorption in infants, with infantile colic as a manifestation of cows' milk allergy. Serum samples were obtained 30 and 60 minutes after an intake of human milk and the levels of α-lactalbumin were then measured using a competitive radioimmunoassay. Both breast-fed and formula-fed infants, with infantile colic, had significantly higher serum levels of α-lactalbumin than did appropriate age-matched, healthy control subjects. These findings suggest that the gut mucosa of infants with infantile colic can be at least transiently abnormal.

The pathogenetic role of immunological reactions in food-induced gastroenteropathies

A hypothesis related to the overall pathogenesis of food allergy is depicted in Fig. 7.1.

It is unlikely that immunological type I, II, III, IV (Gell and Coombs) reactions occur in isolation during intestinal or systemic food allergies. For clarity these mechanisms will be separated and discussed individually.

Immediate hypersensitivity reaction (Type 1) of small bowel and colon (Intestinal anaphylaxis, IgE-mediated) (Fig. 7.2).

During evaluation of mechanisms of intestinal hypersensitivity reactions, it is important to distinguish between the primary sensitisation phase and the mechanisms that cause clinical symptoms, after re-exposure to the sensitizing antigen. Most commonly, IgE-mediated reactions (intestinal anaphylaxis) have been investigated in humans and laboratory rodents (Jarrett, 1984; Perdue et al., 1984, 1991; Turner, Barnet & Strobel, 1990). Frequently, immunological and physiological analyses (in vitro/in vivo), have focused on the effects of intestinal anaphylaxis on gut permeability. Effects on mucosal morphology and physiology, including the protective effects of pharmacological agents on the release of mediators from immune cells (i.e. mast cells) during intestinal anaphylaxis, have also been evaluated (Pearce et al., 1982; Boulton et al., 1988; Miller et al., 1983). Immediate clinical symptoms of intestinal anaphylaxis (diarrhoea, vomiting), after eating a triggering food, are familiar to most medical practitioners (and parents). During a mucosal anaphylactic reaction, proteins can cross the intestinal and vascular barrier in two ways. They can 'leak' into the gut or, under certain circumstances, they are able to pass from the gut lumen into the vascular system. Altered mucosal integrity and function or both, can be assessed under clinical conditions (to some extent), by measuring the urinary excretion ratio of small molecular weight sugars of different sizes. During these conditions, the excretion of lactulose increases, whereas the excretion and absorption of the smaller sugars remain unchanged or decrease. It has to be pointed out here, that macromolecular protein absorption does not

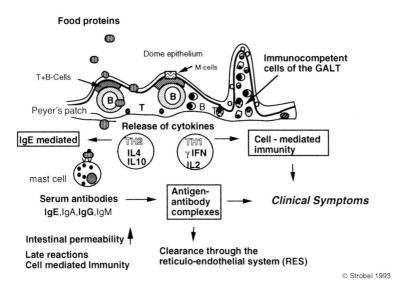

© Strobel 1993

Fig. 7.1. Pathogenesis of food allergic symptoms. Food proteins reach the immunocompetent cells of the gut associated lymphoid tissues (GALT) in small quantities undigested (10^{-4} of administered dose), or after processing and presentation by antigen presenting cells. The poorly understood nature of local antigen processing and presentation through epithelial cell, B-cells, follicular dendritic cells and dendritic cells, generally lead to a suppression of potential hazardous IgE and cell-mediated immune responses, without affecting protective local secretory immunity (IgA/IgM). Under pathological conditions, cell-mediated immune responses play a major role in causing mucosal damage. This cellular immune response, can be locally modified by a particular cytokine release pattern and preferential activation of Th2 cells, that favour IgE production (mast cell degranulation) and other inflammatory amplification loops, that add to alterations of mucosal morphology and function. Secondary phenomena, such as an increased intestinal permeability and increased formation of circulating antigen-antibody immune complexes, may lead to clinical symptoms that can affect virtually all organ systems.

necessarily correlate with sugar permeability and both have to be assessed separately (Turner *et al.*, 1990).

Recently, intestinal reactivity in patients with an IgE-mediated allergic response to inhalant allergens and 'IgE negative' individuals with cows' milk allergy, have been studied with a segmental perfusion technique in adults.

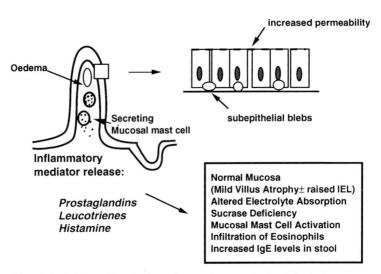

Fig. 7.2. IgE mediated alterations of normal physiological gastro-intestinal functions and associated mucosal damage (modified after Strobel, 1990).

As markers of local antigen-specific release, mast cell mediators and eosinophil products, were measured in the perfusate. In addition, substances that could also originate from plasma such as histamine, albumin and hyaluronan were measured. Interestingly, clinically milk intolerant patients, without measurable specific IgE, also shared raised levels of eosinophilic cationic protein, albumin and hyaluronan over 2 hours, as did patients with IgE mediated inhalant allergies. This finding suggests that early phase 1 reactions may occur without any obvious involvement of IgE mechanisms (Knutson *et al.*, 1993).

In an experimental setting, the release of mucosal mast cell specific enzymes (e.g. rat mast cell specific protease II (RMCPII), or tryptase in humans), are one marker of intestinal anaphylaxis. Analysis of serum levels, of these mediators, can be used as indicators for primary IgE-mediated reactions, at least under strictly controlled experimental conditions (Turner *et al.*, 1990; Miller *et al.*, 1983). The usefulness of measuring the release of mast cell mediators, under clinical conditions, remains to be evaluated. Preformed, or newly generated mediators of inflammation and cytokines released, or produced, from mast cells, or other cells, can amplify the pathogenic process and are able to attract other inflammatory cells i.e. eosinophils, granulocytes and monocytes. In animals, the regulation of IgE antibody production seems to be under a delicate cytokine control network, whereby IL4 augments IgE production and interferon-γ has a suppressive activity.

Recent studies (and current dogma) of food allergic patients, with eczema, indicate that most cells infiltrating the skin lesions are CD4+ T lymphocytes, that are allergen specific (TH$_2$ cells (Sampson, 1993)). Activated TH$_2$ cells secrete a variety of cytokines (IL3-IL6, IL10), which promote IgE production (IL4) and up-regulate IgE receptors and down-regulate TH$_1$ activity although this view has lately been challenged by Kondo et al. (1993) who suggests a predominantly antigen-specific TH$_1$ response in blood-borne lymphocytes of food allergic, eczematous patients.

Similar studies have not been performed in food allergic patients with gastrointestinal symptoms and most changes seen and investigated in IgE-triggered intestinal reactions focus on morphological and physiological changes as outlined below (Perdue et al., 1984, 1991; Turner et al., 1990; Miller et al., 1983):

Mast cell counts (mucosa)	reduced (++)
Mucosal histamine content	reduced
Absorption of H$_2$O and electrolytes	reduced
Mucosal enzymes (sucrase)	reduced
Villus height	usually unchanged
Crypt depth	usually unchanged
Uptake of proteins	increased
Lactulose/rhamnose ratio	increased
Rat mast cell protease II levels	increased (++)

The effect of so-called 'mast-cell stabilising' drugs in the prevention of presumably IgE-mediated clinical symptoms, has been disappointing, despite the obvious involvement of mucosal mast cells. Reports about the usefulness of orally administered, poorly absorbed disodium cromoglycate for treatment of food allergies have been conflicting (André, André & Colin, 1989; Freier & Berger, 1973; Sogn, 1986). In my experience, only a small number of food allergic children will respond to this form of treatment. Although successful in some, the mode of action remains unknown. Identification and elimination of the food(s) in question, represent the most successful form of therapy in these children. In severely handicapped, multiple, food allergic children, a trial with disodium cromoglycate is indicated (100–200 mg, 15–20 minutes before each meal suspended in a glass of warm water).

IgE-induced, food sensitive colitis

Colitic symptoms, such as rectal loss of fresh blood and colonoscopic changes of an erythematous, friable mucosa with petechiae and occasional

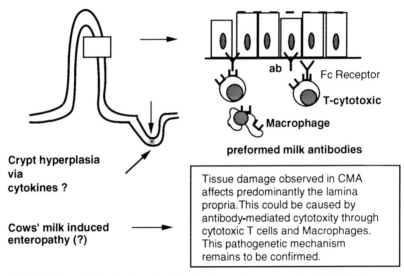

Fig. 7.3. Hypothetical role of antibody dependent cytotoxity (ADCC) mechanisms in cows' milk allergy (CMA) (modified after Strobel, 1990).

ulcerations, have been described in milk allergic infants. These changes seen in children under 2 years were cured by milk elimination (Grybowski, 1967) and reappeared on challenge (Jenkins *et al.*, 1984). Distinction between ulcerative colitis and Crohn's disease is important. A response to a milk elimination may not accurately distinguish between these disease entities and histological examination of the mucosa is mandatory. In milk-induced colitis, there is often an atopic family history, a dense eosinophilic infiltrate and an increased number of IgE-bearing cells (most likely mast cells).

Antibody-dependent cytotoxicity (ADCC) (Type II) (Fig. 7.3)

Antibody-dependent cytotoxicity is characterised by the effects of natural killer (NK) cells and T-lymphocytes, which possess a high affinity immunoglobulin receptor (Fcg), which is used for target cell recognition. These immunological mechanisms are not restricted by the recognition pathway via the histocompatibility complex HLA-DR (Class II antigens). Large, granular, lymphocytes (LGL), which can be identified in the lamina propria and gut epithelium, display several of these activities *in vitro*. ADCC activity has also been reported *in vitro* in infants with cows' milk protein induced gastroenteropathy, without other clinical responses to milk (Saalman *et al.*, 1991).

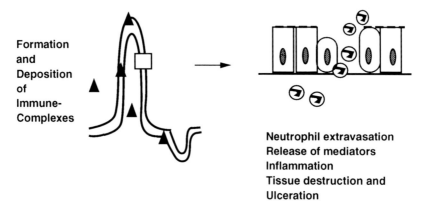

Fig. 7.4. Evidence of immune complex-mediated (Arthus) mucosal damage in humans is circumstantial in inflammatory bowel disease (Halstensen *et al.*, 1990). Its pathogenetic role in intestinal food allergic disease is unclear (modified after Strobel, 1990).

Immune complex (Arthus type) disease (Type III) (Fig. 7.4)

Production of anti-food antibodies, in children, is a physiological response and not generally correlated with disease. Over 80% of all children, receiving cows' milk, have developed cows' milk antibodies by the age of 2–3 years. Increased levels of food specific antibodies, in serum or secretions, are more frequently found in individuals with clinical symptoms of food sensitivity. Immune complex (IC) deposition in tissues, and their histological demonstration, can be a sign of an underlying immunologically mediated (e.g. renal) disease. It would still be premature to suggest that the IC identified on intestinal sections of patients, with inflammatory bowel disease or with food-sensitive enteropathies, represent the immunological cause for the mucosal damage. There is, however, increasing evidence for a putative role of local immune complement activation on the basis of immunohistochemical evidence, in patients with ulcerative colitis (Halstensen *et al.*, 1990). However, injection of preformed IC into experimental animals, for example, did not lead to histological changes that are considered markers of inflammatory bowel disease (i.e. granulocyte infiltration) (Kirkham *et al.*, 1986). In another model, intraluminal antigen exposure in sensitised pigs, resulted in a massive influx of polymorphs, without morphological damage (Bellamy & Nielson, 1974). The contribution of other pathogenetic processes, e.g. local vasculitic processes, in the generation of mucosal injury, remains unclear.

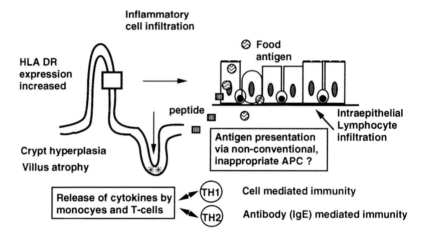

Exact function of α,β and γ,δ, TCR positive IEL unknown

Fig. 7.5. There is good experimental evidence in humans and laboratory rodents that cell-mediated, delayed hypersensitivity mechanisms operate in food sensitive diseases, resulting in villus atrophy. APC = antigen presenting cell; TCR = T cell receptor. See also Fig. 7.1 (modified after Strobel, 1990).

(Delayed-type) hypersensitivity reactions (Type IV) (Fig. 7.5)

Cell-mediated, delayed-type hypersensitivity (DTH) reactions, represent a major immunological pathway responsible for severe mucosal damage (Mowat, 1987; Strobel, Mowat & Ferguson 1985; Strobel & Ferguson, 1986; Strobel, 1990; MacDonald & Spencer, 1988). DTH effects on intestinal morphology have been investigated in detail during immunologically mediated rejection of transplanted bowel or during a graft versus host reaction (GvHR) after bone marrow transplantation (MacDonald & Spencer, 1988; Mowat, Borland & Parrott, 1986; Ferguson, 1987). In both events, the small intestinal mucosa is the major target organ but changes are seen throughout the whole length of the intestinal tract. The extent of mucosal damage can be modulated by varying the number of incompatible cells injected into the recipient. The degree of histoincompatibility between the donor and recipient pair (difference in major and/or minor histocompatibility antigens), also determines the extent of mucosal damage. The striking similarities of these histological changes, with intestinal abnormalities observed in food protein-induced gastroenteropathies, has led to the suggestion that a T-lymphocyte-mediated process, also plays an important role in the pathophysiology of villus atrophy in humans.

Studies during a cell-mediated GvHR in humans and additional evidence from experimental work in rodents, indicate that a first sign, of this mucosal immune response, is an increase of lymphocytes within the intestinal epithelium. If the GvH *reaction* progresses to a GvH *disease*, the IEL infiltration is frequently followed by an increase in crypt cell turnover and an increase of the crypt depth (Strobel & Ferguson, 1986; MacDonald & Spencer, 1988; Mowat *et al.*, 1986; Ferguson, 1987). Depending on the age of the animal or the histo*in*compatibility of donor and recipient pair, mucosal damage can continue to villus atrophy. The crucial role of lymphocytes, in the generation of mucosal changes in humans, has been investigated and confirmed in experiments using intestinal foetal explants of different gestational age (MacDonald & Spencer, 1988). To summarise these experiments, it seems that epithelial damage, and even destruction of the explant after mitogen stimulation, was only observed in the mucosa of foetuses that had already been populated with T lymphocytes, at about 14–18 weeks of gestation but not before. Addition of inhibitors of T-cell function, e.g. cyclosporin A or FK 506, to the culture system, also inhibited intestinal damage.

The role of 'enteropathic' cytokines

Convincing experimental evidence that direct cytotoxicity mechanisms play an important role in damaging the mucosa is lacking and it is tempting to speculate that immunological-mediated damage is triggered by systemic, or more likely *local* release of mediators (cytokines). These 'enteropathic' cytokines may attack or affect intraepithelial lymphocytes and could also act on fibroblast and intestinal crypt stem cells. Alterations of the cytokine activity of intestinal mucosa of patients with inflammatory bowel diseases (IBD) have been reported, but for methodological reasons remain highly variable and contradictory at this moment (Fiocchi, 1991; Beagley & Elson, 1992).

Recent studies have provided substantial evidence that lymphocytes within the lamina propria, differ from lymphocytes in other tissues and in the circulation. Mucosal lymphocytes are phenotypically distinct and show evidence of activation and recent memory induction. On activation, lamina propria lymphocytes have a high level of expression of mRNA for the production of IL2, IL4, IL5 and γ IFN. Although the high level of expression of IL4, IL5 is similar to mouse Th2 clones [review (Beagley & Elson, 1992; Mosman & Coffman, 1989)] there is no good evidence, at present, that normal human lymphocytes exist with a similar functional pattern to murine Th1 or Th2 clones. Activation or imbalance, or both of these delicate local cytokine pathways, could finally trigger mechanisms, which lead to mucosal damage. Once these mechanisms have been activated, possibly in an antigen-specific fashion, mere withdrawal of the specific trigger, may not always be sufficient to reverse or halt the disease process. It is conceivable that clinical examples which are compatible with this hypothesis include, diet-resistant coeliac disease, autoimmune gastroenteropathies and the intractable diarrhoea of infancy syndrome.

Outlook

It is tempting to speculate that the future will bring treatment regimens that are likely to re-induce tolerance to (food) antigens in a specific fashion. This could be achieved either by identifying and using 'tolerogenic' epitopes (Peng, Turner & Strobel, 1990) which are active alone or when coupled to self-proteins, possibly in combination with a short course of blocking monoclonal antibodies able to induce suppression or anergy (Qin et al., 1993). Until then, two of the basic questions concerning food allergies remain unanswered. These are:

- How can a primary sensitisation be prevented and
- How can clinical (and immunological) tolerance be restored in the sensitised child?

References

André, C., André, F. & Colin, L. (1989). Effect of allergen ingestion challenge with and without cromoglycate cover on intestinal permeability in atopic dermatitis, urticaria and other symptoms of food allergy. *Allergy*, **44**, S41–7.
Axelsson, I., Jakobsson, I., Lindberg, T., Polberger, S. Benediktsson, B. & Räihä, N. (1989). Macromolecular absorption in preterm and term infants. *Acta Paediatrica Scandinavica*, **78**, 532–7.
Beagley, K. & Elson, C. (1992). Cells and cytokines in mucosal immunity and inflammation. *Gastroenterology Clinics of North America*, **21**, 347–66.
Bellamy, J. E. C. & Nielson, N. O. (1974). Immune-mediated emigration of neutrophils into the lumen of the small intestine. *Infections and Immunology*, **9**, 615–20.
Bengtsson, U., Rognum, T. P., Brandtzaeg, P. (1991). IgE-positive duodenal mast cells in patients with food-related diarrhea. *International Archive in Allergy and Applied Immunology*, **95**, 86–91.
Bishop, J. M., Hill, D. J. & Hosking, C. S. (1990). Natural history of cow milk allergy: clinical outcome. *Journal of Pediatrics*, **116**, 862–7.
Bock, S. A. (1987). Prospective appraisal of complaints of adverse reactions to foods in children during the first 3 years of life. *Paediatrics*, **79**, 683–8.

Bock, S. A. & Atkins, F. M. (1990). Patterns of food hypersensitivity during sixteen years of double-blind placebo-controlled food challenges. *Journal of Pediatrics*, **117**, 561–7.

Boulton, P., Shields, J. G., Strobel, S., Levinsky, R. J. & Turner, M. W. (1988). Modulation of intestinal hypersensitivity in the rat by the anti-allergic drugs beclomethasone dipropionate and disodium cromoglycate. *Medical Science Research*, **16**, 811–12.

Cant, A. J., Bailes, J. A. & Marsden, R. A. (1985). Cow's milk, soya milk and goat's milk in a mother's diet causing eczema and diarrhoea in her breast fed infant. *Acta Paediatrica Scandinavica*, **74**, 467–8.

Cooper, E. S., Whyte, A. C. A., Finzi-Smith, J. S., MacDonald, T. T. (1992). Intestinal nematode infections in children: the pathophysiological price paid. *Parasitology*, **104**(Suppl.); 91–103.

Dreborg, S. (1989). Skin tests used in type I allergy testing (position paper of the Sub-Committee on skin tests of the European Academy of Allergy and Clinical Immunology (ed. D. S. Dreborg). *Allergy*, **44** (Suppl. 10), 1–59.

Esteban, M. M. (1992). Adverse food reactions in childhood: concept, importance and present problems. *Journal of Pediatrics*, **121**, S1–S3.

Fälth-Magnusson, K., Kjellman, N. I., Odelram, H., Sundqvist, T. & Magnusson, K. E. (1986). Gastrointestinal permeability in children with cows' milk allergy: effect of milk challenge and sodium cromoglycate as assessed with polyethyleneglycols (PEG 400 and PEG 1000). *Clinical Allergy*, **16**, 543–51.

Ferguson, A. (1987). Models of immunologically-driven small intestinal damage. In *Immunopathology of the Small Intestine*, ed. N. Marsh, pp. 225–252. Chichester: John Wiley and Sons.

Fiocchi, C. (1991). Production of inflammatory cytokines in inflammatory bowel disease. *Immunology Research*, **10**, 239–46.

Freier, S. & Berger, H. (1973). Disodium cromoglycate in gastrointestinal protein intolerance. *Lancet*, **i**, 913–15.

Gerrard, J. W. & Shenassa, M. (1983). Sensitization to substances in breast milk: recognition, management and significance. *Annals of Allergy*, 4738.

Grybowski, J. D. (1967). Gastrointestinal milk allergy in infants. *Paediatrics*, **40**, 354–62.

Halstensen, T. S., Mollnes, T. E. Garred, P., Fausa, O. & Brandtzaeg, P. (1990). Epithelial deposition of immunoglobulin G and activated complement (C3b and terminal complement complex) in ulcerative colitis. *Gastroenterology*, **98**, 1264–71.

Hattevig, G., Kjellman, B., Johansson, S. G. O. & Björkstén, B. (1984). Clinical symptoms and IgE responses to common food proteins in atopic and healthy children. *Clinical Allergy*, **1**, 551–9.

Høst, A. & Halken, S. (1990). A prospective study of cow milk allergy in Danish infants during the first 3 years of life. Clinical course in relation to clinical and immunological type of hypersensitivity reaction. *Allergy*, **45**, 587–96.

Høst, A., Husby, S. & Osterballe, O. (1988). A prospective study of cows' milk allergy in exclusively breast-fed infants. Incidence, pathogenetic role of early inadvertent exposure to cows' milk formula, and characterization of bovine milk protein in human milk. *Acta Paediatrica Scandinavica*, **77**, 663–70.

Husby, S. (1988). Dietary antigens: uptake and humoral immunity in man. *Acta Pathologica Microbiologica et Immunologica Scandinavica*, (Suppl. 1), 1–40.

Husby, S., Høst, A. & Hansen, L. G. (1991). Characterization of cow milk proteins in human milk: kinetics, size distribution, and possible relation to atopy. *Advances in Experimental and Medical Biology*, 310.

Jarrett, E. E. (1984). Perinatal influences on IgE responses. *Lancet*, **2**, 797–9.

Jenkins, H. R., Pincott, J. R., Soothill, J. F. & Milla, P. J. (1984). Cause of infantile colitis. *Archives of Diseases of Childhood*, **59**, 326–9.

Katz, A. J., Twarog, F. J., Zeiger, R. S. & Falchuk, Z. M. (1984). Milk-sensitive and eosinophilic gastroenterology: similar clinical features with contrasting mechanisms and clinical course. *Journal of Allergy and Clinical Immunology*, **174**, 72–8.

Kay, A. B. & Lessof, M. H. (1992). Royal College of Physicians' Report. Committee on Clinical Immunology and Allergy.

Kirkham, S. E., Bloch, K. J., Bloch, M. B., Perry, R. P., Walker, W. A. (1986). Immune complex-induced enteropathy in the rat. I. Clinical and histological features. *Digest of Disease Science*, **31**, 737–43.

Kjellman, N. I. M., Hattevig, G., Fälth-Magnusson, K. & Björkstén, B. (1989). Epidemiology of food allergy: with emphasis on the influence of maternal dietary restrictions during pregnancy and lactation on allergy in infancy. In *Food Intolerance in Infancy: Allergology, Immunology and Gastroenterology*, ed. R. N. Hamburger, pp. 105–114 (Carnation Nutrition Education Series; vol 1).

Knutson, T., Bengtsson, U., Dannaeus, A. *et al.* (1993). Intestinal reactivity in allergic and nonallergic patients: an approach to determine the complexity of the mucosal reaction. *Journal of Allergy and Clinical Immunology*, **91**, 553–9.

Kolmannskog, S., Florholmen, J., Flaegstad, T., Kildebo, S. & Haneberg, B. (1986). The excretion of IgE with feces from healthy individuals and from others with allergy and diseases affecting the intestinal tract. *International Archives in Allergy and Applied Immunology*, **79**, 357–64.

Kolmannskog, S., Jansson, S., Haggblom, L., Mentzing, L. O., Hvidsten, D. & Haneberg, B. (1991). Immunoglobulin E in the feces of children and adolescents from some tropical and subtropical countries. *International Archives in Allergy and Applied Immunology*, **95**, 316–21.

Kondo, N., Fukutomi, O., Agata, H. *et al.* (1993). The role of T lymphocytes in patients with food-sensitive atopic dermatitis. *Journal of Allergy and Clinical Immunology*, **91**, 658–68.

Lothe, L. & Lindberg, T. (1989). Cows' milk whey protein elicits symptoms of infantile colic in colicky formula-fed infants: a double-blind crossover study. *Pediatrics*, **83**, 262–6.

MacDonald, T. T. & Spencer, J. (1988). Evidence that activated mucosal T cells play a role in the pathogenesis of enteropathy in human small intestine. *Journal of Experimental Medicine*, **167**, 1341–9.

Miller, H. R. P., Woodbury, R. G., Huntley, J. F. & Newlands, G. F. G. (1983). Systemic release of mucosal mast cell protease in primed rats challenged with *Nippostrongylus brasiliensis*. *Immunology*, **49**, 471–9.

Mosman, T. R. & Coffman, R. L. (1989). Th1 and Th2 cells: different patterns of cytokine excretion lead to different functional properties. *Annual Review in Immunology*, **7**, 145–73.

Mowat, A. M. (1987). The regulation of immune responses to dietary antigens. *Immunology, Today*, **8**, 93–8.

Mowat, A. M., Borland, A. & Parrott, D. M. V. (1986). The delayed type hypersensitivity reaction in the small intestine. VII. Induction of the intestine phase of the murine graft versus host reaction by Lyt 2-T cells activated by I-A alloantigens. *Transplantation*, **41**, 192–8.

Pearce, F. L., Befus, A. D., Gauldie, J. & Bienenstock, J. (1982). Mucosal mast cells. II. Effects of anti-allergic compounds on histamine secretion by isolated intestinal mast cells. *Journal of Immunology*, **128**, 2481–6.

Peng, H. J., Turner, M. W. & Strobel, S. (1990). The generation of a 'tolerogen' after the ingestion of ovalbumin is time-dependent and unrelated to serum levels of immunoreactive antigen. *Clinical and Experimental Immunology*, **81**, 510–15.

Perdue, M. H., Chung, M. & Gall, D. G. (1984). Effect of intestinal anaphylaxis on gut function in the rat. *Gastroenterology*, **86**, 391–7.

Perdue, M. H., Forstner, J. F., Roomi, N. W. & Gall, D. G. (1984). Epithelial response to intestinal anaphylaxis in rats: goblet cell secretion and enterocyte damage. *American Journal of Physiology*, **247**, G632–7.

Perdue, M. H. & Gall, D. G. (1986). Rat jejunal mucosal response to histamine and anti-histamines *in vitro*. Comparison with antigen-induced changes during intestinal anaphylaxis. *Agents Actions*, **19** (1–2); 5–9.

Perdue, M. H., Masson, S., Wershil, B. K. & Galli, S. J. (1991). Role of mast cells in ion transport abnormalities associated with intestinal anaphylaxis. Correction of the diminished secretory response in genetically mast cell-deficient W/Wv mice by bone marrow transplantation. *Journal of Clinical Investigations*, **87**, 687–93.

Pike, M. G., Heddle, R. J., Boulton, P., Turner, M. W. & Atherton, D. J. (1986). Increased intestinal permeability in atopic eczema. *Journal of Investigative Dermatology*, **86**, 101–4.

Qin, S., Cobbold, S. P., Pope, H. *et al*. (1993). 'Infectious' transplantation tolerance. *Science*, **259**, 947–77.

Saalman, R., Carlsson, B., Fällström, S. P., Hanson, L. A. & Ahlstedt, S. (1991). Antibody dependent cell-mediated cytotoxicity to β-lactoglobulin coated cells with sera from children with cows' milk protein allergy. *Clinical and Experimental Immunology*, **85**, 446–52.

Sampson, H. A. (1993). Food antigen-induced lymphocyte proliferation in children with atopic dermatitis and food hypersensitivity. *Journal of Allergy and Clinical Immunology*, **91**, 549–51.

Sanderson, I., Walker, W. (1993). Uptake and transport of macromolecules by the intestine: possible role in clinical disorders (an update). *Gastroenterology*, **104**, 622–39.

Sogn, D. (1986). Medications and their use in the treatment of adverse reaction to foods. *Journal of Allergy and Clinical Immunology*, **78**, 238–43.

Strobel, S. (1990). Immunologically mediated damage to the intestinal mucosa. *Acta Paediatrica Scandinavica*, **356**, S46–S57.

Strobel, S. (1993). Epidemiology of food sensitivity in childhood – with special reference to cows' milk allergy in infancy. In *Epidemiology of Clinical Allergy*, ed. M. L. Burr, pp. 119–130. (Hanson LÅ, Shakib F, ed. Monographs in allergy; vol 31).

Strobel, S., Mowat, A. M. & Ferguson, A. (1985). Prevention of oral tolerance induction to ovalbumin and enhanced antigen presentation during a graft-versus-host reaction in mice. *Immunology*, **56**, 57–64.

Strobel, S. & Ferguson, A. (1986). Modulation of intestinal and systemic immune responses to a fed protein antigen, in mice. *Gut*, **27**, 829–37.

Turner, M. W., Barnet, G. & Strobel, S. (1990). Mucosal mast cell activation patterns in the rat following repeated feeding of antigen. *Clinical and Experimental Allergy*, **20**, 421–7.

Walker, W. A. (1981). Intestinal transport of macromolecules. In *Physiology of the Gastrointestinal Tract*, ed. L. R. Johnson, J. Christensen & M. L. Grossman, pp. 1271–1289. vol 61. New York: Raven Press.

Walker, W. A. (1987). Role of mucosal barrier in antigen handling by the gut. In *Food Allergy and Intolerance*, ed. J. Brostoff & Challacombe, S. 1st edn. pp. 209–222. London: Baillière Tindall.

Walker-Smith, J. A. (1988). *Diseases of the Small Intestine in Childhood*. 3rd ed. London: Butterworths.

Walker-Smith, J. A. (1992). Immunology of gastrointestinal food allergy in infancy and early childhood. In *Immunology of Gastrointestinal Disease*, ed. T. T. MacDonald, pp. 61–74. Dordrecht: Kluwer Academic. (*Immunology and Medicine*, ed. K. Whaley vol 19).

Walker-Smith, J. A., Harrison, M., Kilby, A. Phillips, A. & France, N. E. (1978). Cows' milk sensitive enteropathy. *Archive of Diseases of Childhood*, **53**, 375–82.

Wershil, B. K. & Walker, W. A. (1992). The mucosal barrier, IgE-mediated gastrointestinal events, and eosinophilic gastroenteritis. *Gastroenterology Clinics of North America*, **21**, 387–404.

–8–
Gastrointestinal and liver involvement in primary immunodeficiency

H. C. GOOI

The gastrointestinal tract (GIT) is a major component of the immune system. The embryonic gut is important in the development of both humoral and cellular immunity. The thymus and the bursa of Fabricius are involved in T and B lymphocyte differentiation and maturation, respectively. The thymus is derived from the third and fourth pharyngeal pouch. In avian species the bursa is a sac-like structure arising from the cloaca. The human equivalent of the bursa has not been identified but the gut associated lymphoid tissue has been suggested to play a similar role.

The lining of the GIT is an important body surface which interacts with numerous substances including micro-organisms and dietary antigens. Not only are harmful agents excluded by non-immunological mechanisms and by innate immunity, these substances are processed by the adaptive immune mechanisms which enable the body to recognise and to respond to them. Of the cardiac output, 10% goes to the GIT and the portal venous system returns about 20% of the cardiac output via the liver. Together with the lymphatics there is a sizeable traffic of immune cells circulating through the GIT. It is estimated that these cells are capable of synthesising a few grams of immunoglobulins daily.

The GIT is involved in many ways in primary immunodeficiency diseases (PID). It may be the site of presenting symptoms and signs; GIT pathology may complicate PID and 20–25% of patients with common variable immunodeficiency (CVI) have gastrointestinal involvement. In contrast, in X-linked agammaglobulinaemia (XLA) gastrointestinal disease is uncommon. In severe, combined immunodeficiency (SCID), diarrhoea and malabsorption is a characteristic feature. GIT involvement in PID is therefore dependent on the immune defect but the manner in which these defects lead to gastrointestinal pathology is not clearly understood.

This chapter will discuss gastrointestinal abnormalities on the basis of antibody, cell-mediated, combined, neutrophil and complement deficiency.

A detailed classification of primary immunodeficiency disease has recently been published (Report of a WHO Scientific Group, 1991).

Antibody deficiency syndromes

Upper gastrointestinal tract

The mouth and oesophagus are not commonly involved in antibody deficiency syndromes. Mouth ulcers and fungal infection especially candida are more likely to be associated with neutropenia. Antibody deficient patients need frequent and long-term antibiotics and oral candidiasis unfortunately is a common side-effect.

Stomach

Pernicious anaemia-like syndrome

A pernicious anaemia-like syndrome often complicates CVI, in contrast to XLA where there is no increased incidence of pernicious anaemia (PA). However, this syndrome may occur in IgA deficiency (Spector, 1974).

This syndrome was first reported by Twomey et al., in 1969, who described ten patients with achlorhydria, atrophic gastritis, absence of intrinsic factor and antibodies to gastric parietal cells and intrinsic factor and malabsorption of vitamin B12. This syndrome is rare in children and occurs more frequently in patients who have been treated for longer periods of time. Up to 50% of patients with long standing CVI have achlorhydria even after pentagastrin stimulation but only about half of these have associated reduction of intrinsic factor level (Asherson & Webster, 1980). This complication of antibody deficiency can be distinguished from classical pernicious anaemia by its earlier onset, absent autoantibodies, vitamin B12 malabsorption in the presence of normal gastrin level and atrophic gastritis without a plasma cell infiltrate.

The pathogenesis of this syndrome is not known. It has been suggested that gastric atrophy is secondary to malabsorption and infection in particular *Giardia lamblia*. However, there was no evidence of malabsorption and giardiasis in the 28 patients studied by Asherson and Webster (1980).

The occurrence of a pernicious anaemia-like complication in primary antibody deficiency suggests that cellular immune mechanisms are involved in the pathogenesis of PA. Peripheral blood lymphocyte reactivity, as shown by *in vitro* lymphocyte proliferation and production of macrophage inhibitory factor (MIF), when these are cultured with hog or human intrinsic factor, has been reported in hypogammaglobulinaemic patients (Fixa *et al.*, 1972; Gelfand *et al.*, 1972) and in PA (Whittingham *et al.*, 1975). Though antibodies to gastric parietal cells and intrinsic factor are classically associated with PA and there is an increased incidence of other antibodies, it is not clear whether these antibodies are primary or secondary phenomena.

Malignancy

There is a higher incidence of carcinoma of the stomach in CVI. There were four cases of gastric carcinoma in a series of 50 patients reviewed by Hermans, Diaz-Buxo and Stobo (1976). These occurred 10–33 years after the onset of immunodeficiency. More recently in an analysis of 220 CVI patients in the United Kingdom diagnosed in the years between 1957 and 1975 and followed-up to 1981, there were seven cases of stomach cancer (Kinlen *et al.*, 1985). This is a 47 fold increased incidence and is about five times more frequent than in PA, where the excess incidence is less than tenfold (Mosbech & Videbaek, 1950; Blackburn *et al.*, 1968). In both diseases there is gastric achlorhydria and the increased occurrence of gastric cancer is probably related to this. In CVI there is added immune deficit and these two factors in combination are more important, as the immunosuppressed patients are at no greater risk of gastric cancer (Hanto *et al.*, 1981).

Small and large intestine

Acute or recurrent diarrhoea and malabsorption occurs in over 50% of patients with CVI (Hermans *et al.*, 1976). They may occur in XLA but are much less common. Protracted diarrhoea or repeated acute diarrhoea were noted in 30 out of 64 patients with IgG subclass immunodeficiency studied by Aucouturier *et al.* (1989). They in addition noted that diarrhoea was about ten times more common in those with IgG3 rather than IgG2 deficient patients.

Giardiasis

Earlier reports identified *Giardia lamblia* as the commonest cause of malabsorption. Ament, Ochs and Davis (1973), in their study of 39 patients with primary immunodeficiency diseases, reported 11 patients (ten CVI and one XLA) with giardiasis. Nine patients had gastrointestinal symptoms and in eight, including the XLA patient, *Giardia* was identified. However, *Giardia* may be present in asymptomatic patients, three out of 19 CVI patients in this series. The incidence of giardiasis in CVI in the United Kingdom appears to be lower than that in the United States (Asherson & Webster, 1980). However, in a more recent study of 103 CVI patients in the

United States, giardiasis was not found to be the cause of malabsorption in nine symptomatic patients (Cunningham-Rundles, 1989).

The diagnosis can readily be made by the identification of *Giardia lamblia* in the stools. Negative stools examination does not exclude the diagnosis. In the study mentioned above, the parasite was demonstrated in the stools in only 30% of the cases. The authors recommended examination of Giemsa-stained smears made from intestinal mucus. Histological examination of intestinal biopsies confirmed the diagnosis in all cases. The mucosal involvement is patchy and the histological changes seen varies in severity, from mildly abnormal villus architecture, to total villus atrophy. These changes are reversible with eradication of *Giardia*.

Giardiasis in antibody deficiency syndromes is readily treated with metronidazole. Alternative treatments are tinidazole and mepacrine.

Cryptosporidiosis

Cryptosporidial infection in man was first reported by Nime *et al.* (1976). Subsequent reports indicate that the immunocompromised hosts are at greater risk. Lasser, Lewin and Ryning (1979), reported cryptosporidiosis in an 8 year-old boy with antibody deficiency who did not respond to treatment and when last reported four years later had developed severe malabsorption. Sloper *et al.* (1982), reported a boy with immunoglobulin deficiency with increased IgM, who contracted the parasite when aged 6 years, developed chronic diarrhoea and severe malabsorption despite treatment and succumbed 6 years later. This protozoal parasite is difficult to eradicate and there does not appear to be an effective drug available. However, gamma interferon appears to be a promising agent. A nine year-old boy with CVI under the care of the author developed cryptosporidial diarrhoea and this has not been cured with numerous forms of treatment including oral bovine IgA, raised against Cryptosporidia. However, he has responded to gamma interferon at a dose of 1.5 μg/kg body weight thrice weekly. His stools are now clear of the parasite but diarrhoea of lesser severity persists. It is planned to continue treatment for some time, following which, endoscopy and biopsy will be repeated (see Note added in proof).

Nodular lymphoid hyperplasia

The presence of numerous polyps in the stomach and duodenum, due to lymphoid hyperplasia in a 14 year-old boy with antibody deficiency at autopsy, was first reported by Firkin and Blackburn (1958). The term nodular lymphoid hyperplasia (NLH) was used by Hermans *et al.* (1966), who described eight patients with a syndrome which was designated dysgammaglobulinaemia, associated with nodular lymphoid hyperplasia of the small intestine. NLH may occur in up to 60% of patients with CVI (Ross & Asquith, 1979). However, NLH has been reported in children without antibody deficiency (Fieber & Schaefer, 1966; Capitano & Kirkpatrick, 1970). NLH is not necessarily associated with diarrhoea, malabsorption or giardiasis (Asherson & Webster, 1980), as originally reported by Hermans *et al.* (1966).

The nodules are characteristically 1–5 mm in size, occurring in the small intestine but may be found in the stomach and colon. They appear nodular or polypoid on endoscopy and as filling defects on barium studies. Microscopic examination shows the nodules to be in the lamina propia and consisting of lymphoid follicles, with large germinal centres and prominent mitotic figures and the villi of the overlying mucosa are effaced (Hermans *et al.*, 1966). The relationship between NLH and malignancy is not clear. Hermans *et al.* (1966) reported an increased tendency to the development of GI malignancy in association with NLH. However, no malignancy occurred in ten patients followed up by Asherson and Webster (1980) over 5 years. The author has a patient with NLH for 20 years before the diagnosis of CVI was made and the lesions were benign. NLH may not regress following replacement immunoglobulin therapy.

Bacterial overgrowth and bile salts

There is aerobic and anaerobic bacterial overgrowth in the upper small intestine of patients with CVI (Ament *et al.*, 1973), but the bacterial counts do not reach the levels found in the blind-loop syndrome. Treatment does not alter the bacterial flora. The bacterial overgrowth does not appear to correlate with malabsorption or the GI pathology.

Some of the bacteria, isolated from the upper small intestine of these patients, have the capability to deconjugate bile salts but unconjugated bile salts were not found in the patients studied by Ament, *et al.* (1973). It is not likely that unconjugated bile salts are a contributory factor to the malabsorption seen in patients with antibody deficiency.

Other conditions

Patients with antibody deficiency and malabsorption have been reported to respond to gluten withdrawal (Hughes *et al.*, 1971). The diagnosis of coeliac disease in most instances is unconfirmed, as the patients are not rechallenged with gluten. However, Asherson and Webster (1980) reported a patient who improved clinically following gluten withdrawal and repeat jejunal biopsy showed partial normalisation of villus architecture. Following the re-introduction of gluten, this patient relapsed and this was confirmed by repeat jejunal biopsy.

Crypt abscesses consistent with colitis were noted in the rectal biopsies of six of eight XLA patients and three of 19 CVI patients but these patients were asymptomatic (Ament *et al.*, 1973). Other series have not reported this complication (Hermans *et al.*, 1976, Cunningham-Rundles, 1989).

Liver and gall-bladder disease

In the series of 100 patients with CVI reviewed by Cunningham-Rundles (1989), 13 patients developed hepatitis. Seven patients are believed to have acquired non-A, non-B hepatitis from plasma replacement therapy and two from intravenous immunoglobulin (IVIg], which at that time was still a trial preparation. Five went on to develop chronic hepatitis and another two died of liver failure. Two patients had hepatitis B and both recovered. Twelve patients in a therapeutic IVIg trial, developed non-A, non-B hepatitis (Lever *et al.*, 1984). Most have progressed to chronic liver disease and some have died of this complication (Webster A.D.B. personal communication). Non-A, non-B hepatitis is a serious and sometimes fatal disease, in antibody-deficient patients. However, it must be emphasised that the later generations of IVIg preparations are much safer and have been prepared from plasma that has been more thoroughly screened for pathogens and have added anti-viral treatment during preparation.

Widespread, non-caseating granulomata involving especially the lungs, spleen, lymph nodes and liver, have been observed in common variable immunodeficiency (Rosen & Janeway, 1966). Some of these patients have clinical features and course compatible with sarcoidosis and have been diagnosed as sarcoidosis, with hypogammaglobulinaemia (Bronsky & Dunn, 1965; Davis, Eidelman and Loop, 1970). The enlargement of the spleen, lymph nodes and liver may resolve with replacement immunoglobulin therapy. However, the persistence of the granuloma in the liver, may account for persisting altered liver function. Two patients under the care of the author with CVI, hepatosplenomegaly and abnormal liver function tests but negative HBSAg and HCV RNA (by polymerase chain reaction), had granulomatous hepatitis on liver biopsy.

Intrahepatic sclerosing cholangitis in a child with IgA and IgM deficiency, was first reported by Record *et al.* (1973). Two other family members had died of Gram negative septicaemia and liver histology showed similar lesions. There have been further case reports in immunodeficient patients with sclerosing cholangitis, which may also occur in association with gallstones, ulcerative colitis and AIDS (HIV) with cryptosporidiosis. In all these examples, there has been no clinical evidence of cholangitis but asymptomatic infection cannot be ruled out. It is significant that Hermans *et al.* (1976) reported a 24% prevalence of cholelithiasis in his study of 50 patients with CVI but only one was symptomatic.

Severe combined immunodeficiency

Chronic diarrhoea, malabsorption and infection of the gut by rotavirus and other enteroviruses, coliforms and *Candida*, are characteristic features of severe combined immunodeficiency (SCID). These neonates or young infants are often severely ill and invasive investigations are as a result limited. However, the jejunal biopsies from three SCID infants showed villus atrophy and PAS positive vacuolated macrophages, in the lamina propia (Horowitz *et al.*, 1974). Proctoscopy showed oedematous friable mucosa and crypt abscesses were seen in the rectal biopsies.

Chronic granulomatous disease

Gastrointestinal involvement in chronic granulomatous disease (CGD), occurred in four out of nine patients reported by Ament, Ochs & Davis (1973). This included steatorrhoea, malabsorption and perianal fistula. Small intestinal biopsies showed the presence of vacuolated histiocytes, that were PAS and Sudan black positive.

Granulomata may occur in the intestinal wall and cause gastrointestinal obstruction (Kumararatne, personal communication).

Complement deficiency

GIT involvement is not a feature in complement deficiency. However, vomiting and abdominal pain may occur in hereditary angioedema (C1 esterase inhibitor deficiency). It may present as an acute abdomen and the patient operated on by the unwary.

Acknowledgement

I would like to thank Mrs J.I. Hagger for her help in the preparation of this manuscript.

Note added in proof

This boy unfortunately has relapsed.

References

Ament, M. E. & Ochs, H. D. (1973). Gastrointestinal manifestations of chronic granulomatous disease. *New England Journal of Medicine*, **288**, 382–7.

Ament, M. E., Ochs, H. D. & Davis, S. D. (1973). Structure and function of the gastrointestinal tract in Primary Immunodeficiency Syndromes. A study of 39 patients. *Medicine*, **52**, 227–47.

Asherson, G. L. & Webster, A. D. B. (1980). In *Diagnosis and Treatment of Immunodeficiency Diseases*, 1st edn, ed. G. L. Asherson & A. D. B. Webster, pp. 62–63. Oxford: Blackwell Scientific Publications.

Aucouturier, P., Lacombe, C., Bremard, C., Lebranchu, Y., Seligmann, M., Griscelli, C. & Preud'homme, J. L. (1989). Serum IgG subclass levels in patients with primary immunodeficiency syndromes or abnormal susceptibility to infections. *Clinical Immunology and Immunopathology*, **51**, 22–37.

Blackburn, E. K., Callender, S. T., Dacie, J. V. *et al.* (1968). Possible association between pernicious anaemia and leukaemia: a prospective study of 1625 patients with a note on the very high incidence of stomach cancer. *International Journal of Cancer*, **3**, 163–70.

Bronsky, D. & Dunn, Y. O. L. (1965). Sarcoidosis with hypogammaglobulinaemia. *American Journal of Medical Sciences*, **250**, 11–18.

Capitano, M. A. & Kirkpatrick J. A. (1970). Lymphoid hyperplasia of the colon in children. *Radiology*, **94**, 323–7.

Cunningham-Rundles, C. (1989). Clinical and immunologic analyses of 103 patients with common variable immunodeficiency. *Journal of Clinical Immunology*, **9**, 22–33.

Davis, S. D., Eidelman, S. & Loop, J. W. (1970). Nodular lymphoid hyperplasia of the small intestine and sarcoidosis. *Archives of Internal Medicine*, **126**, 668–72.

Fieber, S. S. & Schaefer, H. J. (1966). Lymphoid hyperplasia of the terminal ileum – a clinical entity? *Gastroenterology*, **50**, 83–98.

Firkin, B. G. & Blackburn, C. R. B. (1958). Congenital and acquired agammaglobulinaemia. *Quarterly Journal of Medicine*, **27**, 187–205.

Fixa, B., Thiele, H. G., Komárkova, O. & Nožička, Z. (1972). Gastric autoantibodies and cell mediated immunity in pernicious anaemia – a comparative study. *Scandinavian Journal of Gastroenterology*, **8**, 237–40.

Gelfand, E. W., Berkel, A. I., Godwin, H. A., Rocklin, R. E., David, J. R., Rosen, F. S. (1972). Pernicious anaemia, hypogammaglobulinaemia and altered lymphocyte reactivity. *Clinical and Experimental Immunology*, **11**, 187–99.

Hanto, D. W., Frizzeria, G., Purtilo, D. T. *et al.* (1981). Clinical spectrum of lymphoproliferative disorders in renal transplant recipients and evidence for the role of Epstein–Barr virus. *Cancer Research*, **41**, 4253–61.

Hermans, P. E., Diaz-Buxo, J. A. & Stobo, J. D. (1976). Idiopathic late-onset immunoglobulin deficiency. Clinical observations in 50 patients. *American Journal of Medicine*, **61**, 221–37.

Hermans, P. E., Huizenga, K. A., Hoffman, H. N., Brown, A. L. & Markowitz, H. (1966). Dysgammaglobulinaemia associated with nodular lymphoid hyperplasia of the small intestine. *American Journal of Medicine*, **40**, 78–89.

Horowitz, S., Lorenzsonn, V. W., Olsen, W. A., Albrecht, R. & Hong, R. (1974). Small intestine disease in T-cell deficiency. *Journal of Paediatric*, **85**, 457–62.

Hughes, W. S., Cerda, J. J., Holtzapple, P. & Brooks, F. P. (1971). Primary hypogammaglobulinaemia and malabsorption. *Annals of Internal Medicine*, **74**, 903–10.

Kinlen, L. J., Webster, A. D. B., Bird, A. G. *et al.* (1985). Prospective study of cancer in patients with hypogammaglobulinaemia. *Lancet*, **i**, 263–6.

Lasser, K. H., Lewin, K. J. & Ryning, F. W. (1979). Cryptosporidial enteritis in a patient with congenital hypogammaglobulinaemia. *Human Pathology*, **10**, 234–40.

Lever, A. M. L., Webster, A. D. B., Brown, D. & Thomas, H. C. (1984). Non-A, non-B hepatitis occurring in agammaglobulinaemic patients after intravenous immunoglobulin. *Lancet*, **ii**, 1062–4.

Mosbech, J. & Videbaek, A. (1950). Mortality from and risk of gastric carcinoma among patients with pernicious anaemia. *British Medical Journal*, **ii**, 390–4.

Nime, F. A., Burek, J. D., Page, D. L., Holscher, M. A. & Yardley, J. H. (1976). Acute enterocolitis in a human being infected with the protozoan Cryptosporidium. *Gastroenterology*, **70**, 592–6.

Record, C. O., Eddleston, A. L. W. F., Shilkin, K. B. & Williams, R. (1973). Intrahepatic sclerosing cholangitis associated with a familial immunodeficiency syndrome. *Lancet*, **ii**, 18–20.

Report of a WHO Scientific Group (1991). Primary Immunodeficiency Diseases. *Immunodeficiency Review*, **3**, 195–236.

Rosen, F. S. & Janeway, C. A. (1966). The gamma globulins III. The antibody deficiency syndromes. *New England Journal of Medicine*, **275**, 709–15.

Ross, I. N. & Asquith, P. (1979). Primary immune deficiency. In *Immunology of the Gastrointestinal Tract*, 1st edn, ed. P. Asquith, pp. 152–182, Edinburgh, Churchill-Livingstone.

Sloper, K. S., Dourmashkin, R. R., Bird, R. B., Slavin, G. & Webster, A. D. B. (1982). Chronic malabsorption due to cryptosporidiosis in a child with immunoglobulin deficiency. *Gut*, **23**, 80–2.

Spector, J. I. (1974). Juvenile achlorhydric pernicious anaemia with IgA deficiency. *Journal of the American Medical Association*, **228**, 334–6.

Twomey, J. J., Jordan, P. H., Jarrold, T., Trubowitz, S., Ritz, N. D. & Conn, H. O. (1969). The syndrome of immunoglobulin deficiency and pernicious anaemia. *American Journal of Medicine*, **47**, 340–50.

Whittingham, S., Youngchaiyud, U., Mackay, I. R., Buckley, J. D. & Morris, P. J. (1975). Thyrogastric autoimmune disease. Studies on the cell mediated immune system and histocompatibility antigens. *Clinical and Experimental Immunology*, **19**, 289–99.

–9–
Secondary immunodeficiency – the acquired immunodeficiency syndrome (AIDS)

JACQUELINE M. PARKIN

Introduction

Much of the current knowledge of the features of secondary immunodeficiency has been learnt from patients with HIV infection and AIDS. This is a reflection of both the scale of this epidemic and the progressive and severe nature of the immune destruction. The result is that HIV infection has become the most common significant immunodeficiency that clinicians are likely to encounter. The gastrointestinal tract is intimately involved in the host–HIV relationship; not only is it a major site of presentation of secondary opportunist infections and tumours, but it is also a primary target for HIV through direct infection of the gastrointestinal and immunological cells within the tract. In addition, the gut is the site of viral entry in acute HIV infection occurring through anal intercourse and vaccine programmes aimed at stimulating mucosal immunity are now viewed as a major goal. This chapter will discuss the immunopathogenic mechanisms of HIV infection, with specific reference to the interactions with the gastrointestinal tract. The concepts of host–pathogen relationships that have been developed are applicable to the many other secondary immunodeficiency states (Table 9.1).

The human immunodeficiency virus (HIV) and AIDS–an overview

It is estimated that 14 million people worldwide are currently HIV infected, and there were 2.5 million documented AIDS cases in early 1993 (WHO 1993). In every country where cases are documented (developed or developing), the annual incidence continues to rise. AIDS affects mainly young people, the virus being transmitted efficiently by sexual intercourse, transplacentally and through the sharing of equipment used for injecting drugs. The result is a disease with great economic, public health, and emotional

Table 9.1. *Causes of secondary immunodeficiency*

Agent	Immunodeficiency caused
Viral	
HIV 1 and 2	Mainly cell-mediated immune deficiency
	Minor dysgammaglobulinaemia, IgG2
	deficiency
Measles	Transient cell-mediated defect
Rubella	Transient cell-mediated defect
EBV	Hypogammaglobulinaemia
Unknown	Common variable
	hypogammaglobulinaemia
Tumours	
HTLV-1 ATCL[a]	Cell-mediated deficiency
Lymphoma	Cell-mediated deficiency
Thymoma	Cell-mediated deficiency
CLL[b]	Dysgammaglobulinaemia
Multiple myeloma	Dysgammaglobulinaemia
Auto-immune diseases	
Sjogren's	Dysgammaglobulinaemia
	IgG2/IgA deficiency
Protein-calorie malnutrition	Cell-mediated deficiency
Protein-losing states	
Nephrotic syndrome	Hypogammaglobulinaemia
Enteropathy	Hypogammaglobulinaemia
Menetrière's disease	Hypogammaglobulinaemia
Drugs	
Corticosteroids	Lymphopenia, decreases cell-mediated
	immunity
	Impaired neutrophil adhesion
Cytotoxics	Neutropenia
Carbamazepine	Neutropenia
Lithium	Neutropenia
Sulphasalazine	Neutropenia
Phenytoin	IgA deficiency
Post bone marrow transplant	
Early	Neutropenia
Late	Cell-mediated deficiency, decreased CD4
	count
	Antibody
Immune complex	Hypocomplementaemia
disease	(consumption)
Liver disease	Hypocomplementaemia
	(reduced production of complement)

[a]ATCL: Adult T cell leukaemia/lymphoma.
[b]CLL: Chronic lymphocytic leukaemia.

impact. These features illustrate why such importance has been placed on research into the pathogenesis and treatment of this condition. The outcome has been an explosion of knowledge of the virology of human and animal retroviruses, as well as insight into the aetiology and treatment of the opportunist infections and tumours that complicate the immunodeficiency. Although the profound clinical and laboratory immunological defects were the features that brought the syndrome of AIDS to attention in 1981 (Gottlieb, Schroff & Schanker, 1981) (Friedman-Kein, Laubenstein & Rubinstein, 1982), the discovery of HIV in 1983 (Barre-Sinoussi, Chermann & Rey 1983) (Gallo, Salahuddin & Popovic, 1984) meant that much of the early research effort focused on the effects of this retrovirus and in the development of specific anti-HIV agents. However, with time, doubts were raised as to whether the direct cytopathic effects of HIV were the sole cause of the cell-mediated immune destruction. It is now considered likely that other mechanisms, such as those due to indirect effects of HIV or its products and immunologically mediated 'auto-immune reactions', also have a role. Thus, the balance of research and therapy, has swung back towards the immunological side of the equation. In order to define the main players in the story, the chapter will start with an overview of the virology of the human immunodeficiency viruses and the host response to these infections.

The virology of human immunodeficiency viruses

Two types of HIV have been described. HIV-1 is the virus found in the vast majority of infected individuals from Europe, Central Africa, Asia, America and Australia. HIV-2 was identified in 1986 (Clavel, *et al.*, 1986*a*), and is endemic in some West African countries, particularly Guinea-Bissau, Cape Verde islands, the Ivory Coast and Senegal (Guenno, Jean & Peghini, 1987; Clavel, 1989). The genomic organisation and core proteins of these two viruses are very similar, the major variation being in the envelope proteins (Clavel, *et al.*, 1986*b*) (Marlink, Ricard & M'Boup 1988). The clinical presentation is indistinguishable (Clavel *et al.*, 1987) (Gody, Ouattara & The 1988), although HIV-2 does appear less pathogenic, both in tissue culture (Evans, Moreau & Odehouri, 1988) (Kong, Lee & Kappes, 1988) and showing slower progression to AIDS (Pepin *et al.*, 1991). The bulk of research has focused on HIV-1, therefore only when differences have been found, will HIV-2 be specifically discussed.

HIV is a retrovirus, so called because it is an RNA virus that transcribes to form a DNA copy, which is the reverse process to normal cellular gene transcription. This is achieved by a virally encoded DNA polymerase, called reverse transcriptase, which initiates the transcription helped by RNAse H, both enzymes being carried within mature virions. The viral genome has three principal genes *env, gag* and *pol*, coding for the precursor envelope protein (gp160 which comprises the envelope gp120, and transmembrane portion, gp41), core proteins (p24, p17 and p15) and the polymerase (reverse transcriptase), protease and endonuclease. Other genes code for regulatory factors of viral replication, tat (trans acting transcriptional), rev (response element), tar, RRE, nef (negative factor), vif (virion infectivity factor), vpr and vpu (Wong-Staal 1989) (Luciw & Shacklett 1993). Many of these gene products are targets for anti-HIV agents; reverse transcriptase inhibitors such as the nucleoside analogues, zidovudine (azidothymidine, AZT), di-deoxyinosine (ddI) and di-deoxy cytidine (ddC), are currently in use and protease and tat inhibitors are into clinical trials. Gene therapy and 'intracellular immunisation' with transdominant proteins, anti-sense elements that can unravel the secondary structure as well as agents to cleave viral RNA within the cell, are also being developed (Johnston & Hoth 1993).

Mechanism of cellular infection by HIV and tissue tropism

HIV-1 infection occurs by the binding of the virus to its specific cellular receptor, the CD4 molecule (Dalgleish, Beverley & Clapham, 1984) (Klatzmann, Champagne & Chameret 1984). This occurs through the gp120 envelope protein (McDougal, Kennedy & Sligh, 1986). This is followed by fusion of the viral envelope and cell membrane and release of HIV into the cytoplasm. The fusion process is dependent on the transmembrane molecule gp41, as mutants lacking this protein bind cells but do not infect (for review see Eales & Parkin 1988). The specific gp120-CD4 interaction defines the cells that are susceptible to infection and therefore the main targets of HIV disease (Maddon, Dalgleish & McDougal 1986). These are predominantly cells of the immune system, CD4+ 'helper' lymphocytes, monocytes, macrophages (Ho, Rota & Hirsh 1986) (Salahuddin, Rose & Groopman 1986) and other antigen-presenting cells such as Langerhan's cells of the skin (Kirkpatrick, Davis & Horsburgh 1984) (Tschachler, Groh & Popovic 1987) and follicular dendritic cells (Armstrong & Horne 1984; Tenner-Racz *et al.*, 1986) as well as the microglia of the central nervous system (Koenig, Gendelman & Orenstein, 1986) (Wiley *et al.*, 1986) (Funke *et al.*, 1987) (Table 9.2(*a*)). CD4–ve cells, including cells of the gastrointestinal tract (Nelson *et al.*, 1988), can also be infected by HIV, through putative second receptors that have not been fully defined (Table 9.2(*b*); Cheng-Mayer 1990). Alternatively, infection of some cells may occur through interaction of opsonised viral particles, as complement and specific antibody enhance infectivity of HIV in some assay systems, through phagocytosis or pinocytosis (Reisinger, Vogbtseder & Berzow 1990; Robinson, Montefiori &

Table 9.2. *Cells infectable by HIV*

a) CD4+ve cells	
Immune system	T-helper lymphocytes
	Monocytes/macrophages
	Dendritic cells
Brain	Microglia
Skin	Langerhan's cells
Gastrointestinal tract	Human colorectal cells*
Liver	Kuppfer cells*
b) CD4−ve cells	
Immune System	CD8 lymphocytes
	B-lymphocytes*
Brain	Glial cells
	Astrocytes
	Human neuroblastoma*
	Retina cells
Lung	Fibroblasts
Kidney	Epithelial cells
Gastrointestinal tract	Columnar and epithelial cells
	Enterochromaffin cells
Liver	Human hepatoma*
Bone marrow	Stem cells

*Infectable *in vitro*.
Adapted from Cheng-Mayer, 1990.

Mitchell, 1988). However, the ability of HIV-1 to infect CD4−ve targets is much lower, and the level of viral replication very slow (up to 100-fold less productive). HIV-2 infects both CD4+ve and CD4−ve cells with equivalent efficacy, the non-CD4 receptor is unknown.

The p17 matrix protein is involved in the transfer of the virus through the nuclear membrane. Within the cell, reverse transcription of viral RNA occurs using cellular nucleotides and reverse transcriptase, to form ssDNA. This is separated from the RNA template by RNAseH and further transcription occurs to form dsDNA. The dsDNA is integrated randomly into the host genetic material by the virally encoded integrase. The integration is dependent on cell activation. Quiescent lymphocytes harbour the virus in mainly an unintegrated form in the cytoplasm; on lymphocyte activation, integration occurs. Once integrated, further transcription of viral genes occurs to form mRNA for the regulatory and structural proteins, as well as genomic RNA for the new viral particles. These assemble in the cytoplasm and at the cellular membrane, helped by the p7 matrix protein. The virus buds through the cell membrane which forms the envelope, therefore containing both viral and host cell elements. The protease enzyme is important in the maturation of the virions. If this is inhibited, defective, non-infectious particles are produced. This process of replication, like integration, is markedly accelerated by activation of the cell, possibly through the direct activation of transcription elements by cytokines (Koyanagi *et al.*, 1988) (Barillari *et al.*, 1992). Therefore, activation events, such as antigenic challenge during intercurrent infections and possibly during the allogeneic challenge of pregnancy, may enhance HIV activity. Other cofactors shown to enhance viral replication *in vitro* are, HSV, HHV-6, CMV, HTLV-1 and mycoplasma. In a mouse model, UV light activates HIV *in vivo* (Wallace & Lasker, 1992). Whether these have clinical implications is uncertain, as it would be expected that HIV-infected individuals having differing rates of co-factor exposure, would express different rates of disease progression. This is not the case, progression to AIDS with time shows a remarkably similar profile in all adult risk groups, whatever the risk factor for HIV-infection or geographical location. The only factor that has been consistently shown to enhance progression rates (outside of paediatric cases) is increasing age (Weiss, 1993).

Cytopathic effects of HIV

HIV isolates are commonly highly cytopathic in cell culture and these observations are used to postulate a role for direct cell damage, in the pathogenesis of the immune deficiency of AIDS. However, there are several factors that need to be taken into account when viewing this evidence. The reverse transcriptase of HIV has no proof-reading facility and there is a high rate of inaccurate transcriptions, (about 1 in 100). This means that virus mutation is common and there is great variability, not only between isolates from different individuals, but also within a single individual (the mutations occur predominantly at hypervariable regions of the envelope protein, gp120 and may be an important mechanism in immune escape). As a result, near-patient isolates, that is strains which are not laboratory adapted, due to multiple passages through cell culture, can show very different characteristics (phenotypes). In general, lymphocytotrophic variants are cytopathic (Gallo *et al.*, 1984) (Hoxie *et al.*, 1986), causing syncytium formation (due to fusion of infected and uninfected CD4+ve cells by gp120, expressed on the surface of infected cells) and eventual cell death by lysis. Such syncytium inducing (SI) phenotypes, are associated with rapidly replicating strains and rapid disease progression (Roos *et al.*, 1992). Monocytotrophic viruses are generally non-syncytium inducing (NSI) and have little or no cytopathic effects *in vitro*. It has been postulated that whilst the lymphocytotrophic viruses are important in causing loss of CD4-lymphocytes as a result of the direct cytopathogenicity, the monocytotrophic viruses are important 'factories' being productively infected, but not destroyed. This may be relevant in the central nervous system, where local production of high levels of soluble viral proteins which have neurotoxic effects, would be damaging. However, there is much variation in these findings. HIV-2 is usually less cytopathic in *in vitro* cultures, but aggressive isolates that rapidly cause cell death have been recognised. In addition, the isolates cultured from the peripheral blood of patients may change back and forth, usually from NSI to SI with disease progression, but also in the opposite direction (personal observation). It is likely that most HIV-positive individuals have a mixture of phenotypes and that it is the predominant, or most rapidly replicating one that is picked up in the cell culture. The breeding of severe combined immunodeficiency (SCID) mice, that can be reconstituted with human immunological elements 'SCID-hu', has enabled the study of pathogenicity of HIV in a small animal model. The initial results are interesting, as they show no correlation between *in vitro* cytopathogenicity and CD4-cell depletion *in vivo* and raise further questions on the role of direct viral cytopathic effects on cell loss (Aldrovandi *et al.*, 1993).

The immune response to HIV

The immune system makes a vigorous cellular and humoral response to structural, regulatory and enzyme elements of HIV (Connick & Schooley 1993). During established infection, approximately 1% of peripheral blood B-cells are specific for HIV. Seroconversion usually occurs within 6 weeks of exposure, although longer periods have been documented where individuals are polymerase chain reaction (PCR) positive for many months, before antibodies are detectable. Although neutralising antibodies are produced (Robert-Guroff, Brown & Gallo, 1985), their importance to the initial control of HIV infection is uncertain, as HIV p24 antigen and infectious virus in blood are lost before neutralising antibody can be detected (Ariyoshi *et al.*, 1992). The 'control' of HIV replication occurs in association with the development of anti-core antibodies, but whether there is a causal relationship is unknown. Against this, is the observation that patients with common variable hypogammaglobulinaemia who are unable to mount an antibody response, appear to control HIV replication in the early stages, making it unlikely that the humoral response is the main factor. HIV-specific T-cells are detectable, reacting with several of the viral proteins. CD8-lymphocytes from HIV-infected individuals are effective in controlling HIV replication *in vitro* (Walker, Moody & Stites 1986) and it is likely that cytotoxic T-lymphocytes (Tc) contribute to the reduction in peripheral blood HIV burden during these early stages. However, there have not been extensive studies of Tc function during acute HIV infection to confirm this. The initial immune response to HIV appears to be crucial in determining the future course of the disease. Those who make only low levels of antibody, in particular anti-p24 (anti-core) are much more likely to have a rapid progression to immunodeficiency, than those who make high titre responses (Weber, Clapham & Weiss 1987). Those who show decreasing levels of anti-p24 antibody, are also more likely to develop HIV antigenaemia and progress clinically (Lange, Paul & Huisman 1986) (Lange *et al.*, 1986) (Kenny *et al.*, 1987).

Following seroconversion, there is a variable period of clinical latency in which the individual is asymptomatic, p24 antigen is undetectable and the viral burden in the peripheral blood low (only 1 in 10 000 to 1 in 50 000 lymphocytes infected by PCR analysis (Ho, Moudgil & Alam 1989)). However, at this stage defects in immune function are already detectable (Murray *et al.*, 1984) and progressive CD4-cell depletion is usually observed (Lau *et al.*, 1992). This apparent discrepancy between progressive immuno-deficiency in the face of HIV 'latency', has recently been solved by studies showing that much of the early HIV infection of the immune system is contained within the follicles of the lymph nodes (Embretson *et al.*, 1993) (Panteleo *et al.*, 1993). Within this micro-environment there is trapping of HIV virions by the processes of the follicular dendritic cells (FDC). This process occurs in lymphoid tissue at any site, including the gut-associated lymphoid tissue. The FDC are in close communication with CD4+-lymphocytes to which HIV infection can be transmitted. The lymph tissue often shows marked follicular hyperplasia due to the influx of CD8-positive cells into the germinal centres (Janossy *et al.*, 1985). It is assumed that these cells are HIV-specific, cytotoxic lymphocytes reacting to the foreign antigen. Although HIV production may be limited at this stage, up to 25% of lymph node cells are infected, as demonstrated by PCR for DNA. The demonstration of persistent viraemia throughout HIV infection, shows that HIV never achieves true latency within the human host (Piatak, Saag & Yang, 1993). With time, the architecture of the lymph nodes becomes effaced, with involution of the germinal centres and destruction of the fibroblastic supporting structure. This may be a result of the cytopathic effect of HIV or

Table 9.3. *Immunological defects associated with HIV infection*

T-Lymphocytes
CD4-lymphocyte depletion
CD4-lymphocyte dysfunction
Decreased proliferation to soluble antigen, mitogen
Decreased interleukin-2 and gamma-IFN production
Defective signalling
Chronically elevated intracellular calcium levels
Defective delayed-type hypersensitivity skin test
Defective cytotoxic function

B-lymphocytes
Polyclonal activation
   Hypergammaglobulinaemia
   Autoantibody production
   Circulating immune complexes
Decreased response to neoantigen
IgG2 deficiency

Other
Antigen presenting cell dysfunction
? defective natural killer cell function
Raised levels, acid-labile alpha-interferon

proteins released, secondary to inflammatory actions of cytotoxic T-cells and cytokines such as tumour necrosis factor. During the stage of lymph node involution or loss of lymphadenopathy as noticed on clinical examination, HIV-related disease often progresses rapidly. During the same time, the viral load in the blood and percentage of infected cells increases steadily, possibly due to the loss of local viral control at the lymph node sites.

Immunopathogenesis of HIV

There are many immunological abnormalities associated with HIV infection (Table 9.3; Seligmann, Chess & Fahey, 1985). Of these, possibly the most important and certainly the most characteristic of AIDS, is the severe and progressive CD4-lymphocyte decline. The CD4+ve lymphocyte is the orchestrating cell of the immune response. This recognises antigen in the context of class II positive antigen presenting cells and then switching on T-dependent B-cell responses, T cytotoxic and T suppressor, natural killer cell and macrophage microbicidal responses, by the secretion of immunologically active cytokines, mainly interferon gamma, interleukins (IL) 2 and IL-

Table 9.4. *Mechanisms of CD4 cell depletion in HIV infection*

Direct effects of HIV on infected cells
  Direct lysis
  Syncytia formation and lysis
  Accumulation of unintegrated viral DNA

Destruction of HIV infected cells or uninfected cells coated with gp120 by
    HIV-specific immune response
  HIV-specific cytotoxic T-cells
  HIV-specific antibody-dependent cytotoxic cells (ADCC)

Non-specific CD4-cell loss
  Anti-lymphocyte antibodies
  Apoptosis
  Molecular mimicry of HIV and MHC

---

4. The loss, of this central cell alone, would therefore cause a secondary effect on all these other cell types, with loss of regulation of the immune response. The postulated mechanisms of the CD4-cell loss are described in the following section. In addition, direct infection of other immunological cells, in particular antigen preventing cells (APC) by HIV, impairs their ability to present antigen to CD4-cells (Eales *et al.*, 1987) (Meyaard, Schuitemaker & Miedema 1993). Excess HIV proteins produced and secreted by infected cells, have direct immunosuppressive effects on lymphoproliferation. In addition, gp120 polyclonally activates B-cells (Schnittman, Clifford-Lane & Higgins, 1986), leading to hypergamma-globulinaemia (Clifford-Lane *et al.*, 1983) and raised levels of immune complexes (Euler *et al.*, 1985). These overactivated cells are unable to mount a response to neoantigens (Ammann *et al.*, 1984) (Ballet *et al.*, 1987). The hypergammaglobulinaemia is due to raised levels of the IgG1 and IgG3 subclasses and many patients are actually deficient in IgG2, which may explain the susceptibility to infection with encapsulated bacteria (Parkin *et al.*, 1987*a*) (Parkin *et al.*, 1988).

CD4-Lymphocyte depletion

Although the direct cytopathic effect of HIV on its target CD4+ lympho-cytes as described above, may account for some cell loss, the small number of infected cells, and the lack of correlation in animal models between viral cytopathogenicity and CD4-depletion, lead to the proposal that other mechanisms are involved (Table 9.4).

Loss of CD4-lymphocytes by HIV-specific Tc or antibody dependent cytotoxic cells (ADCC) and other immunological mechanisms

As described above, during HIV infection there is a broad anti-HIV Tc response. However, although the removal of infected cells is advantageous, it is postulated that uninfected CD4+ lymphocytes may also be attacked, as soluble gp120 which is present in serum, can bind to the CD4-molecule of any cells, which could become targets for gp120-specific Tc cells. Antibody-dependent cytotoxic cells could also function in this way. In addition, gp120-antibody complexes are found in the circulation and coating cells of HIV-infected patients. These complexes could either bind to CD4-cells via gp120, or to any cells bearing FcR for immunoglobulin and once again cause them to become innocent targets of the immune response. It is important to consider these responses in the pathogenesis of immunodepletion, as any vaccination scheme using gp120 as all or part of the immunogen, would induce both humoral and cellular reactions. Such a response may prevent infection, but could be detrimental in those already infected. During HIV infection, there is also induction of anti-CD4 antibodies (Chams *et al.*, 1988) and also anti-CD4 cytotoxic cells (of T cell lineage, but often not showing MHC restriction). However, this 'bystander destruction' theory cannot be the whole answer, as progressive loss of CD4-cells occurs, even with the decline of Tc to undetectable levels. These cells may have a role at early stages of HIV disease.

Apoptosis

An intriguing phenomenon that has recently been described in HIV infection, is the reversion of mature peripheral blood lymphocytes to the immature response of apoptosis ('programmed' or 'stimulation-induced' cell death). Instead of proliferation, up to 40% of circulating, mature T cells, in those with HIV infection, undergo apoptosis on mitogen, superantigen, or T-cell receptor stimulation (Groux *et al.*, 1992) (Gougeon *et al.*, 1991) (Meyaard *et al.*, 1992). The cause of this change in programming during HIV infection, is under intense investigation at present. Studies using HIV-infected cell lines, where up to 90% of cells have integrated viral genome, have shown that HIV itself causes apoptosis (Laurent-Crawford *et al.*, 1991) (Terai *et al.*, 1991). However, the large proportion of lymphocytes affected *in vivo* is several-fold greater, than the 0.1–0.01% of CD4+ lymphocytes that are likely to be directly infected with HIV. In addition, the findings of some investigators that CD8 cells are also affected, makes an indirect mechanism more plausible. A central theme to induction of programmed cell death, is inappropriate/incomplete cellular signalling and the demonstration that the phosphoinositol pathway is generally abnormal in lymphocytes from those with HIV infection and may be of importance (Nye, Knox & Pinching, 1991; Nye, Riley & Pinching 1992). Ameissen and Capron (1991) have made the interesting suggestion that circulating gp120 may act in a similar way to CD4 antibodies, which have been shown to prime lymphocytes for programmed cell death on subsequent antigen stimulation (Newell et al., 1990). This may explain the predominant CD4-lymphocyte loss. Extrinsic signals are also abnormal in HIV infection and loss of second signals due to cytokine 'starvation', especially IL-2 deficiency may be partly to blame. Tumour necrosis factor-α is also a powerful inducer of apoptosis and levels are raised in HIV infection due to increased production by monocytes and macrophages. Macrophages and other antigen-presenting cells could also potentially induce apoptosis, by failing to deliver an appropriate second signal during antigen presentation, due to the HIV-related loss of class II expression.

Apoptosis is initiated by binding of the antigen receptor, in an appropriately primed cell. In addition to specific antigen, this is also achieved by superantigen, each of which binds to multiple T-cell receptors (TCR) of the same Vβ family. It has therefore been proposed that concurrent infectious agents, such as mycoplasma or even HIV itself (mouse retroviruses have been shown to possess superantigen activity), may act as superantigens and enhance cellular loss by apoptosis.

If the cell death induced in vitro, also occurs in vivo after antigen stimulation, then exposure of T-lymphocytes to their specific TCR ligand, would lead to deletion of the responsive clone. Repeated exposures to infectious agents and potentially tumour cells, would therefore lead to progressive loss of cellular immunity, more infections would develop and a vicious cycle established. Of importance, specific cytotoxic T lymphocyte (CTL) immunity to HIV itself would decline.

Molecular mimicry

Several investigators have shown close homology between HIV envelope proteins and MHC class I and II (Golding et al., 1988) and gp120 antibodies that cross-react with the beta-2-microglobulin free MHC class I have been well described (Elliot 1991). The HLA homologous epitopes are mainly within the gp41-binding site of gp120. This homology has potential to induce humoral and cellular auto-immune responses and could explain the many auto-immune phenomena that have been described (Morrow & Parkin 1993).

The gastrointestinal tract in HIV infection

The gastrointestinal tract may act as the receptive site for primary infection, as an HIV-producing tissue for transmission of infection and as the site of HIV-related disease due to the direct effects of HIV on the organ, or as a result of opportunist infections and tumours. In a broader frame, there are similarities and differences between HIV disease and other inflammatory bowel conditions in terms of cytokine production, cellular infiltrates and mucosal abnormalities, that may give valuable information on the mechanisms of gastrointestinal disease outside of HIV infection.

The rectum as a site of initial HIV infection

Penetrative anal intercourse between men, is a major route of transmission of HIV in the developed world. The mucosa is relatively thin, therefore rectal trauma during sexual intercourse may lead to tears, allowing HIV in semen to penetrate into the lamina propria. This could lead to direct infection, as colonic cells are susceptible to HIV (Nelson et al., 1988; Fantini, Yahi & Chermann, 1991). However, it is more likely that lymphocytes and organised lymphoid tissue present within the lamina propria, are the main target (Jarry et al., 1990). The specialised 'M' cells that cover the luminal surface of lymphoid tissue and whose role is to transport antigen from the gut to be presented to the lymphocytes, may enhance infection. The gut-associated lymphoid tissue (GALT) within the rectum is certainly a site for viral replication, as lymphoid aggregates, containing follicles with B-cells and follicular dendritic cells trapping HIV, have been documented (Jarry et al., 1990). Whether this is part of the primary infection, or as a result of secondary spread of HIV is unknown. However, this effective transport mechanism to lymphoid tissue is potentially of benefit paradoxically, as vigorous immune responses are mounted to simian immunodeficiency virus (SIV) vaccines given rectally (Lehner et al., 1992). The circulating of lymphocytes between the various parts of the mucosa-associated lymphoid tissue (MALT), means that the immunological responses to such vaccines are widespread.

Concurrent infections of the rectum and genital tract are known to enhance infection risk of persons for HIV. This reflects the increased target cells which would be recruited to sites of inflammation, and decreased resistance due to ulceration. There have been a small number of cases of HIV infection transmitted via rectal intercourse, when there has been a delay of many months before seroconversion has occurred. It is postulated that the lymphoid tissue may have been the initial site of infection and that HIV was contained and controlled within the aggregates. With time, greater viral replication may have led to systemic spread and a generalised antibody response. In a similar way, genital infections also increase the infectivity of an individual who is already HIV-positive, probably due to the increased viral production that occurs when lymphocytes are recruited and activated. The colorectum may be responsible for 'bidirectional' production of HIV; a study using variants of the colorectal tumour cell line, HT29-D4, showed that while mucous-secreting cells replicate and produce selected strains of HIV through their apical (luminal) membranes, HT29 cells with absorptive phenotype, produce HIV basolaterally (to the serosal surface) (Fantini *et al.*, 1991).

HIV enteropathy

HIV enteropathy refers to a chronic, pathogen-negative, diarrhoea occurring in individuals with HIV infection. Many HIV-positive individuals have features of small intestine disease and sub-total villous atrophy on small bowel biopsy (Gillin *et al.*, 1985). However, the level of malabsorption is out of proportion to these relatively minor changes; decreased xylose, glucose and rhamnose absorption and increased gut permeability has been shown, in HIV-positive individuals, at various stages of HIV infection. Although the villous crypt ratio is greater in HIV-positive patients, compared to coeliac disease patients, the HIV-positive patients show greater malabsorption. Deficiency in brush border enzymes has been suggested as a contributory mechanism.

Despite the fact that some of the cases of 'HIV enteropathy' ultimately turn out to have an underlying infection, tumour, drug-related or allergic cause, there is now a significant body of evidence to show that HIV directly causes intestinal damage. Whatever the route of the initial infection, HIV is soon established within the immunological cells of the lamina propria of the small and large bowel. Studies have shown a 30–70% infection rate for lymphocytes and macrophages at this site. HIV has also been detected in the enterochromaffin and crypt cells, as well as in biopsies from the oesophagus, and stomach. There do not appear to be 'bowel-specific' strains of HIV, although monocytotropic strains replicate better in gastrointestinal tract cells (Moyer *et al.*, 1990) and isolates from the bowel and blood of the same individual may show a differential cell range, cytopathic effects, and susceptibility to neutralisation (Barnett *et al.*, 1991). It is likely that these variants are similar to the many quasi-species that can be detected in the blood and the tissue used for culture will select those able to replicate best in the particular cell line.

Observation of apoptosis of the gut crypt cells (that are known to harbour

HIV), without evidence of other infections, suggests that direct cytopathogenicity occurs at this site. However, the scarcity of infected cells makes this unlikely to be the major mechanism of the enteropathy. There are changes in the immunological cells within the gut during HIV infection. A decrease in CD4-cell numbers (that was often more pronounced than the peripheral blood depletion), and an increase in CD8-cells has been documented by colonoscopic biopsy techniques. All the CD4 cells demonstrated have been 45RO+ ('memory' phenotype). The CD8 population show reduced 45RO+ and CD29+, compatible with non-differentiated cells. However, the study of subsets in the gastrointestinal tract is hampered by sampling error, as lymphoid follicle cells tend to harbour 'naive' (CD45RA) cells and lamina propria memory (CD45RO) lymphocytes. The role of these cells, in causing or protecting from disease is not clear. Potentially of greater relevance to the enteropathy, is the abnormal cytokine secretion patterns within the bowel of HIV-infected persons with diarrhoea. It is possible that the high levels of pro-inflammatory cytokines such as, IL-1β, TNF-α, IL-2, IL-6 and IL-8, are cytopathic, through increasing inflammation and permeability and thereby play a role in pathogenesis.

HIV may have other direct effects, outside of the immune cells within the gastrointestinal tract. Marked abnormalities in the autonomic nerve fibres of the jejunum have been noted at all stages of HIV infection. The study by Griffin et al. (1988) of 11 patients (symptomatic, and asymptomatic), showed all to have extensive damage to nerve bundles, which were swollen, with loss of normal axonal organelles. This is potentially entirely due to HIV infection of the nerve cells, as the main damage was around the crypts in the jejunum, where HIV is localised and it occurred early in HIV disease, before secondary infections and malnutrition would have complicated the picture. This autonomic damage may also have a role in the chronic diarrhoea of HIV infection.

The population with the most marked gastrointestinal presentations of HIV disease, are African patients, where 'slim' is used to describe the characteristic weight loss and debilitation (Serwadda, Mugerwa & Sewankambo, 1985) (Biggar, 1986). However, this group is heterogeneous and lack of diagnostic facilities in developing countries, makes exclusion of underlying causes difficult. In a study of diarrhoea in Lusaka, in HIV-positive patients with Slim disease, 50% had oesophageal candidiasis; 60% had hypochlohydria (of unknown aetiology, but potentially related to decrease in aldosterone), which could lead to bacterial overgrowth and diarrhoea; and 5% had gastric Kaposi's sarcoma. Chronic diarrhoea was also associated with raised levels of IgA HIV-specific antibody in stool. This could represent a heightened immune response, to a greater burden of gut-associated HIV.

Opportunist infections and tumours of the gastrointestinal tract in HIV infection—features of disease in the immunocompromised host

In general, phagocytes (especially neutrophils and monocytes), together with the humoral factors (complement and antibody), protect against extracellular organisms (predominantly bacteria, Table 9.5). In contrast, the cell-mediated system which is abnormal in AIDS (consisting of cytotoxic T cells, ADCC, NK and macrophages), controls intracellular organisms such as viruses, facultative intracellular bacteria, fungi and protozoa, as well as providing tumour surveillance.

The main features, of immunodeficiency, are opportunist infections (i.e. atypical infections either due to normally non-pathogenic organisms, or atypically severe disease with known pathogens) and opportunist tumours. Infections are often multiple and the clinical presentation may be atypical due to the lack of inflammatory response, which is often the cause of symptoms. For example, AIDS patients with cryptococcal meningitis, usually have no photophobia or neck stiffness and have very few white cells in the CSF. The same is true for histopathological studies. *Mycobacteria tuberculosis* infection may be associated with absent or only poorly formed granuloma. It must also be recognised that in an individual who is immuno-suppressed, tests of the immune system cannot be used to diagnose infections. Therefore, antibody responses to a new infection, or to a reactivation of old latent disease, may not be elicited and testing these can only lead to confusion if negative results are obtained. Biopsy or other direct means of diagnosis are essential.

The infections, that occur, will reflect both newly acquired disease and also re-activation of latent infections, that may have been acquired many years ago. This means that the present and past microbiological environment of the host is of importance and diseases that may have been acquired many years before from distant countries, may recrudesce as immunodeficiency intervenes. In this respect antibody responses can be helpful in documenting which infections a patient has been exposed to in the past.

The gastrointestinal tract presentations of HIV infection

The gastrointestinal manifestations of HIV-related immunodeficiency are listed in Table 9.6. Different infections tend to occur at different disease stages (Fig. 9.1). Early in HIV-infection, when immunodeficiency is slight, the infections that occur are with relatively high-grade pathogens that cause disease, even in the immunocompetent host, such as herpes simplex, mucocutaneous candidiasis or tuberculosis. Kaposi's sarcoma also tends to

Table 9.5. *Characteristic infections/tumours associated with immune deficiencies*

	Defects		
	Polymorphonuclear leucocytes (PMN)	Antibody/Complement (C')	Cell-modified immunity (CMI)
Viruses		Echovirus Polio	Herpes HSV 1 and 2 VZV EBV CMV Adenovirus Polyoma: BK, JC Papilloma
Bacteria		Mycoplasma	
	S. epidermidis *S. aureus*	*S. aureus* Pneumococcus	Salmonella
	E. coli Klebsiella Pseudomonas Anaerobes	*H. influenzae* Moraxella Meningococci	Listeria

		Mycobacteria
		TB
		Mycobacterium avium intracellular complex (MAC)
		Nocardia
Fungi	Candida	Candida
	(disseminated)	(muco-cutaneous)
	Aspergillus	Cryptococcus
		Histoplasma
Protozoa		*Pneumocystis carinii**
		Toxoplasma
		Cryptosporidia
Tumours		non-Hodgkin's (NHL) (B-cell lymphoma)
		Kaposi's sarcoma
Other		Graft-virus host diseases (GVHD)

*RNA analysis suggests this organism to be more related to fungi genetically, but phenotypically it behaves as a protozoan.

Table 9.6. *Main HIV-associated diseases within the gastro-intestinal tract*

Mouth
Candida, pseudomembranous, hypertrophic
Hairy oral leukoplakia (EBV-related)
Herpes simplex types 1 and 2
Idiopathic ulceration

Oesophagus and stomach
Candida oesophagitis
EBV-related ulceration (solitary, central oesophagus)
CMV ulcers (solitary, lower third oesophagus)
HSV (multiple ulcers)

Small bowel
HIV enteropathy
Mycobacterium avium intracellulare complex
Cryptosporidium
Microsporidium
Isospora

Liver
Mycobacterium avium intracellulare complex
    and tuberculosis
Bacilliary angiomatosis (*R. hensellae*)
Viral hepatitis, including HIV

Disseminated infection:
    pneumocystis
    histoplasmosis
    Penicillium marfenii
    bacterial septicaemia

Biliary tract/pancreas
Sclerosing cholangitis/ampullary stenosis
    CMV
    Cryptosporidiosis
    Microsporidiosis

Colon
Colitis
    CMV
    ? Adenovirus
    Campylobacter
    Clostridium difficile

Mycobacterium avium intracellulare complex and tuberculosis
Salmonella
Blastocystis hominis

Proctitis/peri-anal
HSV
CMV
Wart virus
Kaposi's sarcoma and non-Hodgkin's lymphoma can occur at any site.

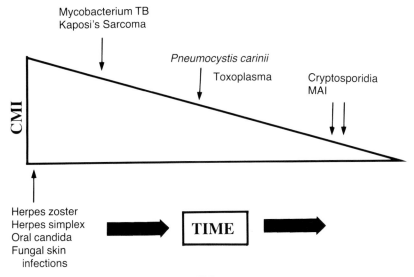

Fig. 9.1.   Immune response to HIV.

develop in patients whose immune systems are still relatively well maintained. Thus, these conditions will often be the major initial gastrointestinal presentations, outside the HIV enteropathy. In advanced disease, disseminated infections with organisms of low pathogenicity can occur, especially *Mycobacterium avium intracellulare* complex (MAC), cytomegalovirus, cryptosporidia and microsporidia and most are confined to patients with a CD4 count less than 100 cells/cm^3. Lymphoma shows two patterns, with central nervous system involvement, usually occurring late in HIV-disease, (1991) and with a poor prognosis, whereas lymphoma outside the CNS may occur in relatively early HIV-infection and respond well to therapy.

The majority of infections that develop can be treated initially. However, most therapies suppress, rather than eradicate, the organisms and long-term maintenance or secondary prophylaxis is required, to prevent relapse. As the immune system becomes progressively depleted, then the lack of help for anti-microbials, allows the infections once again to recur.

Drug reactions

There is a marked increase in allergic drug reactions in HIV-positive patients, in particular to sulphonamides, but also to ciprofloxacin, grizeofulvin, isoniazid, pyrazinamide and rifampicin. Skin reactions and abnormal liver function are the most common features. This appears to be a feature of many immunodeficiencies and although this may appear a paradox at first, it is not altogether surprising. The role of CD4+ve, T cell types, having particular cytokine secretion patterns, in allergic disease (Th1 that produce gamma-interferon and reduce IgE-production and Th2 that produce IL-4 and enhance IgE production), is becoming clear. In HIV infection, the ability to secrete gamma interferon in response to mitogen or antigen is poor. This loss would be expected to allow the escape of IgE-secreting B-cells and the development of allergic disease. This has been found to be the case, in those with a history of atopic disease. Many will develop recrudescence of symptoms, or worsening of persistent disease. Anecdotally, recombinant gamma-interferon, has been demonstrated to control these symptoms (Parkin *et al.*, 1987*b*). However, many of the reactions are more typical of delayed-type hypersensitivity, than immediate-type hypersensitivity and the mechanism of their induction is less clear. With progressive immune depletion, it appears that these reactions do become less frequent and they may reflect the over-activation of the immune system, that is characteristic of the initial phases of HIV infection.

Non-HIV-related infections and diseases of interest

Many patients with HIV-infection are sexually active, well travelled, or come from parts of the world where other infections are common and it must not be forgotten that HIV-positive individuals may contract non-HIV-related diseases. In the gastrointestinal tract, it is now clear that many gut infections, including *Giardia* and *Entamoeba*, may be sexually transmitted through anal intercourse.

It is interesting that some conditions appear to be very rare in HIV-infected populations, suggesting that an intact cellular immune system is required for their pathogenesis. For example, Crohn's disease and sarcoidosis are not reported, whereas ulcerative colitis may still occur. The similar transmission of hepatitis B and HIV means that dual infections are common in homosexual men and intravenous drug users. The immuno-dysregulation of HIV infection makes patients less able to clear hepatitis B and HIV-positive individuals do not respond to alpha-interferon immunomodulation (Brook *et al.*, 1989). Therefore, there are many HIV-positive, persistent carriers. However, HIV-positive individuals are less likely to have active disease and scarring on histology (Goldin *et al.*, 1990), suggesting a role for cell-mediated immunity in the eradication of infection, but also in the production of disease, once persistent infection is present. This is one of the many examples, where the investigation of patients with HIV infection, is giving clues about the pathogenesis of infection and malignancy and leading to new avenues of research.

References

Aldrovandi, G. M., Feuer, G., Gao, L., Jamieson, B., Kristeva, M., Chen, I. S. Y. & Zack J. A. (1993). The SCID-hu mouse as a model for HIV-1 infection. *Nature*, **363**, 732–6.

Ameissen, J. C. & Capron, A. (1991). Cell dysfunction and deletion in AIDS: the programmed cell death hypothesis. *Immunology Today*, **12**, 102–5.

Ammann, A., Schiffman, G., Abrams, D., Volberding, P., Ziegler, J. & Conant, M. (1984). B-cell immunodeficiency in acquired immune deficiency syndrome. *Journal of American Medical Association*, **251**(11): 1447–9.

Ariyoshi, K., Harwood, E., Chiengsong-Popov, R. & Weber, J. (1992). Is clearance of HIV-1 viraemia at seroconversion mediated by neutralising antibodies? *Lancet*, **340**; 257–8.

Armstrong, J. A. & Horne, R. (1984). Follicular dendritic cells and virus-like particles in AIDS-related lymphadenopathy. *Lancet*, **ii**, 370–2.

Ballet, J.-J., Sulcebe, G., Couderc, L.-J. *et al.* (1987). Impaired anti-pneumococcal antibody response in patients with AIDS-related persistent generalized lymphadenopathy. *Clinical and Experimental Immunology*, **68**, 479–87.

Barillari, G., Buonaguro, L., Fiorelli, V. *et al.* (1992). Effects of cytokines from activated immune cells on vascular cell growth and HIV-1 expression. Implications for AIDS-Kaposi's sarcoma pathogenesis. *Journal of Immunology*, **149**, 3727–34.

Barnett, S. W., Barboza, A., Wilcox, C. M., Forsmark, C. E. & Levy, J. A. (1991). Characterization of human immunodeficiency virus type 1 strains recovered from the bowel of infected individuals. *Virology* **182**, 802–9.

Barre-Sinoussi, F., Chermann, J. C. & Rey, FV. (1983). Isolation of a T-lymphotrophic retrovirus from a patient at risk for acquired immune deficiency syndrome (AIDS). *Science*, **220**, 868–70.

Biggar, R. J. (1986). The clinical features of HIV infection in Africa. *British Medical Journal* **293**, 1453–4.

Brook, M. G., McDonald, J. A., Karayiannis, P. *et al.* (1989). Randomised controlled trial of interferon alpha 2A (rbe) (Roferon-A) for the treatment of chronic hepatitis B virus (HBV) infection: factors that influence response. *Gut*, **30**, 1116–22.

Chams, V., Joualt, T., Fenouillet, E., Gluckman, J.-C. & Klatzmann, D. (1988). Detection of anti-CD4 autoantibodies in the sera of HIV-infected patients using recombinant soluble CD4 molecules. *AIDS*, **2**, 353–61.

Cheng-Mayer, C. (1990). Biological and molecular features of HIV-1 related to tissue tropism. *AIDS*, **4**(suppl. 1), S49–S56.

Clavel, F. (1989). Virological and Clinical Features of HIV-2. *Current Topics in AIDS*, **2**, 69–80.

Clavel, F., Guetard, D., Brun-Vezinet, F., Klazmann D, Champalimaud J. L. & Montagnier, L. (1986*a*). Isolation of a new human retrovirus from West African patients with AIDS. *Science*, **233**, 345–6.

Clavel, F., Guyader, M., Guetard, D., Salle, M., Montagnier, L. & Alizon, M. (1986*b*). Molecular cloning and polymorphism of the human immune deficiency virus type 2. *Nature*, **324**, 691–5.

Clavel, F., Mansinho, K., Chamaret, S. *et al.* (1987). Human immunodeficiency virus type 2 infection associated with AIDS in Africa. *New England Journal of Medicine*, **316**, 1180–5.

Clifford-Lane, H., Masur, H., Edgar, L. C., Whalen, G., Rook, A. H. & Fauci, A. S. (1983). Abnormalities of B-cell activation and immunodeficiency in patients with the acquired immunodeficiency syndrome. *New England Journal of Medicine*, **309**, 453–8.

Connick, E. & Schooley, R. T. (1993). HIV-1 specific immune responses. *HIV Molecular Organisation, Pathogenicity and Treatment*, ed. W. J. W. Morrow and N. Haigwood. Elsevier Science Publishers BV.

Dalgleish, A. G., Beverley, P. C. L. & Clapham, P. R. (1984). The CD4 (T4) antigen is an essential component of the receptor for the AIDS retrovirus. *Nature*, **312**, 763–7.

Document WHO/GPA/CNP/EVA/931 (1993). The HIV/AIDS Pandemic 1993 Overview. Global Programme on AIDS, Geneva.

Eales, L.-J., Farrant, J., Helbert, M. & Pinching, A. J. (1987). Peripheral blood dendritic cells in persons with AIDS and AIDS-related complex: loss of high intensity class II expression and function. *Clinical and Experimental Immunology*, **71**, 423–7.

Eales, L.-J. & Parkin, J. M. (1988). Current concepts in the immunopathogenesis of AIDS and HIV infection. *British Medical Bulletin*, **44**, 38–55.

Elliot E. T. (1991). How do peptides associate with MHC class 1 molecules? *Immunology Today*, **12**, 386–8.

Embretson, J., Zupancic, M., Ribas, J. L. *et al.* (1993). Massive covert infection of helper T lymphocytes and macrophages by HIV during the incubation period of AIDS. *Nature*, **362**, 359–62.

Euler, H. H., Kern, P., Loffler, H. & Dietrich, M. (1985). Precipitable immune complexes in healthy homosexual men, acquired immune deficiency syndrome and the related lymphadenopathy syndrome. *Clinical and Experimental Immunology* **59**, 267–75.

Evans, L. A., Moreau, J. & Odehouri, A. (1988). Characterization of a non cytopathic HIV-2 strain with unusual effects on CD4 expression. *Science*, **240**, 1522–5.

Fantini, J., Yahi, N. & Chermann, J.-C. (1991). Human immunodeficiency virus can infect the apical and basolateral surfaces of human colonic epithelial cells. *Proceedings of the National Academy of Sciences, USA*, **88**, 9297–301.

Friedman-Kein, A. E., Laubenstein, L. J. & Rubinstein, P. (1982). Disseminated Kaposi's sarcoma in homosexual men. *Annals of Internal Medicine*, **96**, 693–700.

Funke, I., Hahn, A., Rieber, E. P., Weiss, E. & Riethmuller, G. (1987). The cellular receptor (CD4) of the human immunodeficiency virus is expressed on neurons and glial cells in human brain. *Journal of Experimental Medicine*, **165**, 1230–5.

Gallo, R. C., Salahuddin, S. Z. & Popovic, M. (1984). Frequent detection and isolation of cytopathic retroviruses (HTLV-III) from patients with AIDS and at risk of AIDS. *Science*, **224**, 500–3.

Gillin, J. S., Shike, M., Alcock, N. *et al.* (1985). Malabsorption and mucosal abnormalities of the small intestine in the acquired immunodeficiency syndrome. *Annals of Internal Medicine* **102**, 619–22.

Gody, M., Ouattara, S. A. & The, G. (1988). Clinical experience of AIDS in relation with HIV-1 and HIV-2 infection in a rural hospital in Ivory Coast. *AIDS*, **2**, 433–6.

Goldin, R. D., Fish, D. E., Hay, A. *et al.* (1990). Histological and immunohistochemical study of hepatitis B in human immunodeficiency virus infection. *Journal of Clinical Pathology*, **43**, 203–5.

Golding, H., Robey, F. A., Gates, F. T. (1988). Identification of homologous regions in human immunodeficiency virus 1 gp41 and human MHC class II β1 domain. I. Monoclonal antibodies against the gp41-derived peptide and patients sera react with native class II antigens, suggesting a role for autoimmunity in the pathogenesis of acquired immune deficiency syndrome. *Journal of Experimental Medicine*, **167**, 914–23.

Gottlieb, M. S., Schroff, R. & Schanker, H. (1981). *Pneumocystis carinii* pneumonia and mucosal candidiasis in previously healthy homosexual men: evidence of a new acquired cellular immunodeficiency. *New England Journal of Medicine*, **305**, 1425–31.

Gougeon, M. L., Olivier, R., Garcia, S. *et al.* (1991). Mise en évidence d'un process d'engagement vers la mort cellulaire par apoptose dans les lymphocytes de patients infectés par le VIH. *Complete Rentin Academic Sciences Paris. Ser. III Sci. Vie.* **312**, 529.

Griffin, G. E., Miller, A., Batman P. *et al.* (1988). Damage to jejunal intrinsic autonomic nerves in HIV infection. *AIDS*, **2**, 379–382.

Groux, H., Torpie, R. G., Monte, D., Mouton, Y., Capron, A. & Amiesen, J. C. (1992). Activation-induced death by apoptosis in CD4+ T cells from human immunodeficiency virus-infected asymptomatic individuals. *Journal of Experimental Medicine*, **175**, 331–40.

Guenno, B. L., Jean, P. & Peghini, M. (1987). Increasing HIV-2 associated AIDS in Senegal. *Lancet*, **ii**, 972–3.

Ho, D. D., Moudgil, T. & Alam, M. (1989). Quantitation of human immunodeficiency virus type 1 in the blood of infected persons. *New England Journal of Medicine*, **321**, 1621–5.

Ho, D. D., Rota, T. R. & Hirsh, M. S. (1986). Infection of monocytes/macrophages by human T-lymphotropic virus type III. *Journal of Clinical Investigations*, **77**, 1712–15.

Hoxie, J. A., Alpers, J. D., Rackowski, J. L. *et al.* (1986). Alterations in T4 (CD4) protein and mRNA synthesis in cells infected with HIV. *Science*, **234**, 1123–7.

Janossy, G., Pinching, A. J., Bofill, M. *et al.* (1985). An immunohistological approach to persistent generalised lymphadenopathy and its relevance to AIDS. *Clinical Experimental Immunology*, **59**, 257–66.

Jarry, A., Cortez, A., Rene, E., Muzeau, F. & Brousse, N. (1990). Infected cells and immune cells in the gastrointestinal tract of AIDS patients. An immunohistochemical study of 127 cases. *Histopathology*, **16**, 133–40.

Johnston, M. I. & Hoth, D. F. (1993). Present status and future prospects for HIV therapies. *Science*, **260**, 1286–93.

Kenny, C., Parkin, J. M., Underhill, G. (1987). HIV antigen testing. *Lancet*, **i**, 565–6.

Kirkpatrick, C. H., Davis, K. C. & Horsburgh, C. R. (1984). Reduced la positive Langerhans cells in AIDS. *New England Journal of Medicine* **311**, 857–8.

Klatzmann, D., Champagne, E. & Chameret, S. (1984). T-lymphocyte T4 molecule behaves as the receptor for human retrovirus LAV. *Nature*, **312**, 767–8.

Koenig, S., Gendelman, H. E. & Orenstein, J. M. (1986). Detection of AIDS virus in macrophages in brain tissue from AIDS patients with encephalopathy. *Science*, **233**, 1089–93.

Kong, L. I., Lee, S. & Kappes, J. C. (1988). West African HIV-2 related retrovirus with attenuated cytopathicity. *Science*, **240**, 1525–9.

Koyanagi, Y., O'Brien, W. A., Zhao, J. Q., Golde, D. W., Gasson, J. C. & Chen, I. S. Y. (1988). Cytokines alter production of HIV-1 from primary mononuclear phagocytes. *Science*, **241**, 1673–5.

Lange, J. M. A., Coutinho, R. A., Krone, W. J. A. *et al.* (1986). Distinct IgG recognition patterns during progression of subclinical and clinical infection with lymphadenopathy associated virus/human T lymphotropic virus. *British Medical Journal*, **292**, 228–30.

Lange, J. M. A., Paul, D. A. & Huisman, H. G. (1986). Persistent HIV antigenaemia and decline of HIV core antibodies associated with transition to AIDS. *British Medical Journal*, **293**, 1459–62.

Lau, R. K. W., Hill, A., Jenkins, P. *et al.* (1992). Eight year prospective study of HIV infection in a cohort of homosexual men- clinical progression, immunological and virological markers. *International Journal STD AIDS*, **3**, 261–6.

Laurent-Crawford, A. G., Krust, B., Muller, S., *et al.* (1991). The cytopathic effect of HIV is associated with apoptosis. *Virology*, **185**, 829–39.

Lehner, T., Bergmeier, A., Panagiotidi, C. *et al.* (1992). Induction of mucosal and systemic immunity to a recombinant simian immunodeficiency viral protein. *Science*, **258**, 1365–9.

Luciw, P. A. & Shacklett, B. L. (1993). Molecular biology of the human and Simian immunodeficiency viruses. In *HIV Molecular Organisation, Pathogenecity and Treatment*, ed. W. J. W. Morrow and N. L. Haigwood. Elsevier Science Publishers BV.

Maddon, P. J., Dalgleish, A. G. & McDougal, J. S. (1986). The T4 gene encodes the AIDS virus receptor and is expressed in the immune system and the brain. *Cell*, **47**, 333–48.

Marlink, R. G., Ricard, D. & M'Boup, S. (1988). Clinical, haematologic and immunologic cross-sectional evaluation of individuals exposed to HIV-2. *AIDS Research Human Retroviruses*, **4**, 137–47.

McDougal, J. S., Kennedy, M. S. & Sligh, J. H. (1986). Binding of HTLV-III/LAV to T4+ T cells by a complex of the 110k viral protein and the T4 molecule. *Science*, **231**, 382–5.

Meyaard, L., Otto, S. A., Jonker, R. R., Mijnste, R. M. J., Keet, R. P. M. & Miedema, F. (1992). Programmed death of T cells in HIV-1 infection. *Science*, **257**, 217–19.

Meyaard, L., Schuitemaker, H. & Miedema, F. (1993). T-cell dysfunction in HIV infection: anergy due to defective antigen-presenting cell function? *Immunology Today* **14**, 161–4.

Morbidity and Mortality Weekly Report (1991). Opportunistic non-Hodgkin's lymphoma among severely immunocompromised HIV-infected patients surviving for prolonged periods on antiretroviral therapy-United States. **40**(34), 591–601.

Morrow, W. J. W. & Parkin, J. M. (1993). Autoimmune mechanisms in the pathogenesis of HIV infection. In *HIV Molecular Organization, Pathogenesis and Treatment*, eds W. J. W. Morrow and N. Haigwood. Elsevier Science Publishers B.V. **Chapter 4**.

Moyer, M. P., Huot, R. I., Ramirez, A., Joe, S., Meltzer, M. S. & Gendelman, H. E. (1990). Infection of human gastrointestinal cells by HIV-1. *AIDS Res Hum Retroviruses*, **6**, 1409–15.

Murray, H. W., Rubin, B. Y., Masur, H. & Roberts, R. B. (1984). Impaired production of lymphokines and immune (gamma) interferon in the acquired immunodeficiency syndrome. *New England Journal of Medicine*, **310**, 883–9.

Nelson, J. A., Wiley, C. A., Reynolds-Kihler, C., Reese, C. E., Margaretten, W. & Levy, J. A. (1988). Human immunodeficiency virus infected bowel epithelium from patients with gastrointestinal symptoms. *Lancet*, **i**: 259–62.

Newell, M., Haughen, L. J., Maroun, C. R. & Julius, M. H. (1990). Death of mature T cells by separate ligation of CD4 and the T-cell receptor for antigen. *Nature*, **347**, 286–9.

Nye, K. E., Knox, K. A. & Pinching, A. J. (1991). Lymphocytes from HIV-infected individuals show aberrant inositol polyphosphate metabolism which reverses after zidovudine therapy. *AIDS*, **5**, 413–17.

Nye, K. E., Riley, G. A. & Pinching, A. J. (1992). The defect seen in the phosphotidylinositol hydrolysis pathway in HIV-infected lymphocytes and lymphoblastoid cells is due to inhibition of the inositol 1,4,5-tetrakisphosphate 5-phosphomonoesterase. *Clinical and Experimental Immunology*, **89**, 89–93.

Panteleo, G., Graziosi, C., Demarest, J. F. *et al.* (1993). HIV infection is active and progressive in lymphoid tissue during the clinically latent stage of disease. *Nature*, **362**, 355–8.

Parkin, J. M., Eales, L.-J., Galazka, A. R. & Pinching, A. J. (1987*b*). Atopic manifestations of the acquired immunodeficiency syndrome. Response to interferon gamma. *British Medical Journal*, **294**, 1185.

Parkin, J. M., Helbert, M., Hughes, C. L. & Pinching, A. J. (1988). Immunoglobulin G subclass deficiency and susceptibility to pyogenic infections in patients with AIDS-related complex and AIDS. *AIDS*, **3**, 37–9.

Parkin J. M., Rowland-Hill, C., Shaw, R. J., Scott, K. E. & Pinching, A. J. (1987*a*). Pyogenic infections in patients with AIDS and a possible role for IVIG in the treatment of functional hypogammaglobulinaemia. *Vox Sang*, **52**, 12–13.

Pepin, J., Morgan, G., Dunn, D. *et al.* (1991). HIV-2-induced immunosuppression among asymptomatic West African prostitutes: evidence that HIV-2 is pathogenic, but less so than HIV-1. *AIDS*, **5**, 1165–2.

Piatak, M., Saag, M. S. & Yang, L. C. (1993). High level of HIV1 in plasma during all staging injection determined by competitive PCN. *Science*, **259**, 1749–54.

Reisinger, B. C., Vogbtseder, W. & Berzow, D. (1990). Complement-mediated enhancement of HIV-1 infection of the monoblastoid cell line U937. *AIDS*, **4**, 961–5.

Robert-Guroff, M., Brown, M. & Gallo, R. C. (1985). HTLV-III-neutralizing antibodies in patients with AIDS and AIDS-related complex. *Nature*, **316**, 72–4.

Robinson, W. E., Montefiori, D. C. & Mitchell, W. M. (1988). Antibody-dependent enhancement of human immunodeficiency virus type 1 infection. *Lancet*, **1**, 790–4.

Roos, M. T. L., Lange, J. M., de Goode, R. E. *et al.* (1992). Viral phenotype and increased response to primary human immunodeficiency virus type I injection. *Journal of Infectious Disease*, **165**, 427.

Salahuddin, S. Z., Rose, R. M. & Groopman, J. E. (1986). Human T-lymphotropic virus type III infection of human alveolar macrophages. *Blood*, **67**, 281–4.

Schnittman, S. M., Clifford-Lane, H. & Higgins, S. E. (1986). Direct polyclonal activation of human B cells by the acquired immune deficiency syndrome virus. *Science*, **233**, 1084–6.

Seligmann, M., Chess, L. & Fahey, J. L. (1985). AIDS – an immunologic reevaluation. *New England Journal of Medicine*, **311**, 1276–92.

Serwadda, D., Mugerwa, R. D. & Sewankambo, N. K. (1985). Slim disease: a new disease in Uganda and its association with HTLV-III infection. *Lancet*, **ii**: 849–52.

Tenner-Racz, K., Bofil, M., Schulz-Meyer, A. *et al.* (1986). HTLV-III/LAV viral antigens in lymph nodes of homosexual men with persistent generalised lymphadenopathy and AIDS. *American Journal of Pathology*, **123**, 9–15.

Terai, C., Kornbluth, R. S., Pauza, C. D., Richman, D. D. & Carson, D. A. (1991). Apoptosis as a mechanism of cell death in cultured T lymphoblasts acutely infected with HIV-1. *Journal of Clinical Investigation*, **87**, 1710–15.

Tschachler, E., Groh, V. & Popovic, M. (1987). Epidermal Langerhans cells: a target for THLV-III/LAV infection. *Journal of Investigative Dermatology*, **88** 233–7.

Walker, C. M. Moody, D. J. & Stites, D. P. (1986). CD8+ lymphocytes can control HIV infection *in vitro* by suppressing virus replication. *Science*, **234**, 1563–6.

Wallace, B. M. & Lasker, J. S. (1992). Awakenings . . . UV light and HIV gene activation. *Science*, **257**, 1211–12.

Weber, J. M., Clapham, P. R. & Weiss R. A. (1987). Human immunodeficiency virus infection in two cohorts of homosexual men; neutralising sera and association of anti-gag antibody with prognosis. *Lancet*, **i**, 119–22.

Weiss, R. A. (1993). How does HIV cause AIDS? *Science*, **260**, 1273–9.

Wiley, C. A., Schrier, R. D., Nelson, J. A., Lampert, P. W. & Oldstone, M. B. A. (1986). Cellular localization of human immunodeficiency virus infection within the brains of acquired immunodeficiency syndrome patients. *Proceedings of the National Academy of Sciences USA*, **83**, 7089–93.

Wong-Staal, F. (1989). Molecular biology of human immunodeficiency viruses. *Current Topics in AIDS*, **2**, 81–102.

–10–
Intestinal infections

CHRISTOPHER R. STOKES

Enteric infection is one of the greatest causes of mortality and morbidity in both human and veterinary species. This is a reflection of the magnitude and diversity of the antigenic challenge to the intestine as well as the 'complications' that result from its other physiological roles. That, requires the intestinal tract to have long finger-like villi which not only facilitates the digestion and absorption of nutrients but also provides a large surface area for the interaction with a wide variety of microorganisms and their products.

Important differences exist between the strategies appropriate to the defence from antigen presented via systemic and mucosal routes. Systemic immunity is directed to the active elimination of antigens that have gained entry into host tissues. This is a comparatively rare event and it is appropriate that very powerful mechanisms should be deployed to deal with the intruding material. Such responses may result in collateral damage to the host but by eliminating the provoking material they are self-limiting. In contrast, the immune system of the gut is in constant contact with antigenic material which it is powerless to completely eliminate. Clearly, inflammatory responses under such conditions would be damaging and it is a feature of the gastrointestinal immune system to 'dampen down' such responses. While potentially harmful materials and microorganisms remain within the lumen of the intestine, they represent only a minimal threat to the host. It is only when they come into intimate contact with host tissues that they are capable of causing disease.

Studies of patients with immunodeficiency have indicated an important role for the immune system (Brown *et al.*, 1972) in the maintenance of intestinal integrity. Non-specific defence mechanisms are also capable of influencing events in the intestine and many of the defence strategies adopted involve a synergistic interaction between specific acquired and non-specific mechanisms (for review, see Newby, 1984).

Non-specific defence mechanisms

Within the gastrointestinal tract there are a number of non-specific systems which collectively act to prevent organisms from colonising the intestine (see

Table 10.1. *Non-specific defence mechanisms in the gastrointestinal tract*

Defence mechanism	Anti-microbial activity
Epithelial barrier	Physical barrier
	Rapid turnover of cells and receptors
Gastric pH	Directly bacteriocidal
	Promotes proteolytic breakdown
	Selection of bacterial flora
Peristalsis	Maintains luminal flow and inhibits colonisation
Mucus	Prevents microbial adhesion to epithelium
Biliary and	Inactivation of viruses and certain bacteria
Pancreatic secretions	
	Selection of bacterial flora
	Proteolysis
Microflora	Competition for microbial binding sites
Lactoferrin	Bacteriostatic
Lysozyme	Bactriocidal
Interferon	Anti-viral activity

Table 10.1). Certain of these, such as gastric pH, biliary and pancreatic secretions, lactoferrin, lysozyme and interferon have a direct anti-microbial activity. For others, their effect is indirect. For example, the epithelial surface forms a physical barrier that is continually being renewed. Cells that are generated by division in the crypts, migrate up the villus wall, mature and are shed long before they become effete. The scale of epithelial cell turnover is at considerable cost in terms of energy, and in humans it has been estimated that between 20 and 50 million cells are shed from the intestine each minute (Croft *et al.*, 1968). This ensures that no damaged cells remain and provide a focus for infection and also that the enterocytes provide only a minimal period for pathogens to adhere and infect cells, affording an 'escalator', moving against the infectious agent. The process of removal is greatly facilitated by the continuous flow of luminal contents as brought about by peristalsis and the flow of mucus. The latter is capable of entrapping bacteria and nematodes, so much so, that certain highly successful enteric bacteria, such as *Vibrio cholera*, produce mucolytic enzymes that enable them to reach the epithelial cell surface (Hoskins & Zamcheck, 1968). The mucus layer possesses regions that mimic the receptor sites for bacteria on epithelial cells. For example, in pigs it has been shown that 987P+ enterotoxigenic *E. coli* (ETEC) bind not only to a 33–39 kD villus

epithelial receptor, but also a <17 kD component in mucus (Dean, 1990). In experimental models and also in a few clinical and field situations, the administration of specific receptor analogues has had a protective effect. The indigenous microflora are also able to resist colonisation by pathogenic microorganisms. For example, 'normal' mice require an oral dose of approximately 10^6 *Salmonella enteritidis* to cause infection, whilst following a single dose of streptomycin, the number required is reduced to as few as ten (Bohnoff & Miller, 1962).

Specific immune mechanisms in gut infection

In response to non-invasive enteric infections, such as those caused by *Vibrio* cholera and enterotoxigenic *E. coli*, sIgA appears to be the main, although perhaps not the only protective molecule (Holmgren & Svennerholm, 1983). The predominance of IgA-producing plasma cells in the lamina propria of the intestine, the secretory component-dependent mechanism by which it is transported into the gut lumen and its relative resistance to normal intestinal proteases, make antibodies of this isotype uniquely well suited to protect the intestinal mucosal surface (Mestecky & McGhee, 1987). The immunological activities of sIgA are essentially non-inflammatory, thus avoiding any simultaneous damage to the mucosal surface. Its protective function is provided through immune exclusion, preventing the binding of bacterial and viral pathogens, bacterial toxins, and other molecules potentially harmful to epithelial cells. In experimental models, sIgA has also shown to mediate antibody-dependent T-cell mediated cytotoxicity and to interfere with the utilisation of essential bacterial growth factors such as iron. Although there is clear evidence for memory in the sIgA system, it has been observed that the duration of gastrointestinal responses is relatively short (Evans *et al.*, 1980), lasting for only months in humans (Quiding *et al.*, 1991).

In the protective response to invasive enteric infections (e.g. *Salmonella*, *Shigella*), cell-mediated mucosal reactions, including MHC restricted cellular cytotoxicity (CTL), natural killer cell activity and antibody-dependent cellular cytotoxicity, have all been implicated (Tagliabue *et al.*, 1985). Experimental studies have indicated that intestinal T cells may modulate the kinetics of epithelial cell renewal (Ferguson & MacDonald, 1977: MacDonald & Spencer, 1992) and it has been suggested that this may have a physiological role in eliminating infected cells. Such a process may include a more rapid loss of cells and an associated increase in the number of goblet cells. Gastrointestinal T cell populations are heterogeneous and vary in their distribution. Within the epithelium, intra-epithelial lymphocytes (IEL) are predominantly of a $CD3^+CD2^+CD8^+$ phenotype and their granular appearance together with the presence of granzymes and perforine is consistent with a cytotoxic role (Mcl.Mowat, 1990). Murine IELs have potent NK activity against enteric viruses (Carmen *et al.*, 1986) and cells isolated from reovirus infected mice will lyse reovirus infected cells in a MHC restricted fashion (Taterka, Cuff & Rubin, 1992). Mouse IEL have also been shown to inhibit the growth of *Salmonella* and *Shigella*, a process which was enhanced by the presence of sIgA (Tagliabue *et al.*, 1984). Lymphokine secretion by IEL has been studied and reported to include gamma-IFN, TNFα, IL-3, GM-CSF and under certain conditions IL-2 (for review, see Mcl.Mowat, 1990). With respect to protection, most attention has been focused on gamma-IFN, which has been shown to inhibit the receptivity of epithelial cells for *Shigella* (Holmgren, Fryklund & Larsson 1989).

The lamina propria is highly cellular and in some species greater than 40% of these cells may express T cell markers. Of the CD4 T cells in the lamina propria, very few express the Leu-8 or CD45RA antigens, suggesting that they may have mainly helper activity. The majority of cells are CD45RO$^+$ve indicating a high proportion of memory or recently activated cells (for review, see James, 1992). Further evidence of activation may be gleaned from the expression of IL-2R and HLA-DR molecules. Approximately half of the lamina propria T cells express CD28, suggesting that cells with cytolytic function are present. In contrast, very few lamina propria cells are CD16$^+$ve, a phenotype associated with NK activity in peripheral blood. Lamina propria cells can be activated to secrete high levels of IL-4, IL-5 and IL-6, with lower levels of IL-2 and gamma-interferon. Despite displaying many of the phenotypic features of cytotoxic cells, to date, there is little functional data to indicate that lamina propria lymphocytes do fulfil this role.

Intestinal infections

Enteric infections associated with bacteria, viruses and parasites are a world health problem accounting for at least one billion episodes of diarrhoea and up to 10 million deaths in the Third World each year. Pre-school children are particularly vulnerable and in a number of developing countries, diarrhoeal diseases account for as many as 25–33% of all mortality in this age group. With the exception of rotaviruses, which are responsible for a high proportion of diarrhoeal episodes in children below the age of two, the predominant pathogens causing acute diarrhoeal disease are bacteria.

Bacterial enteropathogens

Enterotoxigenic and enteropathogenic *E. coli*, *Shigella*, *Vibrio cholera*, *Campylobacter* and *Salmonella* are all major human pathogens (Farthing &

Keusch, 1989). Infectivity of different enteric bacteria shows considerable variation with as few as 10^1 to 10^2 *Shigella* organisms capable of establishing infection, whereas 10^8 to 10^9 *E. coli* may be required. In order for an enteropathogen to establish infection, it must be able to colonise the intestine and adherence of the microorganism to the intestinal epithelium, is a critical step in this process. Adherence is dependent on receptor-ligand interactions and it is reasonable to assume that all enteropathogens possess distinct fimbrial, or outer membrane protein attachment factors (adhesins or colonisation factors). Mannose specific, type 1 fimbriae, are associated with several bacterial species (Dugid, Clegg & Wilson, 1979), but for many *E. coli* strains the carbohydrate binding specificity does not depend on the presence of mannose in the receptor structure. For example, strains of *E. coli* which cause diarrhoea in neonatal calves, lambs and piglets have been shown to carry a plasmid encoded antigen, K99, which recognises the ceramide structure [NeuAcÁ(2–3)GalNacβ(1–4)Galβ(1–4)] (Faris, Lindahl & Wadstrom 1990). Such structures are typical of host receptors, which commonly consist of oligosaccharides present in glycoconjugates on epithelial cell surface, or possibly also in the mucus layer. The expression of many of the host receptors is dependent upon the age of the animal and the degree of maturation of the enterocyte and this in part may explain differences in susceptibility to infection.

Once bacteria adhere to the epithelium, they may exert their pathological processes by a variety of mechanisms. Cholera and enterotoxigenic *E. coli*, do not invade or damage enterocytes, but secrete enterotoxins that bind to specific epithelial receptors, leading to a watery diarrhoea and dehydration (for review, see Holmgren & Svennerholm, 1992). The heat-labile enterotoxin (LT) of *E. coli* and cholera toxin are antigenically and immunologically very closely related (Gyles 1971) and consist of two polypeptide subunits, A and B, which are present in the stoichiometric ratio of 1A:5B (Dallas & Falkow, 1979). The B subunit mediates binding of the toxin to the receptor, GM1 gangliosides on the cell surface (Critchley *et al.*, 1982). The A subunit (which is made up of two, A1 and A2 peptides, linked by a disulphide bond) is involved in the stimulation of adenyl cyclase and there is increased formation of cyclic AMP (Gill & Richardson, 1980). This results in increased secretion of fluid and electrolyte by the crypt cells and cells on the side of villi in the small intestine. *E. coli* also produce heat stable enterotoxins (ST), which cause their diarrhoeagenic effects by activating the particulate form of intestinal guanylate cyclase and increasing the intracellular concentration of cyclic GMP (Hughes *et al.*, 1978). Taken together bacterial enterotoxins may be responsible for as many as 50% of all diarrhoeal disease worldwide.

Pathogenicity of other bacteria, involves invasion into or through the intestinal epithelium. Some, such as *Shigella*, produce damage to the epithelium, with ulceration and blood loss. Others, including *Campylobacter* and non-typhoid salmonella, do not cause direct damage, but generate severe tissue-damaging inflammatory responses in the lamina propria and Peyer's patches (Kopecko, Venkatesan & Buysse, 1989).

Enteroviruses

Rotavirus infection is the most common cause of severe diarrhoea in infants and young children worldwide, resulting in an estimated 140 million cases and 1 million deaths per year. The most important mode of transmission of rotavirus is thought to be the faecal–oral route, but it is possible that airborne or droplet routes may also play a role. In susceptible individuals, the virus is highly infectious with a minimal infective innoculum of as few as ten particles, whereas an individual may shed as many as 10^{12} particles per ml of faeces. The virus selectively infects and kills mature enterocytes in the small intestine, without infecting the immature crypt cells. Virus infection results in exfoliation of mature enterocytes, with resultant stunted villi. These stunted villi have a reduced capacity to absorb fluid and there is a net loss of fluid and electrolytes from the small intestine (for review see Taterka *et al.*, 1992). It has been shown that similar pathological changes may be induced by local cell mediated immune responses in the intestine and it has been postulated that these may also be of importance in causing the malabsorption. Studies of experimental infection of lambs with rotavirus have clarified this question, as it was found that the increase in epithelial cell proliferation, was secondary to virally induced damage to mature enterocytes and therefore not dependent on the host response to infection (Snodgrass *et al.*, 1981).

Intestinal parasites

Over the past decade, there has been a growing appreciation of the importance of giardiasis in man. *Giardia lamblia* is a protozoan parasite that is well adapted to the upper small intestine (for review, see Farthing, 1990). The cyst form is highly resilient in the environment and, in human volunteer studies, it has been found that as few as ten cysts are capable of initiating infection. The low pH of the stomach is thought to promote exacystation and the trophozoites localise preferentially in the upper small intestine, initial attachment possibly being mediated by a specific lectin on the parasite that is revealed by host proteases. Whilst lectin-associated binding may serve to initially localise the *Giardia*, subsequent mechanical attachment is by a ventral sucker disc. Bile has a trophic effect on growth and raising the pH stimulates encystation, promoting the shedding of cysts and trophozoites in the faeces. The pathogenesis of the diarrhoea and malabsorption is multifactorial, involving both luminal factors and mucosal damage (Katelaris &

Farthing 1992). On the one hand, *Giardia* have been shown to consume bile salts (so contributing to fat malabsorption) and alter pancreatic exocrine function, resulting in reduced tryptic, chymotryptic and pancreatic lipase activity. It has also been suggested that *Giardia* may induce a motility disturbance (possibly mediated by prostaglandin E_2), with rapid transit and decreased absorptive time. In patients infected with *Giardia lamblia*, villous and crypt hypertrophy can produce malabsorption in severe cases. There are also marked increases in the numbers of IEL, some which can be seen extruding into the lumen (Owen, Nemanic & Stevens, 1979). The protective significance of this is unclear, since although spontaneous cytotoxicity of mouse IEL against *Giardia* has been reported, electron microscopy would indicate that trophozoites of *Giardia* are phagocytosed by macrophages and not killed by IEL.

Vaccines against enteropathogens

The concept of local intestinal immunity and of immunisation via the oral route is not new and was well documented by Besredka (1927) in a series of investigations published during the first three decades of this century. Despite this, progress has been slow and there are a number of reasons that can be put forward to explain why this is so. Most relate to the observations that mucosal responses are most effectively induced by mucosal presentation of antigen and the complex array of antigens that are presented to the intestinal immune system. In particular, with respect to the latter, it is noteworthy that the vast majority of antigens presented to the gastrointestinal immune system (i.e. dietary antigens) impose no direct threat and, that any harm that may result, is largely as a consequence of the host's inappropriate (allergic) response to them. Therefore, it is not unreasonable to consider that the first response of the intestinal immune system is a 'low grade' response, that might 'down-regulate' subsequent responses to that antigen. Such a response, a small local IgA response, with orally induced systemic humoral tolerance, together with local and systemic tolerance of cell mediated responses, whilst being beneficial in the handling of a harmless dietary constituent is clearly an inappropriate response to a potential pathogen. It is against this background, that the search for a vaccine to protect against mucosal infection, must be sought.

Parenteral immunisation

Parenteral immunisation has been used in an effort to overcome the inherent problems associated with stimulation via the oral route. Studies in rats have indicated that under certain conditions, it is possible to access Peyer's patches via the serosal surface (Pierce & Gowans, 1975: Husband & Gowans, 1978). This has been achieved when complete Freund's adjuvant (CFA) is used and, although this approach has been extended to immunise sheep and pigs (Husband, Beh & Lascelles 1979), the complications associated with the use of CFA by the intraperitoneal route, make it not acceptable generally. In an attempt to overcome this, the properties of other adjuvants (saponin, muramyl dipeptide), formulated in either vegetable oil emulsion or liposome vehicles, have been investigated with encouraging results (Husband, 1993).

Studies in experimental animals suggested that with various combinations, systemic and oral immunisation might be used in order to generate a mucosal response. This approach has been extended to human populations by Svennerholm et al. (1977), who showed that parenteral immunisation with *cholera*, resulted in an sIgA response in the breast milk of Pakistani women from a cholera endemic area, but not in Swedish women who had not previously encountered the organism. Similarly people who had recovered from cholera or diarrhoea caused by ETEC producing heat-labile enterotoxin, responded with a vigorous gut mucosal IgA antitoxin response, to a dose of orally administered CTB, that was below the threshold to elicit any response in naive individuals (Holmgren et al., 1988).

Oral immunisation

In general, the conclusion that responses which are protective in the gastrointestinal tract are best stimulated by mucosal presentation of antigen, remains valid. The process of immunisation is complicated by a number of factors, many of which have been already discussed. Based on these, it is possible to identify those characteristics which may be beneficial for a mucosal vaccine. First, live organisms are more effective than non-replicating antigen; secondly, the response to non-replicating antigens is highly dose dependent; thirdly, an ability to adhere to the intestinal epithelium and activate adenylate cyclase; fourthly, targeting via Peyer's patches, and finally an ability to survive in the harsh environment of the gastrointestinal tract. The majority of these features are best illustrated with respect to the development of an oral cholera vaccine. Oral vaccines based on heat and formalin-killed *Vibrio cholera*, either in combination with or without the GM1 binding B subunit, have been used in large-scale clinical trials in Bangladesh, the results of which have shown that both may confer long-lasting protection against cholera, with over 60% protection over a three year follow-up (Clemens et al., 1990). Interestingly, the long-term protective efficacy was greater in those individuals who were over five years of age when vaccinated, indicating that age and possibly 'immunological experience', may be of importance in determining the outcome of this type of vaccine.

The use of these killed vaccines was not associated with any of the adverse reactions, which are occasionally observed with live preparations. By recombinant DNA technology, a *V. cholera* strain deleted of the A subunit gene has been produced. Vaccination of volunteers with this strain resulted in only minimal diarrhoeal side-effect and elicited good antibacterial and antitoxic immune responses, along with significant protection against challenge (Levine *et al.*, 1988; Levine & Kapper 1993)). Live, attenuated, oral vaccines have also been developed for other enteropathogens including *Shigella* sp. and *Salmonella typhi*. With *Shigella*, two approaches have been used (Lindberg & Pal, 1993]. The first, involving the construction of hybrid strains, based largely on the expression of O antigens of *Shigella*, in either *E. coli*, or attenuated *Salmonella*, are largely at the developmental phase (Baron *et al.*, 1987). The second, based on the production of Shigella mutants, which are either substrate dependent (e.g. Aro-, aromatic amino acids or ThyA, thymine) or temperature sensitive, have already been used in monkeys and have provided protection against experimental challenge (Lindberg *et al.*, 1990). Work with live, oral, *Salmonella typhi* vaccines, is more advanced. In particular, a gal-epimerase-deficient mutant Ty21a, has been derived by chemical mutagenesis (Germanier & Fuer, 1975) and incorporated in enteric coated capsules. Clinical trials have resulted in varying degrees of protection, but ranging up to 66% over a five-year period in Chilean schoolchildren (Levine, 1989).

Live, attenuated vaccines have also been used to protect against enteroviruses. Oral immunisation with tissue culture, attenuated, rotaviruses of bovine and rhesus origin, have been found to provide significant clinical protection, from severe gastroenteritis in Finnish children, during the first two to three years of life (Vesikari, 1993).

There are many who would view an extension of the use of live vaccines with some reluctance and therefore the need remains to develop delivery systems, that potentiate the response to fed, non-replicating antigens. At this time, there are two approaches which are the focus of particular attention. Cholera toxin (CT) has the property of not only being a potent stimulator of IgA anti-CT responses, but also of acting as an adjuvant for IgA responses, to an unrelated protein antigen, fed at the same time (Elson & Ealding, 1984). There are two properties of CT which may underlie this activity. Firstly, the ability of the B subunit to bind and cross link the ganglioside GM1, may alter cell function and adhere CT to the intestinal epithelium (Holmgren, 1973). Secondly, the A subunit may enter the cell, where it acts by catalysing the ADP-ribosylation of the stimulator G-protein (Gs) of the adenylate cyclase complex and results in up-regulation of cyclic AMP (Gill & Woolkalis 1988). The relative importance of each of these properties is unclear, partly as a result of conflicting results obtained in experiments with animals of differing microbial health status and where immunisation has been via mucosal surfaces, other than the gut. In the intestine of mice, it has generally been found that the effectiveness of CTB as an adjuvant is considerably less than that of CT, but that, when small sub-optimal amounts of CTB and CT were fed together, they had a synergistic effect (Wilson, Clarke & Stokes 1990). To date, most of the studies of the mucosal adjuvant properties of CT have been confined to rodents, but there is evidence that it may be active in other species. In this regard, it is encouraging that there has been considerable progress in the development of more acceptable presentation systems for CTB and heat labile entero-toxin of *E. coli* and other bacterial toxins, as carriers for oral immunisation (Nashar *et al.*, 1993). Recently, there has been considerable interest in the use of biodegradable microparticles to entrap antigen for oral immunisation (Eldridge *et al.*, 1991; O'Hagen *et al.*, 1993). These offer considerable potential, in that they may protect antigen from the hostile environment of the gut, as well being preferentially localised in Peyer's patches. Import-antly, with regard to the possible future transfer of the encouraging experimental data obtained in rodents to clinical trials in man, is the fact that these preparations are already widely used as drug delivery systems for administration to humans. Other non-living carrier systems have been tested for mucosal delivery of antigen and a number hold out considerable promise. Besides those already mentioned, immunostimulating complexes (ISCOMS) and protein carriers such as the core antigen of hepatitis B virus and Ty particles of yeast, are the focus of attention at present (Randall, 1989; Morein *et al.*, 1987). Currently, it is clear that no one system fulfils all the necessary criteria of acceptability and it is likely that this may well be found in a combination of the above. A growing appreciation that protection from HIV infection may well require a mucosal response, is likely to be a considerable incentive in achieving this.

Future control of enteric infections, requires successfully negotiating a number of steps. It has always been the case that many of these stages (for example identification and localisation of the infectious agent) have required and will continue to require, studies in the target species, in this case man. Advances in *in vitro* culture systems, also means that an under-standing of a number of the mechanisms, of microbial and immunopathoge-nesis, can also be achieved without the use of animal models. The relative lack of progress, in developing mucosal vaccines, has in the past been largely a consequence of the empirical approach and current and future experi-ments in other species may be of considerable benefit, in this regard. In particular, it is to be expected that they may contribute to an understanding of the cellular and molecular mechanisms of induction of mucosal responses, to the wide variety of antigens presented and that this in turn will provide a rational basis for the development of vaccines. What must be clearly apparent from this discussion, is that providing protection from intestinal infection, will not come as a by-product of studies of systemic immunity, but only as a consequence of detailed analysis of this unique immunological compartment.

References

Baron, L. S., Kopecko, D. J., Formal, S. B. *et al.* (1987). Introduction of *Salmonella flexneri* 2a type and group antigens into oral typhoid vaccine strain Ty21a. *Infection and Immunity*, **55**, 2797–801.

Besredka, A. (1927). *Local Immunisation*. Baltimore, USA: Williams & Wilkins.

Bohnoff, M. & Miller, C. P. (1962). Enhanced susceptibility to *Salmonella* infections in streptomycin treated mice. *Journal of Infectious Diseases*, **111**, 117–27.

Brown, W. R., Savage, D. C., Dubois, R. S., Alp, M. H., Mallory, A. & Kern, F. (1972). Intestinal microflora of immunoglobulin-deficient and normal human subjects. *Gastroenterology*, **62**, 1143–52.

Carmen, P. S., Ernst, P. B., Rosenthal, K. L., Clark, D. L., Befus, A. D. & Bienenstock, J. (1986). Intraepithelial leukocytes contain a unique sub-pupulation of NK-like cytotoxic cells active in the defence of gut epithelium to enteric murine coronavirus. *Journal of Immunology*, **136**, 1548–53.

Clemens, J. D., Sack, D. A., Harris, J. R. F. *et al.* (1990). Field trial of oral cholera vaccines in Bangladesh: report from three year follow-up. *Lancet*, **335**, 270–73.

Critchley, D. R., Steuli, C. H., Kellie, S., Ansell, S. & Patel, B. (1982). Characterisation of the cholera toxin receptor on Balb/c 3T3 cells as similar to, or identical with GM1. *Biochemical Journal* **204**, 209–19.

Croft, D. N., Loehry, C. A., Taylor, J. F. N. & Cole, J. (1968). DNA and cell loss from small intestinal mucosa. *Lancet*, **ii**, 70–3.

Dallas, W. & Falkow, S. (1979). The molecular nature of heat-labile enterotoxin (LT) of *Escherichia coli*. *Nature*, **277**, 406–7.

Dean, E. A. (1990). Comparison of receptors for 987P pilli of enterotoxigenic *Escherichia coli* in small intestines of neonatal and older pigs. *Infection and Immunity*, **58**, 4030–35.

Dugid, J. P., Clegg, S. & Wilson, M. I. (1979). The fimbrial and non-fimbrial haemagglutinins of *Escherichia coli*. *Journal of Medical Microbiology*, **12**, 213–27.

Eldridge, J. H., Staas, J. K., Meubroek, J. A. *et al.* (1991). Biodegradable microspheres as a vaccine delivery system. *Molecular Immunology*, **28**, 287–94.

Elson, C. J. & Ealding, W. (1984). Generalised systemic and mucosal immunity after mucosal stimulation with cholera toxin. *Journal of Immunology*, **132**, 2736–41.

Evans, P. A., Newby, T. J., Stokes, C. R., Patel, D. & Bourne, F. J. (1980). Antibody responses of the lactating sow to oral immunisation with *Escherichia coli*. *Scandinavian Journal of Immunology*, **11**, 419–29.

Faris, A., Lindahl, M. & Wadstrom, T. (1990). GM2-like glycoconjugate as possible erythrocyte receptor for the CFA/1 and K99 hemagglutinins of enterotoxigenic *Escherichia coli*. *FEMS Microbiology Letters*, **7**, 265–9.

Farthing, M. J. G. & Keusch, G. T. (eds.) (1989). *Enteric Infection. Mechanisms, Manifestations and Management*. Chapman & Hall, London, UK.

Farthing, M. J. G. (1990). Immunopathology of Giardiasis. *Springer Seminars in Immunopathology*, **12**, 269–82.

Ferguson, A. & MacDonald, T. T. (1977). Effects of local delayed hypersensitivity on the small intestine immunology of the gut. *Ciba Foundation Symposia*, **46**, 305–27.

Germanier, R. & Fuer, E. (1975). Isolation and characterisation of *Gal* E mutant Ty21a of *Salmonella typhi*: a candisate strain for a live oral typhoid vaccine. *Journal of Infectious Diseases*, **131**, 553–8.

Gill, D. M. & Richardson, S. H. (1980). Adenosine diphosphate-ribosylation of adenylate cyclase catalysed by heat-labile enterotoxin of Escherichia coli: comparison with cholera toxin. *Journal of Infectious Diseases* **141**, 64–70.

Gill, D. M. & Woolkalis, M. (1988). [^{32}P] ADP-Ribosylation of proteins catalyzed by cholera toxin and related enterotoxins. *Methods in Enzymology*, **165**, 235–45.

Gyles, C. L. (1971). Heat-labile and heat-stable forms of the enterotoxin from *E. coli* strains enteropathogenic for pigs. *Annals of NY Academy of Science* **276**, 314–22.

Holmgren, J. & Svennerholm, A.-M. (1983). Cholera and the immune response. *Progress in Allergy*, **33**, 106–19.

Holmgren, J. & Svennerholm, A.-M. (1992). Bacterial Enteric infection and vaccine development. *Gastroenterology Clinics of North America* **21**, 283–302.

Holmgren, J. (1973). Comparison of the tissue receptors for *Vibrio cholera* and *Escherichia coli* enterotoxins by means of ganglosides and natural cholera toxoid. *Infection and Immunity*, **8**, 851–9.

Holmgren, J., Fryklund, J. & Larsson, H. (1989). Gamma-interferon-mediated down regulation of electrolyte secretion by intestinal epithelial cells: a local immune mechanism? *Scandinavian Journal of Immunology*, **30**, 499–503.

Holmgren, J., Svennerholm, A.-M., Gothefors, L. *et al.* (1988). Enterotoxigenic *Escherichia coli* diarrhoea in an endemic area prepares the intestine for an amanestic immunoglobulin A Antitoxin response to oral cholera B Subunit vaccination. *Infection and Immunity*, **56**, 230–3.

Hoskins, L. C. & Zamcheck, N. (1968). Bacterial degradation of gastrointestinal mucins. 1. Comparison of mucus constituents in the stools of germ-free and conventional rats. *Gastroenterology*, **54**, 210–17.

Hughes, J. M., Murand, F., Chang, B. & Guerrant, R. L. (1978). Role of cyclic GMP in the action of heat-stable enterotoxin of *Escherichia coli*. *Nature*, **271**, 755–6.

Husband, A. J. & Gowans, J. L. (1978). The origin and antigen-dependent distribution of IgA-containing cells in the intestine. *Journal of Experimental Medicine*, **148**, 1146–60.

Husband, A. J. (1993). Novel vaccination strategies for the control of mucosal infection. *Vaccine*, **11**, 107–12.

Husband, A. J., Beh, K. J. & Lascelles, A. K. (1979). IgA containing cells in the ruminant intestine following intraperitoneal and local immunisation. *Immunology*, **37**, 597–601.

James, S. J. (1992). Mucosal T cell function. *Gastroenterology Clinics of North America*, **21**, 597–612.

Katelaris, P. H. & Farthing, M. J. G. (1992). Diarrhoea and malabsorption in giardiasis: a multifactorial process? *Gut*, **33**, 295–7.

Kopecko, D. J., Venkatesan, M., Buysse, J. M. (1989). Basic mechanisms and genetic control of bacterial invasion. In *Enteric Infection: Mechanisms Manifestation and Management*. (eds.) M. J. C. Farthing & G. T. Keusch. London, UK: Chapman & Hall. p. 41.

Levine, M. M. (1989). Development of vaccines against bacteria. In *Enteric Infections: Mechanisms, Manifestations and Management*. (eds.) M. J. G. Farthing & G. T. Keusch. London, UK: Chapman & Hall. p. 495.

Levine, M. M., Herrington, D., Losonsky, G. *et al.* (1988). Safety, immunogenicity, and efficacy of recombinant live oral cholera vaccines, CVD 103 and CVD 103-HgR. *Lancet*, **ii**, 467–70.

Levine, M. M. & Kapper, J. B. (1993). Live oral vaccines against cholera: an update. *Vaccine*, **11**, 207–12.

Lindberg, A., Karnell, A., Pal, T. *et al*. (1990). Construction of an auxotrophic *Shigella flexneri* strain for use as a live vaccine. *Microbial Pathogenetic*, **8**, 433–40.

Lindberg, A. A. & Pal, T. (1993). Strategies for the development of potential *Shigella* vaccines. *Vaccine*, **11**, 168–79.

MacDonald, T. T. & Spencer, J. (1992). Cell-mediated immune injury in the intestine. *Gastroenterology Clinics of North America*, **21**, 367–86.

Mcl.Mowat, A. (1990). Human Intraepithelial lymphocytes. *Springer Seminars in Immunopathology*, **12**, 165–90.

Mestecky, J. & McGhee, J. R. (1987). Molecular and cellular interactions involved in IgA biosynthesis and immune response. *Advances in Immunology*, **40**, 153–245.

Morein, B., Lovgren, K., Hoglund, S. & Sandquist, B. (1987). The ISCOM: an immunostimulating complex. *Immunology Today*, **8**, 333–8.

Nashar, T. O., Amin, T., Marcello, A. & Hirst, T. R. (1993). Current progress in the development of the B subunits of cholera toxin and *Escherichia coli* heat-labile enterotoxins as carriers for the oral delivery of heterologous antigens and epitopes. *Vaccine* **11**, 235–40.

Newby, T. J. (1984). Protective immune responses in the intestinal tract. In *Local Immune Responses of the Gut*, (ed.) T. J. Newby & C. R. Stokes. pp. 143–198. Boca Raton USA: CRC Press Inc.

O'Hagen, D. T., McGee, J. P., Holmgren, J. *et al*. (1993). Biodegradable microparticle for oral immunisation. *Vaccine*, **11**, 149–54.

Owen, R. L., Nemanic, P. C. & Stevens, D. P. (1979). Ultrastructural observations on Giardiasis in a murine model. 1. Intestinal distribution, attachment, and relationship to the immune system in *Giardia muris*. *Gastroenterology*, **76**, 757–69.

Pierce, N. F. & Gowans, J. L. (1975). Cellular kinetics of the intestinal response to cholera toxoid in rats. *Journal of Experimental Medicine*, **14**, 1550–63.

Quiding, M., Nordstrom, I., Kilander, A. *et al*. (1991). Intestinal immune responses in humans: oral cholera vaccination induces strong intestinal antibody and interferon-gamma production and evokes local immunological memory. *Journal of Clinical Investigations*, **88**, 143–8.

Randall, R. E. (1989). Solid matrix–antibody–antigen (SMAA) complexes for constructing multivalent subunit vaccines. *Immunology Today*, **10**, 336–9.

Snodgrass, D. R., Ferguson, A., Allan, F., Angus, K. W. & Mitchell, B. (1981). Small intestinal morphology and epithelial cell kinetics in lamb rotavirus infections. *Gastroenterology*, **76**, 477–503.

Svennerholm, A.-M., Holmgren, J., Hanson, L. A. *et al*. (1977). Boosting of secretory IgA antibody responses in man by parenteral cholera vaccination. *Scandinavian Journal of Immunology*, **6**, 1345–9.

Tagliabue, A., Boraschi, D., Villa, L., Keren, D. F., Lowell, G. H., Rappuoli, R. & Nenconi, L. (1984). IgA dependent cell-mediated activity against enteropathogenic bacteria: distribution, specificity and characterisation of the effector cells. *Journal of Immunology*, **133**, 988–92.

Tagliabue, A., Nenconi, L., Caffarena, A., Villa, L., Boraschi, D., Cazzola, G. & Cavalieri, S. (1985). Cellular immunity against *Salmonella typhi* after live oral vaccine. *Clinical and Experimental Immunology*, **62**, 242–7.

Taterka, J. A., Cuff, C. F. & Rubin X. (1992). Viral gastrointestinal infections. *Gastroenterology Clinics of North America*, **21**, 303–30.

Vesikari, T. (1993). Clinical trials of live oral rotavirus vaccines: the Finnish experience. *Vaccine*, **11**, 255–61.

Wilson, A. D., Clarke, C. J. & Stokes, C. R. (1990). Whole cholera toxin and B-Subunit act synergistically as an adjuvant for the mucosal immune response of mice to keyhole limpet haemocyanin. *Scandinavian Journal of Immunology*, **31**, 443–51.

–11–
Lymphomas

A. C. WOTHERSPOON and P. G. ISAACSON

Introduction

The gastrointestinal tract is the commonest site of primary extra-nodal lymphoma, accounting for 30–50% of cases (Freeman, Berg & Cutler, 1972, Otter *et al.*, 1989). The lymphomas are almost exclusively non-Hodgkin's type, primary gastrointestinal Hodgkin's disease being extremely rare. There is considerable geographic variation in the incidence of primary gastrointestinal lymphoma: the highest incidence is in the Middle East where 25% of all lymphomas arise in the gastrointestinal tract. In Western countries, gastrointestinal lymphoma comprises 4–18% of all non-Hodgkin's lymphoma, but this incidence may be increasing (Hayes & Dunn, 1989, Azab *et al.*, 1989).

Primary nodal lymphoma involves the gastrointestinal tract as a secondary phenomenon in up to 25% of cases (Fischbach *et al.*, 1992). Strict criteria have therefore been applied for the diagnosis of primary gastrointestinal lymphoma, requiring that the lymphoma be limited to the gastrointestinal tract and contiguous lymph nodes (Dawson, Cornes & Morson, 1961). While ensuring that such lymphomas truly arise in the gastrointestinal tract such a strict definition excludes the possibility of disseminated primary gastrointestinal lymphoma and skews survival data towards a favourable prognosis. The recognition that some primary gastrointestinal lymphomas are morphologically and immunophenotypically distinct has, to a certain extent, circumvented this problem.

With the possible exception of cerebriform T cell lymphoma, any lymphoma listed in the standard lymphoma classifications may arise in the gastrointestinal tract. In terms of frequency, however, the types of lymphoma occurring in the peripheral lymph nodes and the gastrointestinal tract are quite different. A classification of gastrointestinal lymphomas is given in Table 11.1.

In Western countries, the stomach is the commonest site of primary gastrointestinal lymphoma, followed by the small intestine. In the Middle East, however, this distribution is reversed. In both areas, primary oesophageal, colonic and rectal lymphoma account for a minority of cases.

Gastrointestinal lymphoma is most commonly staged using a modification of the Ann Arbor system (Musshoff, 1977). In stage I_E (where E signifies an

Table 11.1. *Primary gastrointestinal non-Hodgkin's lymphoma*

B CELL
1. Lymphomas of mucosa associated lymphoid tissue (MALT)
   a   Low grade B cell lymphoma of MALT
   b   High grade B cell lymphoma of MALT with or without a low grade component
   c   Immunoproliferative small intestinal disease (IPSID)

2. Malignant lymphoma, mantle cell type (lymphomatous polyposis)

3. Burkitt's lymphoma

4. Low and high grade lymphomas corresponding to peripheral lymph node equivalents

T CELL
1. Enteropathy associated T cell lymphoma (EATL)

2. Other types unassociated with enteropathy

RARE TYPES

---

extra-nodal site), the lymphoma is confined to the wall of the stomach or intestine. Stage II implies involvement of regional lymph nodes, which may be contiguous (stage II_{1E}) or non-contiguous (stage II_{2E}). Stage III refers to involvement of lymph nodes on both sides of the diaphragm, the spleen (stage III_S) or both (stage III_{E+S}). In stage IV there is dissemination to the bone marrow or to other non-lymphoid organs.

Low grade B cell lymphoma of mucosa associated lymphoid tissue (MALT)

In Western countries, lymphomas of mucosa-associated lymphoid tissue (MALT) occur most frequently in the stomach, an organ normally devoid of MALT. Histologically identical intestinal (Marchi *et al.*, 1990, Radaszie-wicz, Dragosics & Bauer, 1992) and oesophageal lymphomas (Isaacson & Spencer, 1987) do occur, but are rare. The highest concentration of MALT in the normal individual, the Peyer's patches of the terminal ileum, is a rare site of primary MALT lymphoma. This apparent paradox is explained by the observation that lymphomas frequently arise in MALT that is acquired as part of an autoimmune disease or possibly in response to infection (Hyjek, Smith & Isaacson, 1988, Hyjek & Isaacson, 1988, Wotherspoon *et al.*, 1991).

Primary gastric lymphomas appear to arise from MALT that has been acquired in response to *Helicobacter pylori* infection (Wotherspoon *et al.*, 1991). It has been shown that lymphoid follicles are found in the gastric mucosa only in the presence of concurrent or recent infection by *Helicobacter pylori*, when they are present in approximately 50% of cases (Wyatt & Rathbone, 1988. Stolte & Eidt, 1989). Further studies of the chronic gastritis associated with *Helicobacter pylori* infection showed that these lymphoid follicles were frequently associated with collections of intraepithelial B cells in a pattern reminiscent of MALT (Wotherspoon *et al.*, 1991). Further evidence that lymphoma arises from this acquired MALT is provided both by the finding of *Helicobacter pylori* organisms adjacent to over 90% of primary gastric B cell lymphomas (Wotherspoon *et al.*, 1991) and by the observation of high gastric lymphoma prevalence in an area with an associated high prevalence of *Helicobacter* gastritis (Doglioni *et al.*, 1992). The relationship between *Helicobacter pylori* and gastric lymphoma is therefore similar to that proposed for gastric adenocarcinoma (Parsonnet *et al.*, 1991). Whether there are similar pre-conditions for the origin of MALT lymphomas elsewhere in the gastrointestinal tract is not known.

Low grade MALT lymphoma occur predominantly in individuals over 50 with a peak incidence in the seventh decade, although an increasing number of cases are being reported in younger patients. The male:female ratio is approximately 1.5:1. The symptoms are usually non-specific and in the case of gastric MALT lymphoma are usually of dyspepsia. Small intestinal lymphoma often presents with intestinal obstruction, while rectal bleeding is a common presenting symptom in colonic MALT lymphoma. Severe abdominal pain or the presence of an abdominal mass is rare. In cases of gastric lymphoma the tumour usually involves the antrum and the findings at endoscopy are frequently of non-specific gastritis and/or peptic ulcer. Thickened rugae may occasionally be seen but the presence of a mass is unusual. In the intestine any segment may be involved.

Macroscopically, the lymphomas usually appear as flat infiltrative lesions which are sometimes associated with one or more ulcers. The cut surface has a grey homogenous appearance. Larger masses are rare.

Microscopically, reactive non-neoplastic follicles may be prominent. In most cases the lymphoma infiltrates around these and spreads diffusely into the surrounding mucosa (Fig. 11.1). The tumour cells are small to medium sized, with moderately abundant clear or faintly eosinophilic cytoplasm and nuclei, which have an irregular contour and resemble the nuclei of centrocytes. This similarity to the centrocytes of the follicle centre has led to the neoplastic cells of MALT lymphoma being called centrocyte-like (CCL) cells (Fig. 11.2). A small number of transformed blasts are characteristically present amongst the CCL cells. Plasma cell differentiation is present to a variable degree in approximately one-third of cases and is maximal beneath

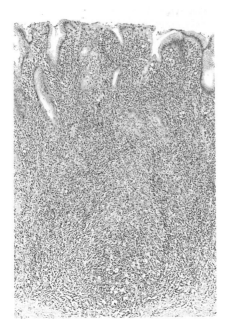

Fig. 11.1. Low grade B cell lymphoma of MALT. The neoplastic centrocyte-like cells infiltrate diffusely within the mucosa and around a residual reactive lymphoid follicle.

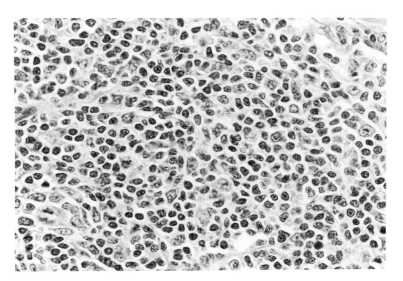

Fig. 11.2. Centrocyte-like cells showing moderately abundant clear cytoplasm and nuclei with irregular contours.

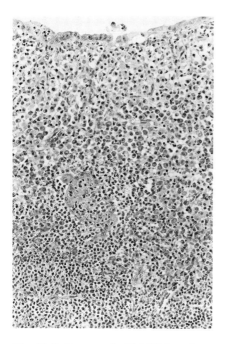

Fig. 11.3. Low grade MALT lymphoma showing marked plasma cell differentiation which is maximal at the luminal surface.

the surface epithelium (Fig. 11.3). In some cases, plasma cells are distorted by accumulations of immunoglobulin, and these may occasionally be found as extracellular tissue deposits.

A characteristic feature of low grade MALT lymphomas is the presence of lymphoepithelial lesions (Fig. 11.4). These are formed by the infiltration of individual crypts by clusters of CCL cells which frequently leads to swelling and eosinophil change in the epithelial cells and eventual disintegration of the crypt epithelium. In some cases, the lesions are few in number and may require a careful search.

The reactive lymphoid follicles are an important component of low grade MALT lymphomas, and the interaction between these and the neoplastic CCL cells is complex, but has been broadly divided into three types (Isaacson *et al.*, 1991). In the first type the reactive follicles are overrun by CCL cells, resulting in a confluent vaguely nodular lymphoma in which small collections of residual follicle centre cells and scattered small, darkly staining mantle cells are seen. In the second type, the follicle centres are selectively replaced either wholly or in part by CCL cells, which results in the expansion of the follicle centres and loss of the characteristic zoning of

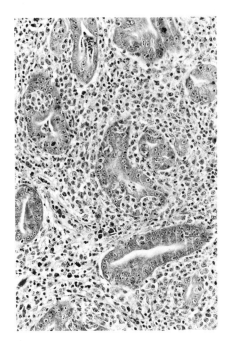

Fig. 11.4. Clusters of centrocyte-like cells infiltrate and destroy individual crypts to form lymphoepithelial lesions.

reactive follicle centres (Fig. 11.5). The CCL cells in the follicle centres are
slightly larger than those of the diffuse infiltrate and frequently show an
increased number of mitoses. In the third type, the intrafollicular CCL cells
show plasma cell differentiation.

Follicular colonisation in MALT lymphomas appears to result from
specific colonisation of reactive follicles by CCL cells. This would be
consistent with a suggested marginal zone lineage for these cells, since
migration into the follicle following antigen stimulation has been shown, in
the rat, to be a normal function of these cells (MacLennan et al., 1990).

Small foci of lymphoma may be present in the mucosa remote from the
main tumour. The smallest of these consist of a single lymphoid follicle
surmounted by CCL cells, which form lymphoepithelial lesions. A recent
study of gastric MALT lymphoma which used a Swiss-roll technique to
embed the whole gastrectomy specimen, allowed the construction of maps
displaying the distribution of the lymphoma (Wotherspoon, Doglioni &
Isaacson, 1992). This showed that in some cases gastric MALT lymphoma is
a multifocal disease and suggests that resection margins are not necessarily
evidence of complete excision and may explain late recurrences seen in a
proportion of cases. The authors have also encountered a number of cases

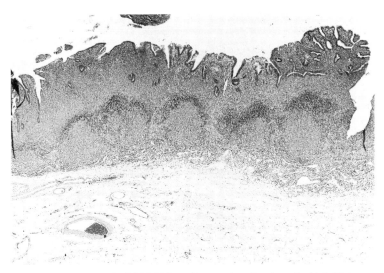

Fig. 11.5. Low grade MALT lymphoma showing lymphoid follicles colonised by neoplastic centrocyte-like cells.

with simultaneous involvement of the stomach and small bowel by low grade MALT lymphoma, in which the neoplastic cells are phenotypically and genotypically identical, but the primary site is unclear.

The characteristic pattern of lymph node involvement consists of an interfollicular infiltrate of CCL cells, which surrounds the follicles occupying the area corresponding to the marginal zone. This infiltrate extends to form confluent sheets and eventually replaces the entire node. There may be selective colonisation of the follicle centres, similar to that seen in the primary tumour. Dissemination beyond the gastrointestinal tract is a later and uncommon complication and bone marrow involvement, although reported, is rare.

The immunophenotype of low grade MALT lymphoma is shown in Table 11.2 and is compared to other nodal low grade B cell lymphomas and to that of marginal zone B cells. There is almost complete immunophenotypic homology between the CCL cell and the marginal zone B cell. Immunostaining with a pan-B cell marker, such as anti-CD20, together with anti-cytokeratin, highlights the lymphoepithelial lesions. Antibodies against CD21 in paraffin sections show an attenuated, follicular dendritic cell network in occupied follicles and demonstrate residual follicle centres. The CCL cells of MALT lymphoma express surface and to a lesser degree cytoplasmic immunoglobulin and show light chain restriction.

Genotypic investigations of MALT lymphomas using both Southern blot analysis and the polymerase chain reaction, have confirmed the presence of

Table 11.2. *Comparison of the immunophenotype of marginal zone B cells with the neoplastic cells of MALT lymphoma, L centroblastic–centrocytic lymphoma, and mantle cell lymphoma*

Antibody	Splenic MZ	Peyer's patch MZ	ML CB/CC	ML Mantle cell	MALT CCL cell
Anti Ig	M, A	M, A	M, D, G	M, D	M, A, (G)
CD 5	−	−	−	+	−
CD 10	−	−	+	−	−
CD 11c	−	−	−	−	−/+
CD 21	+	+	+	+	+
CD 35	+	+	+	+	+
KB61 (CDw32)	+	+	−	+	+
UCL4D12[a]	+	+	−/+	−	+
UCL3D3[a]	−	−	−	+	−

MZ - marginal zone; ML - malignant lymphoma; CB/CC centroblastic/centrocytic; CCL - centrocyte-like.
[a]Smith-Ravin *et al.*, 1990.

immunoglobulin heavy chain gene rearrangement (Spencer, Diss & Isaacson, 1989; Wotherspoon *et al.*, 1990). Neither the *bcl*-1 or *bcl*-2 oncogenes are rearranged in low grade MALT lymphomas (Wotherspoon *et al.*, 1990).

The clinical behaviour of low grade, gastric MALT lymphoma, is characteristic. The lymphoma is seldom disseminated at the time of diagnosis, rarely involves the bone marrow and is associated with a prolonged survival following surgical resection with or without adjuvant radio- or chemotherapy. In a series reported by Cogliatti *et al.* (1991), the survival for low grade, gastric MALT lymphoma was 92% at 5 years and 75% at 10 years. The clinical behaviour of intestinal MALT lymphoma is not as favourable as that of gastric lymphoma, with a 5 year survival of 44–75%. In each site, stage of disease is a factor of major prognostic relevance.

Immunoproliferative small intestinal disease (IPSID)

Immunoproliferative small intestinal disease (IPSID), is a special sub-group of small intestinal MALT lymphoma arising in the upper small intestine, that is restricted in its incidence to certain geographical areas, occurring almost exclusively in the Middle East. An important feature of IPSID is the synthesis of alpha heavy chain, without light chain, by the neoplastic plasma cells; this can be detected in the duodenal juice and/or serum of up to two thirds of cases. Patients presenting with IPSID are usually young adults with profound malabsorption.

The macroscopic appearances of IPSID depend on the stage. In most cases, there is diffuse, even thickening of the small intestinal wall, with enlarged mesenteric lymph nodes. Circumscribed lymphomatous masses may be present, which may be multiple, sometimes producing multiple, small intestinal polyps.

Microscopically, the features of IPSID exemplify all the features of low grade MALT lymphoma, with marked plasma cell differentiation (Fig. 11.6). Three stages of IPSID are recognised (Galian *et al.*, 1977). In stage A, the lymphoplasmacytic infiltrate is confined to the mucosa and mesenteric lymph nodes. In stage B, nodular mucosal lymphoid infiltrates are present and extend below the muscularis mucosa. Stage C, is characterised by lymphomatous masses and transformation to high grade lymphoma. In all stages, the aggregates of CCL cells can be identified around the epithelial crypts and forming lymphoepithelial lesions. Reactive lymphoid follicles vary in number and their colonisation by CCL cells results in the nodular appearances of stage B IPSID (Isaacson *et al.*, 1989). Intrafollicular blast transformation and plasma cell differentiation also occur.

The mesenteric lymph nodes are involved early in the course of IPSID, initially with filling of the sinusoids by mature plasma cells but later with a marginal zone infiltrate of CCL cells, similar to that seen in MALT lymphoma elsewhere.

Immunohistochemical studies of IPSID confirm the synthesis of alpha heavy chain, without light chain, in the plasma cells, CCL cells and transformed blasts. The IgA is always of class IgA1, but occasionally both IgA1 and IgA2 are detected (Isaacson *et al.*, 1989). In cases in which the infiltrate appears to consist entirely of plasma cells, staining with anti-CD20 will reveal clusters of B cells concentrated around the epithelial crypts and forming lymphoepithelial lesions. Gene rearrangement studies in stage A and B IPSID have confirmed immunoglobulin heavy or light chain gene rearrangement (Smith, Price & Isaacson, 1987).

Clinically IPSID runs a prolonged course over many years, rarely spreading out of the abdomen until the terminal stages of the disease, when high grade transformation has occurred. There are numerous reports describing remissions or cure of IPSID in its early stages following the use of broad spectrum antibiotics (Ben-Ayed *et al.*, 1989), although the immunophenotypic and genotypic data suggest that IPSID is a neoplastic disease condition, even in the earliest stages of the disease. The extreme plasma cell differentiation which characterises IPSID, suggests that the lymphoma cells may retain a degree of sensitivity to immune stimulation. By removing the luminal source of immune stimulation, antibiotics may result in the diminu-

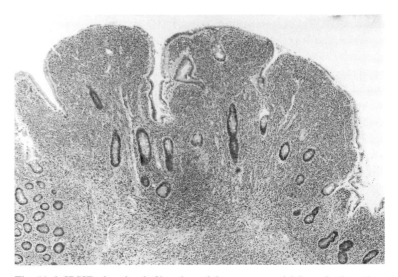

Fig. 11.6. IPSID showing infiltration of the mucosa, with broadening of the villi, predominately by plasma cells.

tion of the plasma cell component of the mucosal infiltrate and symptomatic relief of the malabsorption.

High grade lymphoma of MALT type

Most studies of high grade MALT lymphoma relate to lesions arising in the stomach. High grade primary gastric lymphoma is more frequently reported than the low grade lesion. This difference may be more apparent than real since, until recently, many of the low grade lesions were regarded as florid lymphoid hyperplasia rather than lymphoma. The definition of high grade MALT lymphoma is problematical. Foci of high grade lymphoma may be found in low grade MALT lymphoma, suggesting transformation from low to high grade. The extent of this transformation varies, sometimes being confined to colonised lymphoid follicles, whilst in other cases there are sheets of transformed blasts within a predominantly low grade CCL cell infiltrate. In the absence of an agreed definition of the boundary between high and low grade lesions, we believe that the presence of clusters or sheets of transformed blasts which are not confined to follicle centres, to be indicative of high grade lymphoma.

In a proportion of cases of primary, high grade lymphoma, a low grade component can be identified (Chan, Ng & Isaacson, 1990). There remains a group of cases in which no such component is identifiable. The histological features and clinical behaviour of both primary and secondary high grade lymphoma are not significantly different and so there would seem to be no advantage, at least at present, in classifying such tumours separately.

Histologically, the transformed cells infiltrate in sheets and between glands. Lymphoepithelial lesions are rarely formed by the transformed cells. The blasts may have abundant cytoplasm, with nuclei in which the nucleoli are randomly scattered. Bizarre, often multinucleated, cells are not uncommon.

Immunocytochemistry shows the cells to contain abundant cytoplasmic immunoglobulin, but their immunophenotype is not distinctive. Staining with anti-CD21, may reveal a disrupted follicular dendritic cell network, representing reactive follicle centres which have been overrun and providing further evidence that these tumours originate as low grade lymphomas.

Genotypic studies show immunoglobulin gene rearrangement. No rearrangement of the *bcl*-1 or *bcl*-2 oncogenes is found, but there are reports that c-*myc* rearrangement is found in a high proportion of cases (Raghoebier *et al.*, 1991).

The clinical behaviour of high grade MALT lymphomas is controversial. Some reports suggest that, stage for stage, there is no significant difference between low and high grade MALT lymphoma (Weingrad *et al.*, 1982). Others have shown that high grade lesions have a less favourable behaviour (Joensuu *et al.*, 1987). Cogliatti *et al.* (1991), found that the five year survival for high grade gastric lymphoma was significantly worse than for low grade disease (75% vs 91%), but that there was no difference between primary and secondary high grade lymphoma.

Malignant lymphoma, mantle cell type (centrocytic, lymphomatous polyposis)

Lymphomatous polyposis (also known as multiple lymphomatous polposis) is an uncommon but well recognised disease, mostly found in patients over 50, with an equal sex incidence. Presenting symptoms are of abdominal pain with or without melaena. Barium studies or endoscopy reveal multiple polyps 0.5–2 cm in diameter, which may involve any part of the gastrointestinal tract, but are frequently largest in the ileocaecal region.

Histologically the polyps consist of a diffuse or nodular mucosal lymphoid infiltrate (Fig. 11.7). Characteristically reactive follicle centres are present within the lymphoid infiltrate, which appears to selectively replace the follicle mantle zones. Intestinal glands are displaced, but lymphoepithelial lesions are not seen.

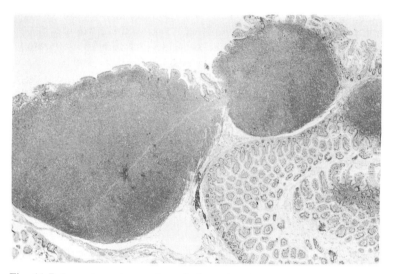

Fig. 11.7. Lymphomatous polyposis (mantle cell lymphoma) showing multiple nodular infiltrates within the mucosa.

Cytologically, the infiltrate consists of a uniform population of small lymphocytes with irregular nuclear contours which are similar to centrocytes. Immunocytochemistry shows these cells to express B cell markers, but also to express CD5, in keeping with a proposed origin from a CD5 positive subpopulation of mantle zone cells (Banks *et al.*, 1992). The cells may also express CD43, and strong expression of immunoglobulin is characteristic. Molecular genetic studies confirm the presence of immunoglobulin gene rearrangement. Rearrangement of the *bcl*-1 oncogene, which is seen in approximately a third of cases of mantle cell lymphomas, is seen in a similar proportion of lymphomatous polyposis cases (Wotherspoon *et al.*, 1990; Williams, Westermann & Swerdlow, 1990).

Clinically, lymphomatous polyposis can be regarded as an intestinal form of mantle cell lymphoma and the mesenteric lymph nodes are frequently involved at diagnosis. Wide dissemination occurs early in the course of the disease, with involvement of liver, spleen and peripheral lymph nodes.

Burkitt's lymphoma

In the Middle East, primary gastrointestinal Burkitt's lymphoma is a common disease of children. Elsewhere, both the endemic (African) form and the non-endemic type of Burkitt's lymphoma commonly involve the gastrointestinal tract and the incidence may be increasing (Lennert & Feller,

1990). The disease is more common in boys and shows a peak incidence between 4 and 5 years of age. There is a predilection for the terminal ileum, but any part of the gastrointestinal tract may be involved.

Macroscopically, the lesions may form a localised obstructing tumour mass, or may involve large segments of the intestine. Mesenteric lymph node and retroperitoneal involvement is frequent.

Histologically, the mucosa is effaced by cohesive sheets of monomorphic blasts of uniform size with round nuclei and two or three central nucleoli. Interspersed between the neoplastic cells are phagocytic histiocytes, giving a characteristic starry-sky appearance.

Immunocytochemically the cells express B cell markers including CD10, but cytoplasmic immunoglobulin is not found. The number of Ki-67 positive proliferating cells is very high, with a median of 80% positive cells.

Cytogenetic and molecular genetic studies of Burkitt's lymphoma have shown the presence of a reciprocal translocation involving the c-*myc* oncogene on chromosome 8, most commonly with the immunoglobulin heavy chain gene locus on chromosome 14 (Manolova *et al.*, 1979). Less frequently, the translocation involves the immunoglobulin light chain gene loci on chromosomes 2 and 22.

The prognosis of Burkitt's lymphoma is largely influenced by the stage of disease at the time of diagnosis. In endemic Burkitt's localised disease has an excellent prognosis with a rapid regression following treatment and a potential for longterm remission. Non-endemic Burkitt's may show a similar initial rapid response but the prognosis is ultimately poor, with relapse within a few months.

Enteropathy associated T cell lymphoma

The association between intestinal lymphoma and malabsorption was first reported in 1937 (Fairley & Mackie, 1937). At that time, it was thought that the lymphoma caused the malabsorption, but it subsequently became clear that the reverse was true (Gough, Read & Naish, 1962). In 1978, Isaacson and Wright characterised the lymphoma associated with coeliac disease as a variant of malignant histiocytosis (Isaacson & Wright, 1978). More recent studies, using immunocytochemistry and molecular biology, have shown this disease to be a T cell lymphoma (Isaacson *et al.*, 1985) and the term enteropathy associated T cell lymphoma (EATL), was coined. There is strong evidence that EATL is related specifically to coeliac disease: the HLA types of the patients, the distribution of the lymphoma, the histology and the immunophenotype of EATL are those of coeliac disease (O'Driscoll *et al.*, 1982). Patients with EATL often demonstrate gluten sensitivity (Swinson *et al.*, 1983) and it has been suggested that a gluten-free diet in coeliacs may be protective against the development of lymphoma (Holmes *et al.*, 1989).

Enteropathy associated T cell lymphoma may complicate established coeliac disease, but frequently follows a short history of adult-onset coeliac disease. In a proportion of cases, there is no preexisting history of coeliac disease, although the histological features of the 'normal mucosa' away from the tumour show the characteristic histology of the disease. A minority of cases have a normal appearing jejunum. The peak incidence of EATL appears in the 6th and 7th decade and the sex incidence is equal. The commonest presentation is with the reappearance of malabsorption, accompanied by abdominal pain, in a patient with a history of coeliac disease, previously responsive to gluten-free diet. Occasionally, patients present with severe gluten insensitive malabsorption, or as an abdominal emergency. There is a further group in whom there is a progressive disease, characterised by malabsorption, ulceration and stricture formation, a condition known as ulcerative jejunitis.

Although most cases of EATL arise in the jejunum, any part of the small intestine may be involved. The tumour is usually multifocal and forms ulcerating nodules or large masses which may be associated. The mesentery is often infiltrated and mesenteric lymph nodes are commonly involved. In most cases, the lymphoma has disseminated at the time of diagnosis, most commonly to the liver, spleen, bone marrow, lung or skin.

The histological features of EATL show marked variation, both between cases and within a single case. The cells may be only slightly larger than mature lymphocytes, or resemble immunoblasts (Fig. 11.8). The most characteristic appearance is that of a highly pleomorphic tumour with numerous multinucleate forms. Intraepithelial tumour cells may be prominent. There is often extensive necrosis and a heavy inflammatory infiltrate, frequently containing many eosinophils. In most cases, the small intestine remote from the tumour shows histological changes identical to those of coeliac disease. The degree of intraepithelial lymphocytosis may be extreme and spill into the lamina propria. In these cases, the lymphocytes are small and lack neoplastic features, but have been shown to be part of the neoplastic clone in at least two cases. Mesenteric lymph node involvement may be predominantly intrasinusoidal, paracortical or both.

The most commonly reported phenotype of EATL is CD3 positive/negative, CD7 positive, CD4 and CD8 negative. Although the cells are CD4 and CD8 negative, they do not express the gamma/delta T cell receptor. The tumour cells react with the monoclonal antibody HML1 (Spencer *et al.*, 1988), which recognizes the normal intraepithelial T cell population and approximately 25% of lamina propria T cells, in contrast to only a few T cells outside the mucosae. On paraffin sections, cases frequently show loss of one or more of the routinely used T cell-related antigens CD3, CD45RO and

(a)

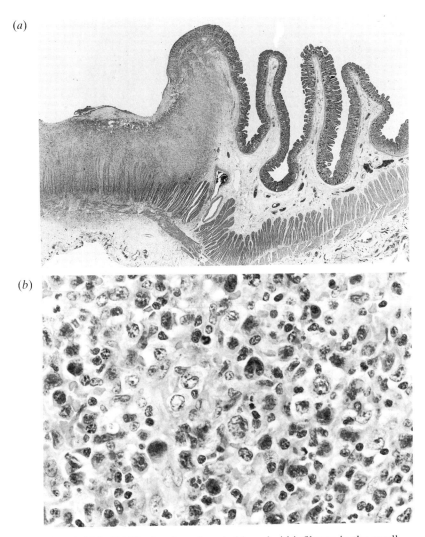

(b)

Fig. 11.8(a). EATL showing ulcerated lymphoid infiltrate in the small bowel extending into the muscularis propria. (b) High power of the infiltrate shows many pleomorphic and multinucleate tumour cells.

CD43. Those cases of EATL composed of large or anaplastic cells are frequently CD30 positive. Genotypic studies of EATL have shown clonal rearrangement of the T cell receptor beta chain (Isaacson *et al.*, 1985).

The clinical course of EATL is unfavourable, except in a minority of cases, in which resection of a localised tumour can be followed by a long remission. In many cases, the lymphoma involves multiple segments of the small intestine, rendering resection impossible, or has disseminated widely prior to diagnosis.

References

Azab, M. B., Henry-Amar, M., Rougier, P. *et al.* (1989). Prognostic factors in primary gastrointestinal non-Hodgkin's lymphoma: a multivariate analysis, report of 106 cases and review of the literature. *Cancer*, **64**, 1208–17.

Banks, P. M., Chan, J., Cleary. *et al.* (1992). Mantle cell lymphoma: a proposal for unification of morphologic, immunologic and molecular data. *American Journal of Surgical Pathology*, **16**, 637–40.

Ben-Ayed, F., Halphen, M., Najjar, T. *et al.* (1989). Treatment of alpha chain disease—results of a prospective study in 21 Tunisian patients by the Tunisian–French intestinal lymphoma study group. *Cancer*, **63**, 1251–6.

Chan, J. K. C., Ng, C. S. & Isaacson, P. G. (1990). Relationship between high-grade lymphoma and low-grade B cell mucosa associated lymphoid tissue lymphoma (MALToma) of the stomach. *American Journal of Pathology*, **136**, 1153–64.

Cogliatti, S. B., Schmid, U., Schumacher, U. *et al.* (1991). Primary B-cell gastric lymphoma: a clinicopathological study of 145 patients. *Gastroenterology*, **101**, 1159–70.

Dawson, I. M. P., Cornes, J. S. & Morson, B. C. (1961). Primary malignant tumours of the intestinal tract. *British Journal of Surgery*, **49**, 80–9.

Doglioni, C., Wotherspoon, A. C., Moschini, A., de Boni, M. & Isaacson, P. G. (1992). High incidence of primary gastric lymphoma in northeastern Italy. *Lancet*, **339**, 834–5.

Fairley, N. H. & Mackie, F. P. (1937). The clinical and biochemical syndrome in lympha-denoma and allied disease involving the mesenteric lymph glands. *British Medical Journal*, **1**, 3972–80.

Fischbach, W., Kestel, W., Kirchner, T., Mossner, J. & Wilms, K. (1992). Malignant lymphomas of the upper gastrointestinal tract. *Cancer*, **70**, 1075–80.

Freeman, C., Berg, J. W. & Cutler, S. J. (1972). Occurrence and prognosis of extranodal lymphomas. *Cancer*, **29**, 252–60.

Galian, A., Lecestre, M. J., Scott, O. J., Bogwel, C., Mutuchansky, C. & Rambaud, J. C. (1977). Pathological study of alpha-chain disease, with special emphasis on evolution. *Cancer*, **39**, 2081–101.

Gough, K. R., Read, A. E. & Naish J. M. (1962). Intestinal reticulosis as a complication of idiopathic steatorrhoea. *Gut*, **3**, 232–9.

Hayes, J. & Dunn, E. (1989). Has the incidence of primary gastric lymphoma increased? *Cancer*, **63**, 2073–6.

Holmes, G. K. T., Prior, P., Lane, M. R., Pope, D. & Allan, R. N. (1989). Malignancy in coeliac disease—effect of a gluten-free diet. *Gut*, **30**, 333–8.

Hyjek, E. & Isaacson, P. G. (1988). Primary B cell lymphoma of the thyroid and its relationship to Hashimoto's thyroiditis. *Human Pathology*, **19**, 1315–26.

Hyjek, E., Smith, W. J. & Isaacson, P. G. (1988). Primary B cell lymphoma of salivary gland and its relationship to myoepithelial sialadenitis. *Human Pathology*, **19**, 766–76.

Isaacson, P. G., Dogan, A., Price, S. K. & Spencer J. (1989). Immunoproliferative small intestinal disease: an immunohistochemical study. *American Journal of Surgical Pathology*, **13**, 1023–33.

Isaacson, P. G., O'Connor, N. T. J., Spencer, J. *et al.* (1985). Malignant histiocytosis of the intestine—a T cell lymphoma. *Lancet*, **ii**, 688–91.

Isaacson, P. G. & Spencer, J. (1987). Malignant lymphoma of mucosa associated lymphoid tissue. *Histopathology*, **11**, 445–62.

Isaacson, P. G., Wotherspoon, A. C., Diss, T. C. & Pan, L. X. (1991). Follicular colonization in B cell lymphoma of mucosa associated lymphoid tissue. *American Journal of Surgical Pathology*, **15**, 819–28.

Isaacson, P. G. & Wright D. H. (1978). Malignant histocytosis of the intestine: its relationship to malabsorption and ulcerative jejunitis. *Human Pathology*, **9**, 661–77.

Joensuu, H., Soderstrom, K. O., Klemi, P. J. & Eerola, E. (1987). Nuclear DNA content and its prognostic value in lymphoma of the stomach. *Cancer*, **60**, 3042–8.

Lennert, K. & Feller, A. C. (1990). *Non-Hodgkin's Lymphomas* (based on the updated Kiel classification), 2nd edn. New York, Berlin, Heidelberg: Springer-Verlag.

MacLennan, I. C. M., Liu, Y. J., Oldfield, S., Zhang, J. & Lane, P. J. L. (1990). The evolution of B-cell clones. *Current Topics in Microbiology and Immunology*, **159**, 37–63.

Manolova, Y., Manolov, G., Kieler, J., Levan, A. & Klein, G. (1979). Genesis of the 14q+ marker in Burkitt's lymphoma. *Hereditas*, **90**, 5–10.

Marchi, M. M., Rota, E., Berlotti, M., Gollini, C. & Signorelli, S. (1990). Primary non-Hodgkin's lymphoma of the esophagus. *American Journal of Gastroenterology*, **85**, 737–41.

Musshoff, K. (1977). Klinische Stadieneinteilung der Nicht-Hodgkin-Lymphome. *Strahlentherapie*, **153**, 218–21.

O'Driscoll, B. R. C., Stevens, F. M., O'Gorman, T. A. *et al.* (1982). HLA type of patients with coeliac disease and malignancy in the west of Ireland. *Gut*, **23**, 662–5.

Otter, R., Bieger, R., Kluin, P. M., Hermans, J. & Willemze, R. (1989). Primary gastro-intestinal non-Hodgkin's lymphoma in a population-based registry. *British Journal of Cancer*, **60**, 745–50.

Parsonnet, J., Friedman G. D., Vandersteen, D. P. *et al.* (1991). Helicobacter pylori infection and the risk of gastric carcinoma. *New England Journal of Medicine*, **325**, 1127–31.

Radasziewicz, T., Dragosics, B. & Bauer, P. (1992). Gastrointestinal malignant lymphomas of the mucosa-associated lymphoid tissue: factors relevant to prognosis. *Gastroenterology*, **102**, 1628–38.

Raghoebier, S., Kramer, M. H. H., van Krieken, J. H. J. M. *et al.* (1991). Essential differences in oncogene involvement between nodal and extranodal large cell lymphoma. *Blood*, **78**, 2680–5.

Smith, W., Price, S. K. & Isaacson, P. G. (1987). Immunoglobulin gene rearrangement in immunoproliferative small intestinal disease (IPSID). *Journal of Clinical Pathology*, **40**, 1291–7.

Smith-Ravin, J., Spencer, J., Beverley, P. C. L. & Isaacson, P. G. (1990). Characterisation of two monoclonal antibodies (UCL4D12 and UCL3D3) which discriminate between human mantle zone and marginal zone B cells. *Clinical and Experimental Immunology*, **82**, 181–7.

Spencer, J., Cerf-Bensussan, N., Jarry, A. *et al.* (1988). Enteropathy-associated T cell lymphoma (malignant histiocytosis of the intestine) is recognised by a monoclonal antibody (HML-1) that defines a membrane molecule on human mucosal lymphocytes. *American Journal of Pathology*, **132**, 1–5.

Spencer, J., Diss, T. C. & Isaacson, P. G. (1989). Primary B cell gastric lymphoma: a genotypic analysis. *American Journal of Pathology*, **135**, 557–64.

Stolte, M. & Eidt, S. (1989). Lymphoid follicles in the antral mucosa: immune response to *Campylobacter pylori*? *Journal of Clinical Pathology*, **42**, 1269–71.

Swinson, C. M., Slavin, G., Coles, E. C. & Booth, C. C. (1983). Coelial disease and malignancy. *Lancet*, **i**, 111–15.

Weingrad, D. N., Decosse, J. J., Sherlock, P., Straus, D., Lieberman, P. H. & Plippa, D. A. (1982). Primary gastrointestinal lymphoma: a 30-year review. *Cancer*, **49**, 1258–65.

Williams, M. E., Westermann, C. D. & Swerdlow, S. H. (1990). Genotypic characterization of centrocytic lymphoma: frequent rearrangement of the chromosome 11 bcl-1 locus. *Blood*, **76**, 1387–91.

Wotherspoon, A. C., Ortiz-Hidalgo, C., Falzon, M. R. & Isaacson, P. G. (1991). *Helicobacter pylori*-associated gastritis and primary B-cell gastric lymphoma. *Lancet*, **338**, 1175–6.

Wotherspoon, A. C., Pan, L. X., Diss, T. C. & Isaacson, P. G. (1990). A genotypic study of low grade B-cell lymphomas, including lymphomas of mucosa associated lymphoid tissue (MALT). *Journal of Pathology*, **162**, 135–40.

Wotherspoon, A. C., Doglioni, C. & Isaacson, P. G. (1992). Gastric B cell lymphoma of mucosa-associated lymphoid tissue is a multifocal disease. *Histopathology*, **20**, 29–34.

Wyatt, J. I. & Rathbone, B. J. (1988). Immune response of the gastric mucosa to *Campylobacter pylori*. *Scandinavian Journal of Gastroenterology*, **23** (suppl. 142), 44–9.

–12–
Small bowel transplantation

R. F. M. WOOD, C. L. INGHAM CLARK and
A. G. POCKLEY

Introduction

With the development of immunosuppressive drugs in the late 1950s there
was interest in the possibility of all forms of organ transplantation. Early
experiments on small bowel transplantation were undertaken by Lillehei in
Minneapolis. He was able to demonstrate from experiments in dogs that
transplantation of the intestine was technically possible (Lillehei, Goott &
Miller, 1959). However, rejection was intense and with the combination of
azathioprine and steroids, even modest prolongation of graft survival could
not be achieved. His work also indicated that, unlike other forms of organ
graft, the small bowel had the potential to cause graft-*versus*-host disease
(GvHD). During the 1960s and 1970s a small number of human intestinal
transplants were performed in desperate cases. With the exception of one
patient who survived for over two months (Fortner *et al.*, 1972), the
remaining individuals all died within days of the operation (Lillehei *et al.*,
1967; Okumura, Fujimari & Ferrari; 1969; Olivier *et al.*, 1969; Alican *et al.*,
1971). In some cases, histology of the graft did not show severe destructive
changes from rejection, and it is now clear that these patients died from
sepsis as a result of bacterial translocation across the gut lumen to the blood
stream. The advent of cyclosporin in the 1980s rekindled interest in small
bowel transplantation leading to clinical programmes in both Europe and
North America.

Graft physiology

A transplanted segment of small bowel is, of necessity, denervated and
deprived of normal lymphatic drainage. The lack of autonomic control leads
to an initial hypersecretion from the crypts. The normal absorptive mechanisms at the villus tip are overwhelmed and there is a net loss of water and
electrolytes into the gut lumen (Watson *et al.*, 1988). This phenomenon has
proved to be a problem in the early stages following both clinical and
experimental transplantation. However, within weeks of grafting adaptation occurs, and electrolyte imbalance has not been commonly seen in

patients with long surviving grafts. Surprisingly, despite the loss of vagal inhibition, motility of the transplanted bowel is not a problem and the intrinsic pacemaker mechanism ensures relatively normal peristalsis (Taguchi et al., 1989). Standard tests of small bowel function, such as maltose absorption, show normal values in well functioning grafts (Lee & Schraut, 1986a).

Experimental studies in the rat with dye injection techniques have demonstrated that fine connections between graft and host lymphatics start to develop within a week of transplantation (Kocandrle, Houttuin & Prohaska, 1966). However, normal handling of fat is impaired (Diliz-Perez et al., 1984) and this is a factor which has to be taken into consideration in designing a suitable diet for the transplant recipient. There may also be difficulties with enteral cyclosporin absorption, since the drug does not dissolve in water and has to be administered in a fat soluble form (Fujiwara, Raju & Grogan, 1987).

Experimental models

The majority of experimental work on small bowel transplantation has been undertaken in the rat. The model used by most groups was developed by Monchik and Russell (1971) and involves transplantation of a heterotopic loop of bowel with two cutaneous stomas. The superior mesenteric artery, on a cuff of aorta, is anastomosed to the abdominal aorta of the recipient, below the level of the renal arteries. The superior mesenteric vein is joined end to side, to the inferior vena cava. Loops can subsequently be connected orthotopically. Initial orthotopic placement is usually associated with a significant rate of mortality and early graft failure (Lee & Schraut, 1986b). In long surviving animals with orthotopic grafts, there will be an increase in serum bile acids, owing to the loss of the normal entero-hepatic circulation. Animals otherwise grow normally and there are no significant differences in other biochemical parameters (Schweizer et al., 1991). The choice of rat strains has a significant bearing on outcome. In the DA (RT1^a) and PVG (RT1^c) strains, the DA animal is a stronger responder than the PVG (Langrehr et al., 1990). Grafts in the PVG → DA direction will therefore be rejected more rapidly than in the DA → PVG direction. The other popular strain combination is the Lewis (RT1^l) and Brown-Norway (RT1^n). By using F1 hybrid offspring of these parental strains, it is possible to have models where rejection and GvHD occur as isolated phenomena (Monchik & Russell, 1971). Thus in the (DA×PVG)F1 → PVG there will be rejection, but no GvHD. In contrast, if parental grafts are transplanted into F1 hybrid recipient strain animals, there will be GvHD but no rejection. There has also been considerable clinical interest in combined liver/small bowel transplantation, as will be discussed later. Models for combined grafting have now been described in the rat (Zhong et al., 1991).

Small bowel transplantation in larger animal models has proved difficult. Strangulated obstruction has been a problem in both canine and porcine transplantation (Nordgren et al., 1984; Pritchard et al., 1985). In addition, high rates of infective complications have also been reported (Craddock et al., 1983).

Immunology

The large lymphoid component of the small bowel distinguishes it from all other forms of organ graft. In addition to the mesenteric lymph nodes and Peyer's patches, there are substantial numbers of lymphocytes in the lamina propria and in the intra-epithelial compartment between the enterocytes lining the villi. Following transplantation, there is a rapid exchange migration of lymphocytes between the donor and recipient (Ingham Clark et al., 1991, 1992a; Lear et al., 1993; Grover et al., 1993). In the rat model, the migration pattern can be studied by using strain-specific monoclonal antibodies to MHC antigens. For example, in the DA/PVG combination, the antibody MN4 is specific for DA Class I (Milton & Fabre, 1985) and OX27 for PVG Class I antigens (Jefferies, Green & Williams, 1985). In unimmunosuppressed animals, donor lymphocytes can be identified in the spleen and Peyer's patches of the recipient within 24 hours of transplantation. The cell migration peaks at day 4 and donor-derived cells then disappear (Lear et al., 1993). The transitory nature of this phenomenon is due to two factors:

1. destruction of the infiltrating cells by local immune reactivity within recipient tissues.
2. lack of repopulation of the recipient by donor cells, as a result of the concomitant destruction of the graft by rejection.

As would be expected in the absence of immunosuppression there is massive infiltration of the graft by recipient lymphocytes (Ingham Clark et al., 1990) and in most strain combinations the villi show evidence of severe damage by day 5 to 6 (Rosemurgy & Schraut, 1986).

The addition of immunosuppression has interesting effects. There is, in fact, an increase in donor cell migration to host lymphoid tissues (Lear et al., 1993), and with stable graft function, although the numbers of migrating cells decline, they persist on a long-term basis (Ingham Clark et al., 1992a). Within the graft, there is a gradual replacement of all donor lymphoid cells by lymphocytes of recipient phenotype (Ingham Clark et al., 1990). In other

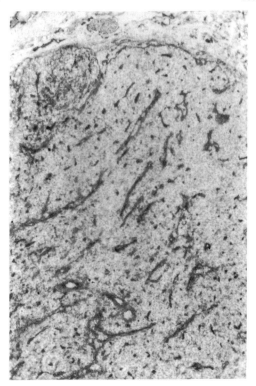

Fig. 12.1. Mesenteric lymph node from a long surviving DA small bowel graft transplanted in a PVG rat. The section has been stained with the monoclonal antibody MN4 which is specific for DA Class I antigen. The positive staining pattern shows that only the stromal supporting structures of the node are of graft origin. The lymphocyte population of the node has been completely replaced by host PVG cells.

organ transplants, the presence of cellular infiltration is taken as the hallmark of rejection. However, in small bowel transplantation, infiltration occurs without evidence of tissue destruction. Fig. 12.1 shows a graft mesenteric node, stained with a monoclonal antibody to identify donor tissue. Only the supporting stroma of the node remains of donor phenotype – all the cells are recipient lymphocytes. This stable chimerism has also been observed in long-surviving recipients of human small bowel transplants (Iwaki *et al.*, 1991). During stable graft function, the gut epithelium alone appears to be spared from infiltration by host cells. However, in developing rejection, before overt mucosal damage is apparent, small numbers of host cells can be identified within the intra-epithelial lymphocyte compartment of the graft (Grover *et al.*, 1993).

The survival of donor cells in recipient tissues, carries the potential for the development of GvHD. In most strain combinations, there are no overt signs of GvHD (hunched posture, redness of paws and ears (Monchik & Russell, 1971)), although a self-limiting GvHD has been described in the Lewis → BN combination (Diflo *et al.*, 1989). In human transplantation, GvHD has rarely been a problem, although it has been described (Grant *et al.*, 1990). Rejection is clearly the dominant immunological force, and the first major episode of rejection tends to wipe out most of the graft lymphocytes which have infiltrated host tissues (Ingham Clark *et al.*, 1993).

The mucosal barrier and mucosal immunity

An intact mucosal surface, with its layer of adherent mucus, is an effective barrier to the translocation of bacteria from the lumen of the bowel, into the portal venous system. Ischaemic damage from preservation and reperfusion injury impairs the defensive mechanism and, if rejection supervenes, there is a major risk of bacterial translocation (Grant *et al.*, 1991; Price *et al.*, 1993). Isolating the transplanted bowel, from the normal faecal stream, is another risk factor for the development of translocation (Price *et al.*, 1991). In experimental studies, the bacterial population, of heterotopically transplanted bowel, is rapidly transformed from normal faecal-type organisms, to commensal bacteria such as *Staph. epidermidis*, which have a particular predilection to translocate (Price *et al.*, 1991). It is probably advantageous to connect the upper end of the graft to the proximal GI tract of the recipient at the time of transplantation, to enable contact between the mucosa and enteric trophic factors. In addition, it may be best not to attempt to flush the donor small bowel of its luminal content, at the time of harvesting (Todo *et al.*, 1993).

The demonstration, that the resident lymphoid population of the graft is replaced by host cells, has raised the question as to whether the graft will retain the potential to make satisfactory immune responses to luminal antigens. The normal mechanism relies on absorption and local processing of luminal antigen, with the production of IgA antibody. Experimental work has shown that, while transplanted bowel retains the ability to produce IgA antibody to antigen to which it has previously been exposed (Xia & Kirkman, 1990*a*), the primary response to a new antigenic challenge may be impaired (Xia & Kirkman, 1990*b*, 1991).

Preservation

Improvements in preservation solutions have meant that organs can now be safely stored for much longer periods than was previously possible.

Given ideal harvesting conditions, kidneys can be kept at 4° C for up to 48 hours and still have an excellent chance of achieving immediate function. In liver transplantation, storage for up to 18 hours is now routine, using University of Wisconsin solution (UW solution). The problem with the small bowel is that it has a delicate mucosal lining and the villus tips are particularly susceptible to ischaemic damage. While the integrity of other organs is solely dependent on the ability of the constituent cells to survive preservation injury, the small bowel has the additional problem of the luminal enzymes, which can rapidly lead to autolysis of the mucosa. So far, preservation of human small bowel has been limited to some 6 to 8 hours, which severely limits the possibilities of pre-operative tissue matching (Schraut, Lee & Tsujinaka, 1986; Nakamura *et al.*, 1993). UW solution has emerged as the universal choice of preservation solution in the current clinical programmes (Todo *et al.*, 1993; Goulet *et al.*, 1990).

Clinical small bowel transplantation

As indicated above, there were no long-term survivors from the attempts at clinical intestinal transplantation, prior to the cyclosporin era. The majority of patients succumbed from overwhelming infection, as the result of bacterial translocation from rejection-damaged mucosa. The improved immunosuppressive potential of cyclosporin, allowed programmes for both isolated small bowel transplantation and combined liver/small bowel grafting to be developed.

Case selection

There are two distinct populations of patients with small bowel failure – children with congenital atresias, gastroschisis, volvulus, necrotising enterocolitis or visceral myopathies (Grosfeld, Rescoria & West, 1986; Caniano, Starr & Ginn-Pease, 1989), and adults with Crohn's disease, volvulus, desmoid tumours or mesenteric infarction (Simons & Jordan, 1969; Mughal & Irving, 1986). Published series suggest that in infants, a minimum of 20 cm of small bowel with the ileocaecal valve, or 40 cm without the ileocaecal valve, is necessary to achieve adequate enteral nutrition (Grosfeld, Rescoria & West, 1986; Wilmore, 1972). In adults, there are sporadic case reports of survival with an extremely short small bowel, but in general most adults with less than 80 cm small bowel, are unable to survive without long-term total parenteral nutrition (TPN) (Allard & Jeejeebhoy, 1989). TPN offers a lifeline for these patients but, while some individuals cope remarkably well, quality of life for many is poor. Approximately half of the patients, who start on parenteral nutrition, will eventually undergo a sufficient degree of intestinal adaptation to allow them to return to oral alimentation, although in some cases additional intravenous fluid supplementation may be necessary (Mughal & Irving, 1986). The process of adaptation can take up to two years and only patients fully dependent on TPN, after allowance for adaptation, should be considered as potential transplant recipients. There are problems with parenteral nutrition during the first year of life. The immature liver has difficulty in dealing with the current formulations of parenteral fluid and this can lead to the development of liver failure by the time the child reaches the age of three to four (Grosfeld, Rescoria & West, 1986; Cooper et al., 1984). At the present time, there are undoubtedly a number of children not appropriate to start on long-term parenteral nutrition and many of these would be suitable candidates for transplantation.

Relative contra-indications to transplantation are, previous multiple abdominal procedures and, in particular, episodes of intra-abdominal sepsis (Wolman et al., 1986). Surveying the population of patients in the United Kingdom currently on home TPN, it has been estimated that the demand for adult intestinal transplantation, is around 20 cases per year. This figure would almost certainly double if all the infants with small bowel failure, were to be offered treatment (Ingham Clark et al., 1992b).

Isolated small bowel transplantation with cyclosporin immunosuppression

A series of eight isolated small bowel transplants were performed by the Paris group, between 1986 and 1990 (Goulet et al., 1990). Although the majority of the transplants survived for many months, only one child has maintained long-term graft function. In Kiel, a total of four transplants were undertaken in adult patients (Deltz et al., 1990). Again, one patient achieved good function for over four years after transplantation. In this case, the graft came from a living related donor. There was close HLA matching and this was probably an important factor in the long survival of the graft. Although the results of isolated small bowel transplantation with cyclosporin represented a major advance, the success rate remained poor in comparison with other forms of transplantation. All recipients experienced multiple rejection episodes and most spent long periods in intensive care.

Combined liver/small bowel transplantation

In 1989, Dr David Grant and his team in London, Ontario, carried out a combined liver and small bowel transplant, in a patient with short gut syndrome, resulting from intestinal resection, following thrombosis of the superior mesenteric artery (Grant et al., 1990). Cyclosporin was used as the major component of the immunosuppressive regimen and despite a stormy post-operative course, the patient survived and remains well with good intestinal function. Interestingly in their initial case, Grant and his colleagues, documented an episode of GvHD. The patient became febrile with the typical skin rash of GvHD. Skin biopsy was confirmatory and, in addition, graft-derived cells of male phenotype were identified in the peripheral blood of the female transplant recipient (Grant et al., 1990). The episode was self-limiting and there has been no evidence of recurrent GvHD in this patient. The success of this case highlighted the potentially protective effect of the liver when combined with a small bowel graft. Previous experimental work by Calne had demonstrated enhanced survival of pig kidney grafts when the animal had also received a liver transplant (Calne et al., 1969). The group in London, Ontario, have gone on to carry out a further four combined grafts. However, only one of these patients has achieved long-term survival. Two of the patients have died from lymphoproliferative disease and one from overwhelming infection (McAlister et al., 1993). These problems are directly related to the high level of immunosuppression required to prevent rejection. As in the Paris and Kiel cases, late rejection has proved to be a problem, requiring additional courses of high dose intravenous steroids and other agents such as the monoclonal antibody OKT3.

Isolated and combined transplantation with FK506

The macrolide immunosuppressive agent FK506 (Ochiai et al., 1987), produced by the Fujisawa Company, has been undergoing clinical trials in liver transplantation since 1988. It was also shown to be successful in preventing rejection of experimental small bowel grafts (Hoffman et al., 1990) and the Pittsburgh group started to use it in clinical small bowel transplantation in 1990. They have reported a series of over 30, isolated and combined, small bowel transplants. The survival rate of both patients and grafts has so far been impressive. In the early post-transplant phase, better results have been obtained from isolated small bowel, compared with combined liver/small bowel grafts (Todo et al., 1993). However, late rejection has been a problem and there has been morbidity and mortality from infection and lymphoproliferative disease. Of the four deaths reported so far, three have involved sepsis (one with GvHD) and one aggressive lymphoproliferative disease.

Future prospects

The results of the clinical cases performed to date, highlight the need for improved control of rejection if small bowel transplantation is to be made more widely available to patients with intestinal failure. The numbers of immunocompetent lymphocytes in the graft can be reduced by irradiation, however, this may have the disadvantage of rendering the mucosa more susceptible to immune attack (Monchik & Russell, 1971; Deltz *et al.*, 1986). An alternative is to pretreat the donor with anti-lymphocyte globulin (Shaffer *et al.*, 1988; Williams *et al.*, 1991), or to perfuse the graft with a pan-T cell monoclonal antibody, conjugated with ricin A chain (Smith *et al.*, 1992; Ingham Clark *et al.*, 1992c). While both these approaches have been shown to be effective in experimental animals, it is unlikely that they would have a profound influence on the outcome in human transplantation. A more practical option, is to look for agents that will suppress the release of effector molecules – such as cytokines – which are largely responsible for the cellular damage to the graft. The eventual aim must be to reduce the level of relatively non-specific immunosuppression which currently places the recipient at high risk of developing infection and lymphoproliferative disease. More research is required to unravel the immunological function of the gut sufficiently, to identify methods of maintaining normal barrier function, while holding the destructive forces of rejection and graft-*versus*-host disease in check.

References

Alican, F., Hardy, J. D., Cayirli, M. *et al.* (1971). Intestinal transplantation: laboratory experience and report of a case. *American Journal of Surgery,* **121**, 150–9.

Allard, J. P. & Jeejeebhoy, K. N. (1989). Nutritional support and therapy in the short bowel syndrome. *Gastroenterology Clinics of North America,* **18**, 589–601.

Calne, R. Y., Sells, R. A., Pena, J. R. *et al.* (1969). Induction of immunological tolerance by porcine liver allografts. *Nature,* **223**, 472–6.

Caniano, D. A., Starr, J. & Ginn-Pease, M. E. (1989). Extensive short-bowel syndrome in neonates: outcome in the 1980s. *Surgery,* **105**, 119–24.

Cooper, A., Floyd, T. S., Ross, A. J., Bishop, H. C., Templeton, J. M. Jr. & Ziegler, M. M. (1984). Morbidity and mortality of short bowel syndrome acquired in infancy: an update. *Journal of Pediatric Surgery,* **19**, 711–18.

Craddock, G. N. Nordgren, S. R., Reznick, *et al.* (1983). Small bowel transplantation in the dog using cyclosporine. *Transplantation,* **35**, 284–8.

Deltz, E., Ulrichs, K., Schack, T., Friedrichs, B., Muller-Ruchholtz, W. & Muller-Hermelink, H. K. (1986). Graft-versus-host reaction in small bowel transplantation and possibilities for its circumvention. *American Journal of Surgery,* **151**, 379–86.

Deltz, E., Schroeder, P., Gundlach, M., Hansmann, M. L. & Leimenstoll, G. (1990). Successful clinical small bowel transplantation. *Transplant Proceedings,* **22**, 2501.

Diflo, T., Maki, T., Balogh, K. & Monaco, A. P. (1989). Graft-*versus*-host disease in fully allogeneic small bowel transplantation in the rat. *Transplantation,* **47**, 7–11.

Diliz-Perez, H. S., McClure, J., Bedetti, C. *et al.*, (1984). Successful small bowel allotransplantation in dogs with cyclosporine and prednisone. *Transplantation,* **37**, 126–9.

Fortner, J. G., Sichak, G., Litwin, S. D. & Beattie, E. J. Jr. (1972). Immunological responses to an intestinal allograft with HLA-identical donor–recipient. *Transplantation,* **14**, 531–5.

Fujiwara, H., Raju, S. & Grogan, J. (1987). Cyclosporin absorption in total orthotopic small bowel transplantation in dogs. *Transplant Proceedings*, **19**, 1125.

Goulet, O., Revillon, Y., Jan, D. *et al.* (1990). Small bowel transplantation in children. *Transplant Proceedings*, **22**, 2499–500.

Grant, D., Wall, W., Mimeault, R., Zhong, R., Ghent, C., Garcia, B. *et al.* (1990). Successful small bowel/liver transplantation. *Lancet*, **335**, 181–4.

Grant, D., Hurlbut, D., Zhong, R., *et al.* (1991). Intestinal permeability and bacterial translocation following small bowel transplantation in the rat. *Transplantation*, **52**, 221–4.

Grosfeld, J. L., Rescoria, F. J. & West, K. W. (1986). Short bowel syndrome in infancy and childhood. *American Journal of Surgery*, **151**, 41–6.

Grover, R., Lear, P. A., Ingham Clark, C. L., Pockley, A. G. & Wood, R. F. M. (1993). Method for diagnosing rejection in small bowel transplantation. *British Journal of Surgery*, **80**, 1024–6.

Hoffman, A. L., Makowka, L., Banner, B. *et al.* (1990). The use of FK506 for small intestine allotransplantation. *Transplantation*, **49**, 483–90.

Ingham Clark, C. L., Cunningham, A. J., Crane, P. W., Wood, R. F. M. & Lear, P. A. (1990). Lymphocyte infiltration patterns in rat small bowel transplants. *Transplant Proceedings*, **22**, 2460.

Ingham Clark, C. L., Price, B. A., Malcolm, P., Lear, P. A. & Wood, R. F. M. (1991). Graft-versus-host disease in small bowel transplantation. *British Journal of Surgery*, **78**, 1077–9.

Ingham Clark, C. L., Price, B. A., Crane, P. W., Lear, P. A. & Wood, R. F. M. (1992*a*). Persistence of allogeneic cells in graft and host tissues following small bowel transplantation. *British Journal of Surgery*, **79**, 424–6.

Ingham Clark, C. L., Lear, P. A., Wood, S., Lennard-Jones, J. E. & Wood, R. F. M. (1992*b*). Potential candidates for small bowel transplantation. *British Journal of Surgery*, **79**, 676–9.

Ingham Clark, C. L., Smith, C. J., Crane, P. W. *et al.* (1992*c*). Reduction of graft-versus-host reactivity after small bowel transplantation: *ex vivo* treatment of intestinal allografts with an anti-T cell immunotoxin. *Clinical and Experimental Immunology*, **88**, 220–5.

Ingham Clark, C. L., Grover R., Pockley, A. G. & Wood, R. F. M. (1993). Delayed-start cyclosporine immunosuppression reduces graft cell migration after small bowel transplantation. *Transplantation*, **56**, 1284–6.

Iwaki, Y., Starzl, T. E., Yagihashi, A. *et al.* (1991). Replacement of donor lymphoid tissue in small-bowel transplants. *Lancet*, **337**, 818–19.

Jefferies, W. A., Green, J. R. & Williams, A. F. (1985). Authentic T helper CD4 (W3/25) antigen on rat peritoneal macrophages. *Journal of Experimental Medicine*, **162**, 117–27.

Kocandrle, V., Houttuin, E. & Prohaska, J. V. (1966). Regeneration of the lymphatics after auto-transplantation and homotransplantation of the entire small intestine. *Surgery, Gynecology and Obstetrics*, **122**, 587–92.

Langrehr, J. M., Lee, K. K. W., Wachs, M. E., Lee, T. K., Stangl, M., Venkataramanan, R. *et al.* Comparison of the effectiveness of cyclosporine A in small-bowel transplantation using different rat strain combinations. *Transplant Proceedings*, 1990, **22**, 2533–5.

Lear, P. A., Ingham Clark, C. L., Crane, P. W., Pockley, A. G. & Wood, R. F. M. (1993). Donor cell infiltration of recipient tissue as an indicator of small bowel allograft rejection in the rat. *Transplant International*, **6**, 85–8.

Lee, K. K. W. & Schraut, W. H. (1986*a*). Structure and function of orthotopic small bowel allografts in rats treated with cyclosporine. *American Journal of Surgery*, **151**, 55–60.

Lee, K. K. W. & Schraut, W. H. (1986*b*). Small-bowel transplantation in the rat: graft survival with heterotopic *vs* orthotopic position. In: *Small-Bowel Transplantation. Experimental and Clinical Fundamentals*. ed. E. Deltz, A. Thiede & H. Hamelmann, pp. 7–13. Berlin: Springer-Verlag.

Lillehei, R. C., Goott, B. & Miller, F. A. (1959). The physiological response of the small bowel of the dog to ischaemia including prolonged in vitro preservation of the bowel with successful replacement and survival. *Annals in Surgery,* **150**, 543–60.

Lillehei, R. C., Idezuki, Y., Feemster, J. *et al.* (1967). Transplantation of the stomach, intestine and pancreas: experimental and clinical observations. *Surgery,* **62**, 721–41.

McAlister, V., Grant, D., Wall, W., Roy, A., Ghent, C., Zhong, R. & Duff, J. (1993). Immunosuppressive requirements for small bowel/liver transplantation. *Transplant Proceedings,* **25**, 1204–5.

Milton, A. D. & Fabre, J. W. (1985). Massive induction of donor-type class I and class II MHC antigens in rejecting cardiac allografts in the rat. *Journal of Experimental Medicine,* **161**, 98–112.

Monchik, G. J. & Russell, P. S. (1971). Transplantation of small bowel in the rat: technical and immunological considerations. *Surgery,* **70**, 693–702.

Mughal, M. & Irving, M. (1986). Home parenteral nutrition in the United Kingdom and Ireland. *Lancet,* **ii**, 383–6.

Nakamura, K., Nalesnik, M., Jaffe, R. *et al.* (1993). Morphological monitoring of human small bowel allografts. *Transplant Proceedings,* **25**, 1212.

Nordgren, S., Cohen, Z., Mackenzie, R., Finkelstein, D., Greenberg, G. R. & Langer, B. (1984). Functional monitors of rejection in small intestinal transplants. *American Journal of Surgery,* **147**, 152–7.

Ochiai, T., Nakajima, K., Nagata, M. *et al.* (1987). Effect of a new immunosuppressive agent, FK 506, on heterotopic cardiac allotransplantation in the rat. *Transplant Proceedings,* **19**, 1284–6.

Okumura, M., Fujimara, I. & Ferrari, A. A. (1969). Transplante del intestino delgrado apresentaceo de um caso. *Review Hospital Clinic Faculty Medicine Sao Paulo,* **24**, 39–54.

Olivier, C. L., Retorri, R., Olivier, C. H., Baur, O. & Roux, J. (1969). Homotransplantation orthotopique de l'intestine grele et des colons droit et transverse chez l'homme. *Journal of Chirolurgy,* **98**, 323–30.

Price, B. A., Cumberland, N. S., Ingham Clark, C. L., Wood, R. F. M. & Lear, P. A. (1991). Bacterial supercolonisation and the potential for translocation following small bowel transplantation. *British Journal of Surgery,* **78**, 1507.

Price, B. A., Cumberland, N. S., Ingham Clark, C. L., Pockley, A. G., Lear, P. A. & Wood, R. F. M. (1993). The effect of rejection and graft-versus-host disease on small intestinal microflora and bacterial translocation after rat small bowel transplantation. *Transplantation,* **56**, 1072–6.

Pritchard, T. J., Madara, J. L., Tapper, D., Wilmore, D. W. & Kirkman, R. L. (1985). Failure of cyclosporine to prevent small bowel allograft rejection in pigs. *Journal of Surgery Research,* **38**, 553–8.

Rosemurgy, A. S. & Schraut, W. H. (1986). Small bowel allografts. Sequence of histological changes in acute and chronic rejection. *American Journal of Surgery,* **151**, 470–5.

Schraut, W. H., Lee, K. K. W. & Tsujinaka, Y. (1986). Intestinal preservation of small-bowel grafts by vascular washout and cold storage. In: *Small-Bowel Transplantation. Experimental and Clinical Fundamentals.* ed. E. Deltz, A. Thiede & H. Hamelmann. pp. 65–73. Berlin: Springer-Verlag.

Schweizer, E., Gundlach, M., Gassel, H. J., Deltz, E. & Schroeder, P. (1991). Effects of two-step small bowel transplantation on intestinal morphology and function. *Transplant Proceedings,* **23**, 688.

Shaffer, D., Maki, T., Demichele, S. J., Karlstad, M. D., Bistrian, B. R., Baloch, K. *et al.* (1988). Prevention of graft-versus-host disease and rejection by sensitised small bowel allografts. *Transplantation,* **45**, 262–9.

Simons, F. E. & Jordan, G. L. Jr. (1969). Massive bowel resection. *American Journal of Surgery*, **118**, 953–9.

Smith, G. J., Ingham Clark, C. L., Crane, P. W., Lear, P. A., Wood, R. F. M. & Fabre, J. W. (1992). *Ex vivo* perfusion of intestinal allografts with anti-T cell monoclonal antibody/ricin A chain conjugates for the suppression of graft-versus-host disease. *Transplantation*, **53**, 717–22.

Taguchi, T., Zorychta, E., Sonnino, R. E. & Guttman, F. M. (1989). Small intestinal transplantation in the rat: effect on physiological properties of smooth muscle and nerves. *Journal of Pediatric Surgery*, **24**, 1258–63.

Todo, S., Tzakis, A., Reyes, J. *et al.* (1993). Intestinal transplantation in humans under FK506. *Transplant Proceedings*, **25**, 1198–9.

Watson, A. J. M., Lear, P. A., Montgomery, A. *et al.* (1988). Water, electrolyte, glucose and glycine absorption in rat small intestinal transplants. *Gastroenterology*, **94**, 863–9.

Williams, J. G., Pirenne, J., Mayoral, J. M. *et al.* (1991). Effect of donor pre-treatment with anti-lymphocyte globulin on small bowel transplantation in rats. *British Journal of Surgery*, **78**, 1176–7.

Wilmore, D. W. (1972). Factors correlating with a successful outcome following extensive intestinal resection in newborn infants. *Journal of Paediatrics*, **80**, 88–95.

Wolman, S. L., Jeejeebhoy, K. N., Stewart, S. & Grieg, P. D. (1986). Experience in home parenteral nutrition and indications for small-bowel transplantation. In: *Small-Bowel Transplantation. Experimental and Clinical Fundamentals*. eds. E. Deltz, A. Thiede and H. Hamelmann. pp. 214–21. Berlin: Springer-Verlag.

Xia, W. & Kirkman, R. L. (1990a). Immune function in transplanted small intestine. Total secretory IgA production and response against cholera toxin. *Transplantation*, **49**, 277–80.

Xia, W. & Kirkman, R. L. (1990b). Immune function in transplanted small intestine. II. SIgA production in cholera-toxin primed rats. *Transplant Proceedings*, **22**, 2481.

Xia, W. & Kirkman, R. L. (1991). Inhibitory effect of cyclosporine on specific secretory IgA production against cholera toxin in small bowel transplantation. *Transplant Proceedings*, **23**, 682.

Zhong, R., He, G., Sakai, Y. *et al.* (1991). Combined small bowel and liver transplantation in the rat: possible role of the liver in preventing intestinal allograft rejection. *Transplantation*, **52**, 550–2.

–13–
Clinical aspects of immunologically mediated intestinal diseases

J. E. SMITHSON and D. P. JEWELL

Introduction

It will be readily apparent from the preceding chapters that there have been enormous advances in recent years in our understanding of the immuno-pathology of the gut. This chapter examines the impact which such advances have made in the clinical management of patients with immunologically mediated intestinal disease. In view of the potential size and complexity of this field the discussion has been necessarily restricted, but it is hoped that the examples covered will serve to illustrate important underlying concepts. The first section of this chapter will deal with selected clinical manifestations of various diseases and the role of immunological processes in their patho-physiology, diagnosis and assessment. This will be followed by an overview of immunomodulatory therapy in current use as well as prospects for the future.

Clinical manifestations, diagnosis and assessment

When the host immune response to antigen is inappropriate or exaggerated and leads to tissue damage, hypersensitivity is said to exist. This is a feature common to many of the diseases considered in this volume. Various aspects of these disorders will now be examined in terms of hypersensitivity according to the four part classification originally proposed by Coombs and Gell in 1963. In this way, certain characteristic clinical features of different intestinal diseases can be related to underlying immune processes. In addition, the role of immunological markers will be considered with respect to diagnosis and disease assessment.

Type I reactions

Type I, or immediate, hypersensitivity arises as a consequence of the interaction of allergen with specific mast cell-bound IgE. Subsequent degranulation leads to the release of various inflammatory mediators including histamine and kinins.

This type of reaction accounts for the typical clinical picture of rapid onset food allergies such as those which may be seen with nuts or shellfish. The florid combination of lip swelling, vomiting and even urticaria and bronchospasm, shortly after ingestion of the offending food, make diagnosis straightforward. If necessary, it can be confirmed by the demonstration of specific IgE by radio-allergoabsorbent testing (RAST) and skin prick tests with the suspected allergen.

Type I reactions may contribute in varying degrees to the pathophysiology of other intestinal diseases. Colitis in infants has an allergic basis in most cases (Jenkins et al., 1984), with milk, soya and wheat proteins the main causes. Eosinophilia is a common feature, both in peripheral blood and mucosal biopsies and IgE antibodies are often present. Amongst adults with distal ulcerative colitis, there appears to be a subgroup in whom there is a disproportionate increase in the numbers of IgE positive plasma cells in the rectal mucosa (Rosekrans et al., 1980). In such patients, dietary manipulation may be useful, but as Wright and Truelove demonstrated in 1965, a milk-free diet will benefit only a minority of colitics. The mast cell stabiliser, disodium cromoglycate, may be of use in some patients with chronic proctitis and a high mucosal eosinophil count when administered topically (Heatley et al., 1975). However, when given orally the drug appears to be less effective either for maintaining remission (Dronfield & Langman, 1978), or for treating chronic persistent disease (Buckell et al., 1978).

The presence of a peripheral blood and tissue eosinophilia, together with increased serum IgE, is characteristic of the rare group of conditions described under the collective term of eosinophilic gastroenteropathy or gastroenteritis (Cello, 1979). The pathological features are suggestive of a Type I process and there appears to be an association with allergic disorders, but dietary treatment is largely ineffective and immunosuppression is usually required.

Type II reactions

This form of hypersensitivity is due to circulating antibody which recognises host antigens. Tissue damage may follow as a consequence of complement activation. Classical examples include Goodpasture's syndrome and autoimmune haemolytic anaemia. However, although autoreactive antibodies can be demonstrated in a number of intestinal diseases, their pathogenetic role remains largely unclear.

The evidence for a direct role of auto-antibody is strongest in the case of pernicious anaemia (PA), which has a marked association with other disorders considered to have an autoimmune aetiology. Typically a number of different antibodies occur in PA which bind to antigens found on parietal cells and intrinsic factor (IF).

IgG to the human parietal cell canaliculus may produce a fall in parietal cell mass and acid secretion in animal studies (Tanaka & Glass 1970; Lopes, Ito & Glass, 1976; Loveridge et al., 1980). More recent work suggests that the major parietal cell antigen recognised by these auto-antibodies is the proton pump itself, inhibition of which leads to achlorhydria (Karlsson et al., 1988; Burman et al., 1989). Antibodies to IF may lead to vitamin B12 malabsorption, either by blocking IF binding of B12, or by preventing ileal uptake of the IF-B12 complex (Rose & Chanarin 1971). However, parietal cell and IF antibodies can also be demonstrated in the serum of a proportion of unaffected relatives and in patients with other organ-specific auto-immune disorders, such as insulin-dependent diabetes and Addison's disease. From a diagnostic point of view, this limits the predictive value of a positive test, which must be backed up by histological and functional studies.

Autoreactive antibodies are also characteristic of coeliac disease. IgA and IgG directed against reticulin and endomysium can be detected both in serum and in jejunal aspirates, especially in untreated patients. It is hard to envisage a direct pathogenetic role for these antibodies, since the target antigens are ubiquitous and not restricted to the small intestine. Nevertheless, they are very useful for diagnostic purposes, because they are highly specific and their titres fall to a level similar to that of healthy controls, following gluten withdrawal and mucosal recovery (Hallstrom, 1989).

The pathological and diagnostic role of auto-antibodies is even less clear in ulcerative colitis (UC), which is only weakly associated with other diseases considered to have an auto-immune aetiology. In actively inflamed mucosa there is a profound increase in the number of plasma cells, particularly those secreting IgG1, suggesting that there may be a primary role for humoral mechanisms in this condition. However, there are few data to substantiate this contention. Many studies have demonstrated the presence of serum antibodies reactive with colonic mucosal components (e.g. Broberger & Perlmann 1959; Wright & Truelove 1966; Hibi et al., 1983; Fiocchi, Roche & Michener 1989; Takahashi et al., 1990), with lymphocytes (Korsmeyer et al., 1974) and with neutrophils (Saxon et al., 1990), but titres do not correlate clearly with disease activity, extent or duration. Recently it has been reported that the anti-neutrophil cytoplasmic antibody (termed pANCA because of the perinuclear pattern seen with immunostaining), is more prevalent in unaffected relatives of patients with UC (Shanahan et al.,

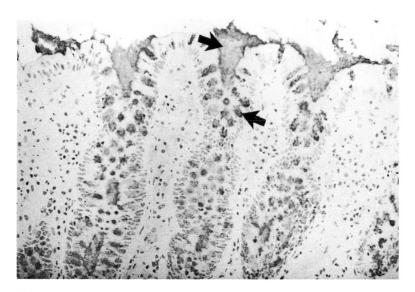

Fig. 13.1. Classical anti-colon antibody. The arrows indicate positive staining of mucin both within goblet cells and free in the crypts in normal colonic mucosa. Immunoperoxidase method, haematoxylin counterstain.

1992) and is positively associated with the HLA-DR2 haplotype (Yang *et al.*, 1992). The authors suggest that pANCA may distinguish between different genetic subsets within the UC population and hence may lead to further clues concerning pathogenesis.

Anti-colon antibodies which react with goblet cell mucin can be induced in experimental animals following immunisation with coliform bacteria, but mucosal inflammation does not follow (Cooke, Filipe & Dawson 1968). In patients with UC this type of antibody has been shown to be cross-reactive with a cell wall component of *E. coli* (Lagercrantz *et al.*, 1968) and may arise as an epiphenomenon of the inflammatory process, since it can also be detected in some patients with infective diarrhoea (Carlsson, Lagercrantz & Perlmann 1977). Examples of anti-colon and anti-neutrophil antibody visualised by immunohistochemical methods are shown in Figs. 13.1 and 13.2.

Somewhat stronger evidence for a pathogenetic role for mucosal IgG in ulcerative colitis has emerged from more recent studies. Halstensen *et al.* (1990), have demonstrated deposition of IgG1 and co-localised activated complement on the apical aspect of colonic superficial epithelium in active UC. The authors argue that this may provide a mechanism for epithelial damage by auto-antibody secreted or perhaps leaking into the colonic lumen. Das and colleagues have reported that mucosal and serum IgG in

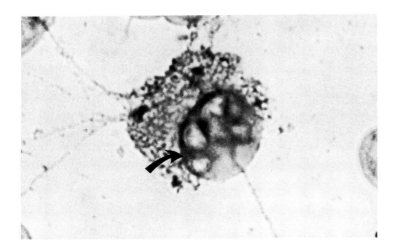

Fig. 13.2. Anti-neutrophil cytoplasmic antibody (ANCA). Note peri-nuclear accentuation of staining (arrow) and granular appearance of cytoplasm with sparing of cell nucleus. Indirect alkaline phosphatase method, fast red substrate. No counterstain. By courtesy of Dr. S. K. Lo.

patients with UC specifically recognises a 40 kD colonic protein (Takahashi & Das, 1985; Takahashi *et al.*, 1990). A recent report from this group suggests that the protein may be tropomyosin, a cytoskeletal component (Das *et al.*, 1993). The demonstration of immunoreactivity in a variety of other tissues using a monoclonal antibody raised against the 40 kD protein (Das, Vecchi & Sakamaki, 1990), provides an attractive mechanism to account for the extra-intestinal manifestations of UC. However, other workers employing comparable techniques have been unable to confirm the presence of similar auto-antibodies (Snook *et al.*, 1991; Cantrell, Prindiville & Gershwin, 1990).

From a diagnostic point of view, the role of autoantibodies in UC remains to be proven. There are wide discrepancies in the reported prevalence of the same antibodies between different laboratories, which probably reflects variation in methods. Until there is standardisation of assays and a better understanding of the nature of the target antigens, there will be little clinical application for antibodies as disease markers in UC.

Type III reactions

When circulating or tissue antibody combines with antigen, immune complexes are formed. Normally these are cleared by the mononuclear phagocyte system, but chronic production of antibody to persisting self or microbial antigens, or repeated exposure to exogenous antigen, may result in immune complex deposition and a subsequent inflammatory response. Widespread disease affecting different organs occurs when immune complexes lodge in small vessels, e.g. in skin, joints and kidney in systemic lupus erythematosus (SLE). Alternatively, the clinical manifestations may be relatively localised, as is the case in extrinsic allergic alveolitis due to chronic local challenge by inhaled foreign antigen. The potential of Type III reactions for producing multi-system disease and their typical pathology, consisting of oedema, haemorrhage, inflammatory infiltrates and eventual tissue necrosis, suggest that they may contribute to the pathogenesis of certain intestinal disorders.

In coeliac disease (CD), extracellular immunoglobulin and complement deposition can be demonstrated in the mucosa of the small intestine within hours of gluten challenge (Shiner & Ballard 1972; Doe, Henry & Booth 1974). Such observations have led to the suggestion that the local interaction of constituents of gluten, with specific antibody, may be primarily responsible for the mucosal lesion in CD. It is not clear why some individuals develop gluten sensitivity, but an attractive hypothesis is that it occurs as a consequence of cross reactivity between homologous protein sequences shared by human adenovirus 12 and A-gliadin, a toxic moiety of gluten (Kagnoff et al., 1987). Humoral mechanisms also appear to be important in dermatitis herpetiformis, which occurs in about 5% of adults with coeliac disease and which displays similar pathophysiology. Circulating immune complexes containing IgA can be detected in many cases and immunofluorescence of skin adjacent to the typical blistering lesions, reveals deposition of IgA in a granular pattern in the dermal papillae.

In a significant proportion of patients with active inflammatory bowel disease, there is accompanying peripheral arthropathy, erythema nodosum and uveitis. The nature and pathology of these extra-intestinal manifestations are suggestive of Type III hypersensitivity and indeed circulating immune complexes (or at least aggregated IgG) can be demonstrated in many cases. Whether Type III reactions are involved in the intestinal lesions of ulcerative colitis and Crohn's disease is harder to establish. However, experimental work has shown that a chronic colitis can be induced in sensitised animals following intravenous administration of preformed immune complexes (Mee et al., 1979).

Type IV reactions

According to the original Coombs and Gell classification, Type IV or delayed hypersensitivity is defined simply in terms of the delay (at least 12 hours), between antigen exposure and the subsequent immune reaction. It is now clear that this type of reaction is not based on a single specific pathophysiological process. Instead it may encompass a variety of different cellular and molecular interactions, but central to all of these is the role of the sensitised T cell. This is easily demonstrated in experimental models where it can be shown that, unlike other forms of hypersensitivity, Type IV reactions may be transferred between animals by lymphocytes but not by serum.

Whilst T cell-dependent processes are common to many of the intestinal disorders considered in this volume, each disease tends to be characterised by a distinct clinical and pathological phenotype. Moreover, the manifestations of a given disorder such as Crohn's disease may vary considerably between different affected individuals. The reasons for such phenotypic diversity are not fully understood, but recent studies of the HLA system and functional T cell subsets in other disease states may provide some clues.

It is well known that there is a clinical spectrum of disease in patients with leprosy, ranging from the tuberculoid form at one extreme, to the lepromatous type at the other. The former is characterised pathologically by a classical delayed hypersensitivity response, with granulomatous skin lesions consisting mainly of T cells and macrophages and few, if any, *M. leprae* bacilli. In contrast, the latter is typified by a strong, albeit ineffectual, humoral response and an abundance of bacilli. Condensing the data from a number of different studies, de Vries (1992) has argued that this dichotomy is determined by host HLA specificities, since HLA-DR3 is associated with tuberculoid disease, whilst HLA-DQ1 is strongly linked with the lepromatous form. It is proposed that these different HLA molecules may present different microbe-derived peptides to discrete subgroups of T cell, which, in turn, then trigger the characteristic individual response. In other words, the type of response mounted by an individual to a given antigen, is determined by inherited HLA alleles. The types of molecular mechanisms which may determine these specific interactions, between HLA molecules and T cells, have been demonstrated recently in an elegant analysis of the known association between possession of the HLA-B53 allele and resistance to severe malaria (Hill *et al.*, 1992).

Various HLA associations have been described in different immune mediated intestinal diseases. The strongest association described to date is that between the HLA-B8,DR3,DQw2 haplotype and coeliac disease, although the possible underlying mechanism remains unknown.

The situation with inflammatory bowel disease is less clear. It has been hypothesized that Crohn's disease and ulcerative colitis might lie at either extreme of a single disease spectrum. By analogy with leprosy, Crohn's disease would represent the 'tuberculoid' form of disease characterised by a patchy granulomatous cell-mediated response, whereas UC is manifested in the form of 'lepromatous' disease, with diffuse mucosal involvement and a marked humoral reaction. In contrast with leprosy however, convincing HLA associations with different types of inflammatory bowel disease have yet to be reported. Recent studies using accurate genotyping techniques have failed to reach agreement on the putative link between the HLA-DR2 allele and UC (Toyoda *et al.*, 1993; Mehal *et al.*, 1993), although two groups have independently identified an association between HLA-DQw5 and Crohn's disease (Toyoda *et al.*, 1993; Neigut *et al.*, 1992). As further immunogenetic studies are carried out and techniques are refined, tighter linkage may be established between HLA alleles and disease subgroups. Ultimately it may become possible to differentiate at a genetic level between different clinical phenotypes such as proctitis and pancolitis. Clearly, this could have important implications for clinical practice.

Animal models designed to express human HLA genes are likely to prove extremely useful tools in determining the role of individual alleles in different conditions. Of relevance to intestinal disease, it was recently shown that transfection of the human HLA-B27 and β2-microglobulin genes into rats, may result in the development in some animals of spontaneous inflammatory disease of the gut and joints, in a pattern similar to that observed in humans who possess this allele (Hammer *et al.*, 1990). Eluci-dation of the mechanisms involved may shed light on the known strong association between HLA-B27 and the development of spondyloarthro-pathy in patients with infectious colitis and inflammatory bowel disease. One attractive hypothesis invoked to explain this link, is that enteric organisms such as *Salmonella* and *Klebsiella* induce auto-reactivity by molecular mimickry, that is, by sharing common determinants with the HLA-B27 molecule (Oldstone, 1987).

If, as suggested above, different HLA specificities lead to the selection of restricted subsets of T cells, how does this bring about different clinical patterns of disease? Based on work in the mouse, Mosmann *et al.* (1986) described two discrete populations of helper T cells which were defined according to the profiles of cytokines which they produced. T_H1 cells synthesised interleukin 2 (IL-2) and gamma-interferon (γ-IFN), cytokines essential for T cell and macrophage activation, whereas T_H2 cells produced B cell growth factors including interleukin 4 (IL-4). Thus, it could be argued that the predominantly cell-mediated processes of cytotoxicity and classical delayed-type hypersensitivity might be driven by T_H1 T cells, whilst the T_H2 subgroup would promote humoral responses.

This concept has been partially validated in studies of cytokine responses in chronic infectious disease. Again, leprosy has proved to be an informative model. Yamamura *et al.* (1991), found that IL-2 and γ-IFN predominated in tuberculoid skin lesions but that IL-4, 5 and 10 were abundant in leproma-tous patients; there appeared to be a reciprocal relationship between the two groups of cytokines. A similar analysis has been reported by the same group in a study of leishmaniasis and it was again shown that clinical disease subgroups could be characterized by their cytokine profiles (Caceres-Dittmar et al., 1993).

Studies of cytokine expression in inflammatory bowel disease have yielded conflicting results to date and this may reflect methodological differences between research groups. However, it is interesting that upregulation of IL-2 (Mullin et al., 1992, Breese et al., 1993) and γ-IFN (Breese et al., 1993), has been reported in active Crohn's disease, but not ulcerative colitis, suggesting that the former may be driven by T_H1 type cells.

From the clinical viewpoint, cytokines released as a consequence of cellular activation, account for certain characteristic features of chronic intestinal disease and give rise to a variety of surrogate markers which are employed to assess activity and response to treatment. For example, IL-1, IL-6 and tumour necrosis factor alpha (TNFα), which are synthesised mainly by cells of the monocyte/macrophage system, are known to induce pyrexia, cachexia and increased hepatic synthesis of acute phase proteins. The latter action is reflected in the erythrocyte sedimentation rate (ESR) and serum C reactive protein (CRP), which provide helpful information in clinical practice. The finding that peripheral blood monocyte production of IL-1β and TNFα was greater in patients with active Crohn's disease than in a group with ulcerative colitis, may account for the more dramatic CRP response characteristic of the former condition (Mazlam & Hodgson 1992). With improved standardised assays it may become possible to employ direct measures of circulating and tissue bound cytokines to direct clinical management, in a way that is tailored to individual patients. Finally, it should be mentioned that many cytokines induce increased leucocyte/endothelial adhesion, which leads to cellular migration into inflamed tissue. This phenomenon is exploited by the developing techniques of isotope-labelled white cell scanning (see Fig. 13.3), which allow non-invasive assessment of the extent and activity of inflammatory bowel disease (Saverymuttu et al., 1982; Giaffer et al., 1993).

Rationale for therapy

In certain types of immunologically mediated intestinal disease, antigens derived from the diet or gut lumen are responsible for initiating and sustaining the harmful immune response. When such antigens are recognised as in food allergy and coeliac disease, the most logical and effective treatment is dietary exclusion to avoid exposure. Although causative antigens have yet to be identified in Crohn's disease, it is clear that dietary therapy may be highly effective in this condition, often inducing remission without recourse to anti inflammatory or immunosuppressant treatment

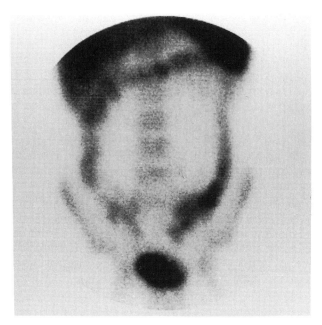

Fig. 13.3. Technetium-99m HMPAO labelled white cell scan showing active ileo-colonic Crohn's disease. By courtesy of Dr M. Weldon.

(O'Morain, Segal & Levi, 1984). Further evidence for the importance of luminal antigens in Crohn's disease, is that a temporary ileostomy which isolates the terminal ileum and colon from the faecal stream, may bring about remission or prevent disease recurrence (Rutgeerts *et al.*, 1991; Harper *et al.*, 1983). This is not the case in ulcerative colitis which typically fails to respond to faecal diversion. Indeed, there are case reports of UC involving neo-vaginas fashioned by plastic surgical techiques from loops of isolated sigmoid colon, in which 'vaginal' inflammation developed concurrently with colitis (Froese, Haggitt & Friend, 1991; Hennigan & Theodorou, 1992).

Therefore, if triggering antigens can not be removed or excluded from the gut, the clinician must resort to therapy which intervenes in the ensuing immune and inflammatory response. The crucial steps in this cascade are analysed below and, in each case, known and potential therapies will be considered. For the purpose of this discussion it is assumed that similar basic mechanisms are operating in a variety of diseases, although the relative contributions of different cell populations will inevitably vary.

Antigen presentation and recognition

The primary event in the majority of immune reactions, is the recognition of antigen in association with an MHC molecule, by a specific T cell receptor. Host and viral antigens which may induce auto-reactivity, are processed and then expressed in the context of Class I MHC molecules, on the surface of nucleated cells such as those of the intestinal epithelium. They may then be recognised by CD8 positive (cytotoxic/suppressor) T cells. Exogenous antigens, derived for example from the gut lumen, are presented after intracellular processing with Class II MHC molecules, by 'professional' antigen presenting cells, including dendritic cells, B cells and macrophages, to CD4 positive (helper) T cells. In addition, the induction of Class II expression by inflamed intestinal epithelium may provide a further route for antigen presentation in disease. These cellular interactions are illustrated in Fig. 13.4.

As yet there are few therapies in man directed specifically against this first stage of the immune response. Corticosteroids, which are effective in a wide variety of immune-mediated intestinal diseases, impair antigen presentation by macrophages in a non-specific fashion; 5-ASA, the active moiety of sulphasalazine, has been shown to reduce HLA-DR expression in a colonic epithelial cell line (Crotty *et al.*, 1992). However, these drugs act at various levels in the immune/inflammatory cascade and it is likely that their predominant actions are to inhibit cellular proliferation and the production of inflammatory mediators (see below).

There is growing interest in the potential for immunotherapy, directed at the interaction between the T cell receptor (TCR) and the antigen-MHC complex. In certain diseases it can be shown that there are predominant T cell subsets which share the same variable elements in the β chain (Vβ) of their TCR. This phenomenon has been recognised both in extrinsic allergic encephalomyelitis, an animal model of auto-immune disease (Urban *et al.*, 1988) and in man. Paliard *et al.* (1991), found that in rheumatoid arthritis, the frequency of Vβ 14 positive cells was higher in synovial fluid than peripheral blood. Posnett *et al.* (1990), describe finding a concentration of Vβ8 positive cells in mesenteric lymph nodes draining bowel affected by Crohn's disease. The significance of these observations is that they may identify an important pathogenic group of T cells, which could be targeted by immunotherapy. Possible strategies include, blocking TCR with peptides or monoclonal antibodies, vaccination with TCR peptides and induction of anergy in the relevant T cell subsets, by tolerisation using superantigens. None of these approaches has yet been employed in man.

The predominantly CD4 positive helper T cell population plays a central role in the immune response; not only do these cells recognise antigen but

ANY NUCLEATED CELL   CYTOTOXIC/SUPPRESSOR T CELL

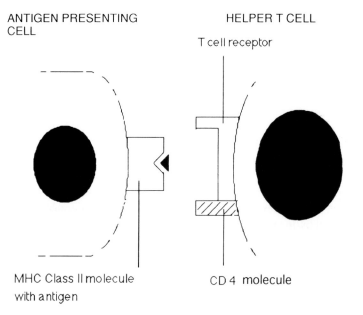

MHC Class I molecule   CD8 molecule
with antigen

ANTIGEN PRESENTING   HELPER T CELL
CELL

MHC Class II molecule   CD 4 molecule
with antigen

Fig. 13.4. Basic molecular mechanisms of antigen presentation and
recognition. Potential sites for intervention are discussed in text.

they also serve to amplify events in the subsequent cascade (see below). Observations that patients with rheumatoid arthritis (Bjilsma *et al.*, 1988) and Crohn's disease (James, 1988), may achieve apparent remission following the development of AIDS, provide support for the therapeutic strategy of depleting or blocking the activity of the helper T cell subset. Anti-CD4 monoclonal antibodies which interfere with antigen recognition, have been shown to be effective in an animal model of auto-immune disease (Brostoff & Mason, 1984). Further encouraging results have been reported in patients with rheumatoid arthritis (Herzog *et al.*, 1989) and in preliminary studies of patients with refractory inflammatory bowel disease (Emmrich *et al.*, 1991).

An alternative approach is to block TCR-MHC interaction, using peptides or monoclonal antibodies which recognise specific HLA molecules. Logically, this strategy would only be applicable in those diseases characterised by strong HLA associations. Again, experimental models are promising (see de Vries, 1992), but these techniques have not been used in humans.

Cellular activation and proliferation

Following antigen recognition by T cells, a cascade of events ensues which serves to amplify the immune response. This phase is the target for the majority of immunomodulatory therapies in current use. It is characterised by the activation and proliferation of effector cells and is illustrated in simplified form in Fig. 13.5. The production of interleukins (especially IL-2) and gamma interferon by activated helper T cells, is pivotal in the orchestration of these events, which are also driven by interleukin 1 (IL-1) synthesised principally by macrophages and peripheral blood monocytes.

Corticosteroids

The potent therapeutic effects of corticosteroids in a variety of immunological diseases are well known, although the underlying biochemical and cellular mechanisms are less well characterised. However, reduction of IL-1 synthesis (Snyder & Unanue, 1982) and interference with lymphocyte trafficking (Parillo & Fauci, 1979), are two immunomodulatory actions likely to be of clinical significance. Because of the systemic side-effects associated with high dose steroids, there is growing interest in the development of compounds with low bioavailability, for treating immune mediated intestinal diseases. Examples include, orally administered fluticasone propionate, which has been studied in patients with untreated coeliac disease (Mitchison *et al.*, 1991) and budesonide (prepared as an enema), for distal ulcerative colitis (Danish Budesonide Group, 1991). New corticosteroids such as these will probably prove to be of most benefit where disease activity is limited to the intestinal mucosa since, by design, their restriction to the gut

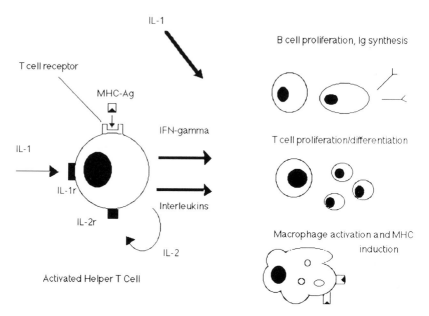

Fig. 13.5. Helper T cell activation and amplification of the immune response. Abbreviations: MHC-Ag (Class I or II molecule complexed with antigen); IL-1r,2r (interleukin 1 and 2 receptors); IFN-gamma (interferon-gamma); Ig (immunoglobulin). See text for therapeutic possibilities.

4renders them unable to influence distant immune activation in the bone marrow, blood and lymphoid tissue.

Anti-metabolites

This group of drugs inhibit cellular division in a non-specific fashion. Their efficacy, in immunologically mediated diseases, is thought to be due to their effect on rapidly proliferating clones of activated lymphocytes.

Azathioprine, and its active metabolite 6-mercaptopurine, are purine analogues which interfere with nucleic acid synthesis. One or both of these agents have been shown to be valuable in the treatment of a wide range of disorders including ulcerative colitis (Jewell & Truelove 1974; Hawthorne *et al.*, 1992), Crohn's disease (O'Donoghue *et al.*, 1978; Present *et al.*, 1980) and in cases of refractory coeliac disease (Hamilton, Chambers & Wynn-Williams, 1976). They are not effective in all patients and their use is limited by toxicity and concern about a possibly increased risk of lymphoreticular malignancy.

Methotrexate is an anti-folate which indirectly inhibits DNA synthesis by blocking dihydrofolate reductase. Early reports of its use in inflammatory bowel disease were favourable (Kozarek *et al.*, 1989; Baron, Truss & Elson, 1991) and further support comes from a small controlled trial (Arora *et al.*, 1992), but pneumonitis, hepatotoxicity and bone marrow suppression are serious potential side-effects.

Therapies directed at lymphocytes and their products

In addition to strategies designed to block antigen recognition (see above), there is considerable potential for treatments which target the activated T cell population and particularly the helper cell subset. Non-selective depletion of circulating T cells by lymphoplasmapheresis, has been claimed to produce steroid independent remission, in patients with chronically active Crohn's disease (Bicks & Groshart, 1989), but a controlled trial has shown no effect for maintaining remission (Lerebours *et al.*, 1991).

The IL-2 inhibitor cyclosporin A (CyA) has revolutionised immunosuppression in organ transplantation and it has been introduced with enthusiasm for the treatment of intestinal disease. The drug appears to block IL-2 gene transcription by inhibiting a specific intra-cellular pathway in activated T cells (Flanagan *et al.*, 1991). Early studies in Crohn's disease were encouraging (Allison & Pounder, 1984; Parrott *et al.*, 1988) but larger controlled clinical trials have yielded conflicting results (Brynskov *et al.*, 1989a; Jewell D. P. & Lennard-Jones J. E., 1994). For severe ulcerative colitis, oral cyclosporin appears to have little effect (Baker & Jewell 1989), but when administered intravenously in a pilot study (Lichtiger & Present 1990) and in a recent clinical trial (Lichtiger *et al.*, 1993), the drug showed substantial promise. To date, the only controlled data indicating a useful effect of oral CyA in ulcerative colitis, are from a group of patients with mild disease who were undergoing a trial for co-existing sclerosing cholangitis (Sandborn *et al.*, 1993a). Rectal preparations of cyclosporin have been reported to provide benefit in some patients with refractory distal ulcerative colitis (Brynskov *et al.*, 1989b; Winter *et al.*, 1994), but relapse occurred commonly on discontinuation of the drug. The most recent controlled study of cyclosporin enema treatment failed to show any significant beneficial effect. (Sandborn *et al.*, 1993b).

Cyclosporin has been employed to good effect in other intestinal diseases. The value of the drug is well established in the field of bone marrow transplantation, where it is used both to prevent and treat graft-versus-host disease (Barrett, 1991). Several reports have also indicated that cyclosporin may be highly effective in cases of paediatric auto-immune enteropathy (Bernstein & Whitington, 1988; Sanderson *et al.*, 1991).

The rapid progress which is being made in the field of cytokine research is likely soon to yield a range of agents, designed to block selective lymphocyte activation pathways. This approach will be particularly appropriate if specific targets can be identified in different disorders, e.g. T_H1 cytokines (discussed above) in Crohn's disease. Already a recombinant IL-1 receptor antagonist has been shown to be effective in an animal model of colitis (Cominelli et al., 1992) and clinical trials should follow.

Another therapeutic avenue awaiting development is the use of mono-clonal anti-idiotype antibodies which would specifically block the binding of auto-antibodies to host antigens. Recent advances in bioengineering have enabled the 'humanisation' of monoclonal antibodies produced in mice, thereby overcoming the problems of immune complex disease and neutrali-sation which have hampered previous trials of antibody treatment, when repeated dosing has been necessary.

Effectors of inflammation

Tissue damage occurs due to the action of the components of the final limb of the immune response, either following direct auto-immune attack or as a by-product of the response to foreign antigen. Inflammatory and cytotoxic mediators are liberated by activated mucosal effector cells, including macro-phages, mast cells and eosinophils; to these are added neutrophils and lymphocytes recruited from the circulation by cytokine-regulated induction of vascular adhesion molecules (see Fig. 13.6). A number of the mediators shown may be induced or synthesised by more than one cell type.

Identification of the major components of the inflammatory cascade and analysis of their inter-relationships, has allowed increased understanding of the mode of action of conventional therapies, such as corticosteroids and salicylates. The efficacy of these drugs was realised as a result of clinical observation and serendipity, but many compounds currently under develop-ment have been designed with a specific intervention in mind.

Of the several anti-inflammatory actions ascribed to corticosteroids, the most significant in clinical terms are likely to be the following: impairment of macrophage function and subsequent inhibition of release of IL-1, IL-6 and TNFα; inhibition of phospholipase A2, resulting in a reduction in the synthesis of arachidonic acid and its derived mediators including leuko-trienes and prostaglandins. Recent data suggest that direct modulation of leucocyte-endothelial adhesion is also likely to be of importance (Cronstein et al., 1992). Similarly, salicylates employed in inflammatory bowel disease appear to owe their efficacy to a multiplicity of actions including reduction in vascular adhesion and chemotaxis, inhibition of IL-1, platelet activating factor (PAF) and leukotriene release, and scavenging of reactive oxygen metabolites (Travis & Jewell, 1993). The action of 5-lipoxygenase (5-LPO) on arachidonic acid leads to the generation of such potent inflammatory species as leukotriene B4 (LTB4), which is a powerful neutrophil chemo-

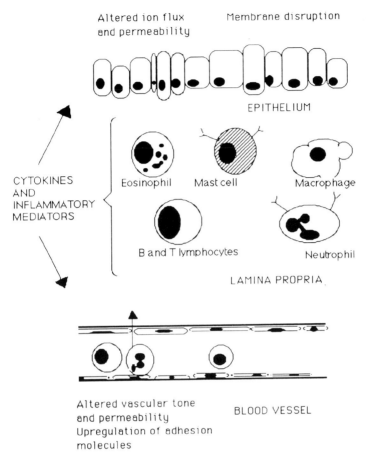

Fig. 13.6. Effectors of inflammation. Important mediators include LTB4, prostaglandins, complement, PAF, histamine, kinins and free oxygen radicals. Locally produced cytokines include Il-1, Il-6 and TNF α. Further detail in text.

attractant. Zileuton (Abbott-64077), a newly designed 5-LPO inhibitor, has shown promise in early clinical trials in ulcerative colitis (Stenson *et al.*, 1991); further compounds in the same class are also undergoing clinical evaluation.

Several other avenues of intervention are being explored, with the result that monoclonal antibodies to TNFα, selective PAF antagonists and specific inhibitors of adhesion molecule expression are all likely to undergo clinical trials soon. A cautionary note, however, might be sounded with respect to the new bio-engineered therapies. Although there is an attractive simplicity to the concept of blocking individual pathways in the immune/inflammatory cascade, the efficacy of conventional treatments such as corticosteroids may be due to the very non-specificity of their actions. This may enable them to overcome the enormous redundancy which is inherent in the cascade and which may allow many inflammatory processes, to by-pass drug inhibition of single pathways.

References

Allison, M. C. & Pounder, R. E. (1984). Cyclosporin for Crohn's disease. *Lancet*, **i**, 902–3.

Arora, S., Katkov, W. N., Cooley, J. *et al.* (1992). A double-blind, randomized, placebo-controlled trial of methotrexate in Crohn's disease. *Gastroenterology*, **102**, A591.

Baker, K. & Jewell, D. P. (1989). Cyclosporin A for the treatment of severe inflammatory bowel disease. *Alimentary Pharmacology and Therapeutics*, **3**, 143–9.

Baron, T. H., Truss, C. D. & Elson, C. O. (1991). Steroid sparing effect of oral methotrexate in refractory inflammatory bowel disease. *Gastroenterology*, **100**, A195.

Barrett, A. J. (1991). Immunosuppressive therapy in bone marrow transplantation. *Immunology Letters*, **29**, 81–7.

Bernstein, E. F. & Whitington, P. F. (1988). Successful treatment of atypical sprue in an infant with cyclosporine. *Gastroenterology*, **95**, 199–204.

Bicks, R. O. & Groshart, K. D. (1989). The current status of T-lymphocyte apheresis (TLA) treatment of Crohn's disease. *Journal of Clinical Gastroenterology*, **11**, 136–8.

Bjilsma, J. W., Derksen, R. W., Huber-Bruning, O. & Borleffs, J. C. (1988). Does AIDS 'cure' rheumatoid arthritis? *Annals of Rheumatological Diseases*, **47**, 350–1.

Breese, E., Braegger, C. P., Corrigan, C. J., Walker-Smith, J. A. & MacDonald, T. T. (1993). Interleukin-2- and interferon-gamma-secreting T cells in normal and diseased human intestinal mucosa. *Immunology*, **78**, 127–31.

Broberger, O. & Perlmann, P. (1959). Autoantibodies in human ulcerative colitis. *Journal of Experimental Medicine*, **110**, 657–74.

Brostoff, S. W. & Mason, D. W. (1984). Experimental allergic encephalomyelitis: successful treatment *in vivo* with a monoclonal antibody that recognizes T-helper cells. *Journal of Immunology*, **133**, 1938–42.

Brynskov, J., Freund, L., Rasmussen, S. N. *et al.* (1989*a*). A placebo-controlled, double-blind, randomized trial of cyclosporine therapy in active chronic Crohn's disease. *New England Journal of Medicine*, **321**, 845–50.

Brynskov, J., Freund, L., Thomsen, O. O., Andersen, C. B., Rasmussen, S. N. & Binder, V. (1989*b*). Treatment of refractory ulcerative colitis with cyclosporin enemas. *Lancet*, **i**, 721–2.

Buckell, N. A., Gould, S. R., Day, D. W., Lennard-Jones, J. E. & Edwards, A. M. (1978). Controlled trial of disodium cromoglycate in chronic persistent ulcerative colitis. *Gut*, **19**, 1140–3.

Burman, P., Mardh, S., Norberg, L. & Karlsson, F. A. (1989). Parietal cell antibodies in pernicious anaemia inhibit H^+K^+-adenosine triphosphatase, the proton pump of the stomach. *Gastroenterology*, **96**, 1434–8.

Caceres-Dittmar, G., Tapia, F. J., Sanchez, M. A. *et al.* (1993). Determination of the cytokine profile in American cutaneous leishmaniasis using the polymerase chain reaction. *Clinical and Experimental Immunology*, **91**, 500–5.

Cantrell, M., Prindiville, T. & Gershwin, M. E. (1990). Autoantibodies to colonic cells and subcellular fractions in inflammatory bowel disease: do they exist? *Journal of Autoimmunity*, **3**, 307–20.

Carlsson, H. E., Lagercrantz, R. & Perlmann, P. (1977). Immunological studies in ulcerative colitis VIII. Antibodies to colon antigen in patients with ulcerative colitis, Crohn's disease and other diseases. *Scandinavian Journal of Gastroenterology*, **12**, 707–14.

Cello, J. P. (1979). Eosinophilic gastroenteritis: a complex disease entity. *American Journal of Medicine*, **67**, 1097–104.

Cominelli, F., Nast, C. C., Duchini, A. & Lee, M. (1992). Recombinant interleukin-1 receptor antagonist blocks the proinflammatory activity of endogenous interleukin-1 in rabbit immune colitis. *Gastroenterology*, **103**, 65–71.

Cooke, E. M., Filipe, N. I. & Dawson, I. M. P. (1968). The production of colonic autoantibodies in rabbits by immunization with *Escherichia coli*. *Journal of Pathology and Bacteriology*, **96**, 125–30.

Cronstein, B. N., Kimmel, S. C., Levin, R. I., Martiniuk, F. & Weissmann, G. (1992). A mechanism for the antiinflammatory effects of corticosteroids: the glucocorticoid receptor regulates leukocyte adhesion to endothelial cells and expression of endothelial–leukocyte adhesion molecule 1 and intercellular adhesion molecule 1. *Proceedings of the National Academy of Sciences, USA*, **89**, 9991–5.

Crotty, B., Hoang, P., Dalton, H. R. & Jewell, D. P. (1992). Salicylates used in inflammatory bowel disease and colchicine impair interferon-gamma induced HLA-DR expression. *Gut*, **33**, 59–64.

Danish Budesonide Group. (1991). Budesonide enema in distal ulcerative colitis. A randomised dose–response trial with prednisolone enema as a positive control. *Scandinavian Journal of Gastroenterology*, **26**, 1225–30.

Das, K. M., Vecchi, M. & Sakamaki, S. (1990). A shared and unique epitope(s) on human colon, skin, and biliary epithelium detected by a monoclonal antibody. *Gastroenterology*, **98**, 464–9.

Das, K. M., Dasgupta, A., Mandal, A. & Geng, X. (1993). Autoimmunity to cytoskeletal protein tropomyosin. A clue to the pathogenetic mechanism for ulcerative colitis. *Journal of Immunology*, **150**, 2487–93.

de Vries, R. R. P. (1992). HLA and disease: from epidemiology to immunotherapy. *European Journal of Clinical Investigation*, **33**, 1–8.

Doe, W. F., Henry, K. & Booth, C. C. (1974). Complement in coeliac disease. In *Coeliac Disease*, (eds.) W. Th. J. M. Hekkens, & A. S. Pena. Stenfert Kroese, Leiden p. 179.

Dronfield, M. W. & Langman, M. J. S. (1978). Comparative trial of sulphasalazine and oral sodium cromoglycate in the maintenance of remission in ulcerative colitis. *Gut*, **19**, 1136–9.

Emmrich, J., Seyfarth, M., Fleig, W. E. & Emmrich, F. (1991). Treatment of inflammatory bowel disease with anti-CD4 monoclonal antibody. *Lancet*, **338**, 570–1.

Fiocchi, C., Roche, J. K. & Michener, W. M. (1989). High prevalence of antibodies to intestinal epithelial antigens in patients with inflammatory bowel disease and their relatives. *Annals of Internal Medicine*, **110**, 786–94.

Flanagan, W. M., Corthesy, B., Bram, R. J. & Crabtree, G. R. (1991). Nuclear association of a T-cell transcription factor blocked by FK-506 and cyclosporin A. *Nature*, **352**, 803–7.

Froese, D. P., Haggitt, R. C. & Friend, W. G. (1991). Ulcerative colitis in the autotransplanted neovagina. *Gastroenterology*, **100**, 1749–52.

Giaffer, M. H., Tindale, W. B., Senior, S., Barber, D. C. & Holdsworth, C. D. (1993). Quantification of disease activity in Crohn's disease by computer analysis of Tc-99m hexamethyl propylene amine oxime (HMPAO) labelled leucocyte images. *Gut*, **34**, 68–74.

Hallstrom, O. (1989). Comparison of IgA-class reticulin and endomysium antibodies in coeliac disease and dermatitis herpetiformis. *Gut*, **30**, 1225–32.

Halstensen, T. S., Mollnes, T. E., Garred, P., Fausa, O. & Brandtzaeg, P. (1990). Epithelial deposition of immunoglobulin G1 and activated complement (C3b and terminal complement complex) in ulcerative colitis. *Gastroenterology*, **98**, 1264–71.

Hamilton, J. D., Chambers, R. A. & Wynn-Williams, A. (1976). Role of gluten, prednisone, and azathioprine in non-responsive coeliac disease. *Lancet*, **i**, 1213–16.

Hammer, R. E., Maika, S. D., Richardson J. A., Tang, J. P. & Taurog, J. D. (1990). Spontaneous inflammatory disease in transgenic rats expressing HLA-B27 and human beta 2m: an animal model of HLA-B27-associated human disorders. *Cell*, **63**, 1099–112.

Harper, P. H., Truelove, S. C., Lee, E. C. G., Kettlewell, M. G. W. & Jewell, D. P. (1983). Split ileostomy and ileo-colostomy for Crohn's disease of the colon and ulcerative colitis. *Gut*, **24**, 106–13.

Hawthorne, A. B., Logan, R. F., Hawkey, C. J., Foster, P. N., Axon, A. T., Swarbrick, E. T., Scott, B. B. & Lennard-Jones, J. E. (1992). Randomised controlled trial of azathioprine withdrawal in ulcerative colitis. *British Medical Journal*, **305**, 20–2.

Heatley, R. V., Calcraft, B. J., Rhodes, J., Owen, E. & Evans, B. K. (1975). Disodium cromoglycate in the treatment of chronic proctitis. *Gut*, **16**, 559–63.

Hennigan, T. W. & Theodorou, N. A. (1992). Ulcerative colitis and bleeding from a colonic vaginoplasty. *Journal of the Royal Society of Medicine*, **85**, 418–19.

Herzog, C., Walker, C., Muller, W. *et al*. (1989). Anti-CD4 antibody treatment of patients with rheumatoid arthritis: I. Effect on clinical course and circulating T cells. *Journal of Autoimmunity*, **2**, 627–42.

Hibi, T., Aiso, M., Ishikawa, M. *et al*. (1983). Circulating antibodies to the surface antigens on colonic epithelial cells in ulcerative colitis. *Clinical and Experimental Immunology*, **54**, 163–8.

Hill, A. V. S., Elvin, J., Willis, A. C. (1992). Molecular analysis of the association of HLA-B53 and resistance to severe malaria. *Nature*, **360**, 434–9.

James, S. P. (1988). Remission of Crohn's disease after human immunodeficiency virus infection. *Gastroenterology*, **95**, 1667–9.

Jenkins, H. R., Pincott, J. R., Soothill, J. F., Milla, P. J. & Harries, J. T. (1984). Food allergy: the major cause of infantile colitis. *Archives of Disease in Childhood*, **59**, 326–9.

Jewell, D. P. & Lennard-Jones, J. E. (1994). Oral cyclosporin for chronic active Crohn's disease: A multicentre controlled trial. *European Journal of Gastrology and Hepatology* (in press).

Jewell, D. P. & Truelove, S. C. (1974). Azathioprine in ulcerative colitis: final report on controlled therapeutic trial. *British Medical Journal*, **4**, 627–30.

Kagnoff, M. F., Paterson, Y. J., Kumar, P. J. *et al*. (1987). Evidence for the role of a human intestinal adenovirus in the pathogenesis of coeliac disease. *Gut*, **28**, 995–1001.

Karlsson, F. A., Burman, P., Loof, L. & Mardh, S. (1988). Major parietal cell antigen in autoimmune gastritis with pernicious anaemia is the acid-producing H^+K^+-adenosine triphosphatase of the stomach. *Journal of Clinical Investigation*, **81**, 475–9.

Korsmeyer, S. J., Strickland, R. G., Wilson, I. D. & Williams, R. C. (1974). Serum lymphocytotoxic and lymphocytophilic antibody activity in inflammatory bowel disease. *Gastroenterology*, **67**, 578–83.

Kozarek, R. A., Patterson, D. J., Gelfand, M. D., Botoman, V. A., Ball, T. J. & Wilske, K. R. (1989). Methotrexate induces clinical and histologic remission in patients with refractory inflammatory bowel disease. *Annals of Internal Medicine*, **110**, 353–6.

Lagercrantz, R., Hammarstrom, S., Perlmann, P. & Gustaffson, B. E. (1968). Immunological studies in ulcerative colitis IV. Origin of autoantibodies. *Journal of Experimental Medicine*, **129**, 1339–52.

Lerebours, E., Modigliani, R., Florent, C., Rene, E. & GETAID (1991). Controlled trial of the efficacy of lymphocyte apheresis in preventing relapse in Crohn's disease patients. *Gastroenterology*, **100**, A224.

Lichtiger, S., & Present, D. H. (1990). Preliminary report: cyclosporin in treatment of severe active ulcerative colitis. *Lancet*, **336**, 16–19.

Lichtiger, S., Present, D. H., Kornbluth, A. & Hanauer, S. (1993). Cyclosporin A in the treatment of severe, refractory ulcerative colitis: a double-blinded placebo controlled trial. *Gastroenterology*, **104**, A732.

Lopes, J. D., Ito, H. & Glass, G. B. J. (1976). Inhibition of parietal and peptic cell proliferation by parietal cell and intrinsic factor antibodies. *Gastroenterology*, **70**, 910.

Loveridge, N., Bitensky, L., Chayen, J., Hausamen, T.-U., Fisher, J. M. & Taylor, K. B. (1980). Inhibition of parietal cell function by human gammaglobulin containing gastric parietal cell antibodies. *Clinical and Experimental Immunology*, **41**, 264–70.

Mazlam, M. Z., & Hodgson, H. J. F. (1992). Peripheral blood monocyte cytokine production and acute phase response in inflammatory bowel disease. *Gut*, **33**, 773–8.

Mee, A. S., McLaughlin, J. E., Hodgson, H. J. F. & Jewell, D. P. (1979). Chronic immune colitis in rabbits. *Gut*, **20**, 1–5.

Mehal, W. Z., Lo, S. K., Wordsworth, P. B., Chapman, R. W. & Fleming, K. A. (1993). HLA DRw52a and Dw2 are not associated with the development of anti-neutrophil antibody type 1 (ANCA 1) in ulcerative colitis (UC). *Gastroenterology*, **104**, A743.

Mitchison, H. C., Gillespie, S., Laker, M., Zaitoun, A., & Record, C. O. (1991). A pilot study of fluticasone propionate in untreated coeliac disease. *Gut*, **32**, 260–5.

Mosmann, T. R., Cherwinski, H., Bond, M. W., Giedlin, M. A., & Coffman, R. L. (1986). Two types of murine helper T cell clone. I. Definition according to profiles of lymphokine activities and secreted proteins. *Journal of Immunology*, **136**, 2348–57.

Mullin, G. E., Lazenby, A. J., Harris, M. L., Bayless, T. M. & James, S. P. (1992). Increased interleukin-2 messenger RNA in the intestinal mucosal lesions of Crohn's disease but not ulcerative colitis. *Gastroenterology*, **102**, 1620–7.

Neigut, D., Proujansky, Trucco, M., Dorman, J. S., Kocoshis, S., Carpenter, A. B. & Ball, E. J. (1992). Association of an HLA-DQB-1 genotype with Crohn's disease in children. *Gastroenterology*, **102**, A671.

O'Donoghue, D. P., Dawson, A. M., Powell-Tuck, J., Bown, R. L. & Lennard-Jones, J. E. (1978). Double-blind withdrawal trial of azathioprine as maintenance treatment for Crohn's disease. *Lancet*, **ii**, 955–7.

Oldstone, M. B. (1987). Molecular mimicry and autoimmune disease. *Cell*, **50**, 819–20.

O'Morain, C., Segal, A. W. & Levi, A. J. (1984). Elemental diet as primary treatment of acute Crohn's disease: a controlled trial. *British Medical Journal*, **288**, 1859–62.

Paliard, X., West, S. G., Lafferty, J. A. *et al.* (1991). Evidence for the effects of a superantigen in rheumatoid arthritis. *Science*, **253**, 325–9.

Parillo, J. E. & Fauci, A. S. (1979). Mechanisms of glucocorticoid action on immune processes. *Annual Reviews of Pharmacology and Toxicology*, **19**, 179–201.

Parrott, N. R., Taylor, R. M., Venables, C. W. & Record, C. O. (1988). Treatment of Crohn's disease in relapse with cyclosporin A. *British Journal of Surgery*, **75**, 1185–8.

Posnett, D. N., Schmelkin, I., Burton, D. A., August, A., McGrath, H. & Mayer, L. F. (1990). T cell antigen receptor V gene usage. Increases in V beta 8+ T cells in Crohn's disease. *Journal of Clinical Investigation*, **85**, 1770–6.

Present, D. H., Korelitz, B. I., Wisch, N., Glass, J. L., Sachar, D. B. & Pasternack, B. S. (1980). Treatment of Crohn's disease with 6-mercaptopurine: a long term randomized double-blind study. *New England Journal of Medicine*, **302**, 981–7.

Rose, M. S. & Chanarin, I. (1971). Intrinsic factor antibody and absorption of vitamin B12 in pernicious anaemia. *British Medical Journal*, **i**, 25–6.

Rosekrans, P. C. M., Meijer, C. J. L. M., Van der Wal, A. M. & Lindeman, J. (1980). Allergic proctitis, a clinical and immunopathological entity. *Gut*, **21**, 1017–23.

Rutgeerts, P., Goboes, K., Peeters, M. *et al.*, (1991). Effect of faecal stream diversion on recurrence of Crohn's disease in the neoterminal ileum. *Lancet*, **338**, 771–4.

Sandborn, W. J., Wiesner, R. H., Tremaine, W. J. & Larusso, N. F. (1993a). Ulcerative colitis disease activity following treatment of associated primary sclerosing cholangitis with cyclosporin. *Gut*, **34**, 242–6.

Sandborn, W. J., Tremaine, W. J., Schroeder, K. W. *et al.* (1993b). A randomized, double blind, placebo-controlled trial of cyclosporin enemas for mildly to moderately active left-sided ulcerative colitis. *Gastroenterology*, **104**, A775.

Sanderson, I. R., Phillips, A. D., Spencer, J. & Walker, S. J. (1991). Response of autoimmune enteropathy to cyclosporin A therapy. *Gut*, **32**, 1421–5.

Saverymuttu, S. H., Peters, A. M., Hodgson, H. J. F., Chadwick, V. S. & Lavender, J. P. (1982). Indium-111 autologous leucocyte scanning: comparison with radiology for imaging the colon in inflammatory bowel disease. *British Medical Journal*, **285**, 255–7.

Saxon, A., Shanahan, F., Landers, C., Ganz, T. & Targan, S. (1990). A distinct subset of antineutrophil cytoplasmic antibodies is associated with inflammatory bowel disease. *Journal of Allergy and Clinical Immunology*, **86**, 202–10.

Shanahan, F., Duerr, R. H., Rotter, J. I. *et al.* (1992). Neutrophil autoantibodies in ulcerative colitis: familial aggregation and genetic heterogeneity. *Gastroenterology*, **103**, 456–61.

Shiner, M. & Ballard, J. (1972). Antigen-antibody reactions in jejunal mucosa in childhood coeliac disease after gluten challenge. *Lancet*, **i**, 1202–5.

Snook, J. A., Lowes, J. R., Wu, K. C., Priddle, J. D. & Jewell, D. P. (1991). Serum and tissue autoantibodies to colonic epithelium in ulcerative colitis. *Gut*, **32**, 163–6.

Snyder, D. S. & Unanue, E. R. (1982). Corticosteroids inhibit murine macrophage Ia expression and interleukin 1 production. *Journal of Immunology*, **129**, 1803–5.

Stenson, W. F., Lauritsen, K., Laursen, L. S. (1991). A clinical trial of zileuton, a specific inhibitor of 5-lipoxygenase, in ulcerative colitis. *Gastroenterology*, **100**, A400.

Takahashi, F. & Das, K. M. (1985). Isolation and characterization of a colonic autoantigen specifically recognized by colon tissue-bound immunoglobulin G from idiopathic ulcerative colitis. *Journal of Clinical Investigation*, **76**, 311–18.

Takahashi, F., Shah, H. S., Wise, L. S. & Das, K. M. (1990). Circulating antibodies against human colonic extract enriched with a 40 kDa protein in patients with ulcerative colitis. *Gut*, **31**, 1016–20.

Tanaka, N. & Glass, G. B. J. (1970). Effect of prolonged administration of parietal cell antibodies from patients with atrophic gastritis and pernicious anaemia on the parietal cell mass and hydrochloric acid output in rats. *Gastroenterology*, **58**, 482–93.

Toyoda, H., Wang, S.-J., Yang, H.-Y. *et al.* (1993). Distinct associations of HLA class II genes with inflammatory bowel disease. *Gastroenterology*, **104**, 741–8.

Travis, S. P. L. & Jewell, D. P. (1993). Salicylates for ulcerative colitis–their mode of action. *Pharmacology and Therapeutics* (in press).

Urban, J. L., Kumar, V., Kono, D. H. *et al.* (1988). Restricted use of T cell receptor V genes in murine autoimmune encephalomyelitis raises possibilities for antibody therapy. *Cell*, **54**, 577–92.

Winter, T., Dalton, H. D., Merrett, M. N., Campbell, A. & Jewell, D. P. (1994). Cyclosporin retention enemas in refractory distal ulcerative colitis. *Scandinavian Journal of Gastroenterology*, **28**, 701–4.

Wright, R. & Truelove, S. C. (1965). A controlled therapeutic trial of various diets in ulcerative colitis. *British Medical Journal*, **2**, 138–41.

Wright, R. & Truelove, S. C. (1966). Auto-immune reactions in ulcerative colitis. *Gut*, **7**, 32–40.

Yamamura, M., Uyemura, K., Deans, R. J. *et al.* (1991). Defining protective responses to pathogens: cytokine profiles in leprosy lesions. *Science*, **254**, 277–82.

Yang, H., Rotter, J. I., Toyoda, H. *et al.* (1992). Ulcerative colitis: a genetic heterogeneous group defined with genetic (DR2) and subclinical markers (anti-neutrophil cytoplasmic antibodies (ANCAs)). *Gastroenterology*, **102**, A716.

–14–
Chronic active hepatitis

P. J. JOHNSON and I. G. McFARLANE

Introduction

Chronic active hepatitis (CAH) is a term used interchangeably to describe both a syndrome and a hepatic histological entity, the defining features of which are a dense portal and periportal lymphoplasmacytic infiltrate with piecemeal necrosis of periportal hepatocytes (Fig. 14.1), which often leads to cirrhosis (Scheuer, 1987; Ludwig, 1992). The syndrome has been recognised for many years (Cullinan, 1936; Amberg, 1942; Waldenstrom, 1950). Infection with the hepatitis B, delta (D) or C viruses are the most clearly defined aetiological agents but the histological features are also seen in a number of other primary liver diseases (Table 14.1) and in idiosyncratic reactions to a wide range of therapeutic drugs. When all of these aetiological factors are excluded there remains a group of patients with idiopathic CAH, some of whom have pronounced 'immunological' features (see below) and are considered to be suffering from 'auto-immune' hepatitis (AIH), while the remainder are often classified as 'cryptogenic'.

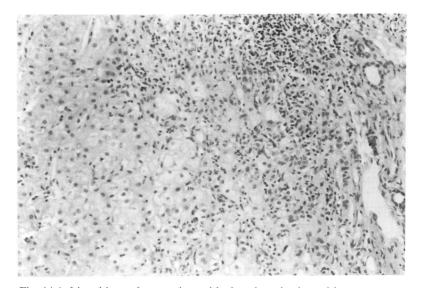

Fig. 14.1. Liver biopsy from patient with chronic active hepatitis.

Table 14.1. *Disorders most often associated with histological features of chronic active hepatitis*

Autoimmune	Autoimmune hepatitis Primary biliary cirrhosis Primary sclerosing cholangitis (Autoimmune cholangiopathy)
Viral	Acute hepatitis A Chronic hepatitis B, C and D infections Other hepatotropic viruses
Metabolic	Alcoholic liver disease Wilson's disease
Drug-induced	Idiosyncratic reactions to a wide range of drugs
Cryptogenic	Distinction from autoimmune hepatitis is not always made (see text)

Persistence of symptoms or signs of liver disease for more than 6 months is a generally accepted arbitrary criterion to establish chronicity, but the majority of patients with CAH are probably asymptomatic – since many already have an established cirrhosis when they first present (Hay *et al.*, 1989; Johnson *et al.*, 1990). When symptoms do arise they are usually related to particularly active disease and lethargy, fatigue (often extreme), anorexia and nausea are prominent. As the liver begins to fail, either because of continuing disease activity, or if the disorder has progressed to the stage of cirrhosis, signs of liver decompensation (jaundice, ascites, peripheral oedema, oesophageal varices, coagulopathy, and encephalopathy) develop. However, most of the clinical features are related to the degree of liver dysfunction rather than to a particular aetiology of CAH. Similarly, the biochemical liver tests, showing a 'hepatitic' pattern of abnormalities, are not specific for different aetiologies of CAH and other investigations, including serum tests for viral markers and auto-antibodies, are required.

Auto-immune hepatitis (AIH)

Clinical features

The patient is classically a young woman who presents with either an acute hepatitic or a chronic, rumbling, illness characterised by lethargy, arthralgia, oligomenorrhoea, fluctuating jaundice and a Cushingoid appearance with striae, hirsutism and acne. Particularly in those with a more protracted onset of symptoms, cutaneous manifestations of chronic liver disease and signs of cirrhosis may be prominent. Not infrequently the patient will be atopic and may even have another auto-allergic condition and there is often a history of auto-immune disorders (rheumatoid arthritis, auto-immune thyroid disease, diabetes, vitiligo) in first-degree relatives.

Laboratory investigations typically reveal serum aminotransferase activity more than ten times the upper normal limit and marked hypergammaglobulinaemia (often in the range 50–100 g/l) due mainly to selective elevation of immunoglobulin G. Antinuclear antibodies (ANA) are found in the sera of about 70% of cases, many of whom, together with the remaining 30%, have smooth muscle auto-antibodies (SMA) (Doniach *et al.*, 1966; Whittingham, Mackay & Irwin, 1966; Whittingham *et al.*, 1966). A small proportion (about 3%) have liver–kidney microsomal auto-antibodies (LKM-1), usually without ANA or SMA (Homberg *et al.*, 1987) and antimitochondrial antibodies (AMA) are said to be detectable in up to 20% of cases (Kenny *et al.*, 1986) although the frequency is much less (about 2%) in our experience (McFarlane, 1993).

It is now recognised, however, that the disease also affects males and that there is an older age group of patients in whom the condition seems to have a more insidious onset and tends to follow a milder course (McFarlane, 1993). In these cases, the aminotransferase activities and hypergammaglobulinaemia may be less markedly abnormal (1.5–3 fold elevations) but the histological changes are usually indistinguishable from (and may be no less severe than) those of the younger patients. The majority of patients of all ages respond to corticosteroid therapy. It is also now recognised that there are patients with a disorder that broadly conforms to 'classical' AIH (comprising about 20% of cases in some series), who present without ANA, SMA or LKM-1 antibodies (although these may develop later in the course of the disease) (Johnson *et al.*, 1990; Czaja, Hay & Rakela, 1990; Czaja *et al.*, 1993*a*).

Humoral and cellular mechanisms

In attempting to define the pathogenetic mechanisms in AIH comparisons have been drawn with other autoimmune diseases, particularly systemic lupus erythematosus (SLE) (Joske & King, 1955; Mackay, Taft & Cowling, 1956, 1959; Aronson & Montgomery, 1959; Bartholomew *et al.*, 1958, 1960; Mackay & Wood, 1962). Among the earliest similarities noted were circulating lupus erythematosus (LE) cells and the ANA giving the same 'homogeneous' pattern of immunofluorescent staining on tissue sections or HEp-2 cells as the ANA in SLE. This relationship to SLE is, however, only superficial, for it is now clear that only about 10–15% of patients have LE cells, that the ANA differ in antigenic specificity from the ANA in SLE, and that such patients do not fall within the spectrum of SLE (Geall, Schoenfield & Summerskill, 1968; Gurian et al., 1985; Worman & Courvalin, 1991; Nishioka, 1993).

The SMA in many AIH patients react with actin filaments (Gabbiani et al., 1973; Lidman et al., 1976; Hamlyn & Berg, 1980) and were considered by some authorities to be pathognomonic of this condition. More recent evidence, however, indicates that, in about 50% of AIH cases with SMA, the antibodies recognise other cytoskeletal proteins (Dighiero et al., 1990) and anti-actin antibodies can also be found in other disorders (Hamlyn & Berg, 1980; Diederichsen & Riisom, 1980). It is unlikely that SMA or ANA are involved in mediating tissue damage, because the antigens with which they react are not normally exposed to the immune system in vivo.

LKM-1 autoantibodies, first described by Rizzetto and colleagues (Rizzetto, Swana & Doniach, 1973), are now known to react specifically with cytochrome P450 IID6 (formerly P450db1) (Manns et al., 1989, 1991) and are distinct from other LKM antibodies (Homberg, Andre & Abuaf, 1984; Beaune et al., 1987; Crivelli et al., 1983). Patients with LKM-1 have been recognised most often in continental Europe and tend to present predominantly in the paediatric age group (Homberg et al., 1987). The question of whether these antibodies are involved in pathogenesis remains controversial (Yamamoto et al., 1993; Loeper et al., 1993; Vergani & Mieli-Vergani, 1993).

The mitochondrial antibodies found in patients with features of AIH are usually of a different specificity to those that are particularly associated with primary biliary cirrhosis (PBC) (see Chapter 15). They identify patients with the so-called 'overlap syndrome' of PBC and AIH, but recent recommendations are that such patients should not be included within the spectrum of AIH (see below).

A wide variety of other auto-antibodies have been described in AIH, including several, such as anti-SLA, anti-LC-1 and anti-LP, that react with various soluble antigens in liver (Manns, 1991; Stechemesser, Klein & Berg, 1993) and others that recognise membrane-bound antigens (McFarlane & Williams, 1985; Swanson et al., 1990; Toda et al., 1990). In addition, almost all patients presenting with AIH have high titres of auto-antibodies reacting with the hepatic asialoglycoprotein receptor (ASGP-R) which, so far, is the only target of auto-reactions in AIH that has been positively identified (McFarlane et al., 1986; Treichel et al., 1990; Poralla et al., 1991). These are of particular interest in terms of pathogenesis because, unlike many of the antigens with which the other auto-antibodies react, the ASGP-R is not only uniquely hepatocyte-specific but also is preferentially expressed on the surfaces of periportal liver cells (Daniels, Smith & Schmucker, 1987; McFarlane et al., 1990a), the prime targets of tissue damage in AIH.

That T lymphocytes form the peripheral blood or livers of AIH patients recognise liver-specific antigens (including ASGP-R) is now well established, and it has been shown that clonally expanded T cells from AIH patients will specifically stimulate autologous B lymphocytes in vitro to produce anti-ASGP-R antibodies (Vento et al., 1986, 1987; O'Brien et al., 1986; Wen et al., 1990; Lohr et al., 1990). These are mainly CD4+ (helper/ inducer) T cells (Vento et al., 1987; Wen et al., 1990; Lohr et al., 1990); direct (CD8+) T cell cytotoxic auto-reactions against hepatocytes do not appear to play a major role in tissue damage in AIH. Rather, all of the considerable evidence available points to an antibody-dependent, non-T cell cytotoxic (ADCC), mechanism (Mieli-Vergani, Civeira & Vergani, 1992; McFarlane, Farrant & Eddleston, 1993) but whether anti-ASGP-R is one of the auto-antibodies directly involved in such ADCC reactions is not yet known.

Genetics and immunoregulation

AIH in north European caucasoids is associated with inheritance of the HLA A1-B8-DR3 haplotype and particularly with the DR3 allotype (Galbraith et al., 1974; Opelz et al., 1977; Mackay & Tait, 1980). Overall, about 50% of patients carry DR3 and there is a secondary association with DR4 which accounts for almost all of the remainder (Donaldson et al., 1991). The majority of the younger patients are DR3+, while DR4 is much more strongly represented among the older age groups (Fig. 14.2). In Japan, where 'classical' AIH in young females is rarely seen, and most patients are in the older age groups, there is no association with DR3 (which is very rare in the normal Japanese population) but a strong association with DR4 (Seki et al., 1990).

These HLA markers are also common in other auto-immune disorders and seem to be associated with an overall heightening of immunoresponsiveness rather than with mechanisms specific to AIH. The T cell recognition of liver-specific antigens discussed above does, however, seem to be more particularly related to the disease and there is evidence indicating that AIH patients have a specific defect in their ability to control the autoreactive response to ASGP-R (O'Brien et al., 1986; Vento et al., 1987). This defect can be traced through families and is inherited in an autosomal, non-HLA-linked mode (O'Brien et al., 1986) but, as familial AIH is very uncommon, it is clear that there must be other factors that precipitate the disease in the susceptible individuals.

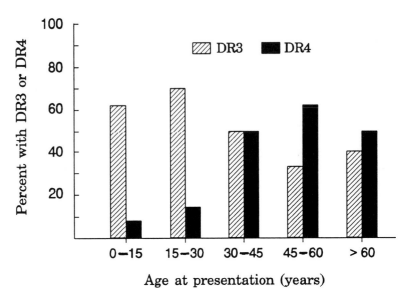

Fig. 14.2. Variations in frequency of HLA DR3 and DR4 allotypes with age at presentation with autoimmune hepatitis (adapted from McFarlane, 1993).

Sub-types

There are continuing attempts to sub-divide AIH according to auto-antibody profiles and other immunological parameters. The first proposed sub-division was between patients with ANA and/or SMA (Type 1) and those with LKM-1 antibodies (Type 2) (Homberg *et al.*, 1987). Recognition that about 20% of patients present without ANA, SMA or LKM-1, i.e. 'cryptogenic' CAH (Hay *et al.*, 1989; Johnson *et al.*, 1990; McFarlane, 1993), but have circulating anti-SLA antibodies and are otherwise indistinguishable from those with typical AIH, has led to a proposal to describe such patients as having Type 3 AIH (Manns *et al.*, 1987). With the finding that a high proportion of southern European patients with chronic hepatitis C virus (HCV) infections have KLM antibodies (see below), has come the suggestion that Type 2 should be further sub-divided into Type 2a (younger, predominantly female patients without HCV) and Type 2b (older, predominantly male cases with HCV) (Johnson & McFarlane, 1993). Very recently, yet another classification: Type 1a (ANA positive), Type 1b (SMA positive), Type 2 (LKM-1 positive) and Type 3 (anti-LP positive) has been proposed (Stechemesser, Klein & Berg, 1993). There is also the question of whether patients with HLA DR3 should be distinguished from those with DR4.

Sub-division according to HLA type might be justifiable, since HLA DR3 and DR4 are very rarely inherited together as a haplotype (Donaldson *et al.*, 1991) and it is possible that these markers identify two genetically distinct groups – the former (DR3+) being younger, more often female, and having more severe AIH and the latter (DR4+) defining older patients with milder disease and including a higher proportion of males. The justification for discriminating between LKM-1 positive (Type 2) and negative (Type 1) patients relates to the very marked preponderance of young females in the Type 2 group, in whom the disease is particularly severe and sometimes associated with insulin-dependent diabetes mellitus (IDDM). The presentation is often acute, even fulminant, with severe histological features and a marked propensity to progress rapidly to cirrhosis. In contrast, the Type 1 group tends to be older, includes males and those with milder disease, seem to be more steroid-responsive, and very rarely have IDDM. But this is a generalisation, for Type 1 patients can also present with severe disease.

Nevertheless, with the exception of LKM-1, none of the auto-antibodies is specific for any of these proposed sub-groups and, indeed, the vast majority of cases in all groups present with anti-ASGP-R autoantibodies and cannot be distinguished on the basis of responsiveness to corticosteroid therapy. Thus, the various proposed sub-divisions do not clearly identify separate groups on a therapeutic or pathogenetic basis. For this reason, an international panel convened to discuss criteria for diagnosis of AIH has recently recommended that, until the situation is clarified, sub-divisions of AIH should be avoided and that patients, with auto-immune markers and evidence of viral infections, should be considered as having both AIH and chronic viral hepatitis (Johnson & McFarlane, 1993).

Extrahepatic manifestations

Skin rashes, myalgia and arthralgia are often prominent features at presentation, and the recurrence of these symptoms during the course of the disease may herald impending relapse. Incapacitating arthralgia frequently develops during withdrawal of corticosteroid therapy, but usually subsides within three months (Stellon *et al.*, 1988). Occasionally, rheumatoid factor is present, but in most cases there is no clue as to the cause of the arthritis. In addition to those features, at least half of the patients will have evidence of disease of organs other than the liver, including thyroid disease, diabetes mellitus (in LKM-1 positive cases), Sjogren's syndrome, Coomb's positive haemolytic anaemia, renal tubular acidosis, fibrosing alveolitis, and glomerular nephritis (Golding, Smith & Williams, 1973; Keating *et al.*, 1987). Indeed, it is not uncommon for patients to be referred from rheumatology, dermatology, endocrinology, and other clinics where their underlying AIH has been revealed during investigation of one of these systemic manifestations.

About 1% of patients with ulcerative colitis appear to have typical AIH, with hypergammaglobulinaemia and non-organ specific auto-antibodies, but more often the liver involvement in this condition falls into the category of small or large duct sclerosing cholangitis. The situation is complicated by the observation that some children with sclerosing cholangitis present with features typical of AIH (Mieli-Vergani *et al.*, 1989).

Response to treatment and prognosis

As noted above, the clinical, laboratory and histological features of all types of AIH respond rapidly to immunosuppressive therapy in the great majority of cases. The standard procedure is to induce remission with moderate doses of prednisolone (0.5 mg/kg body weight per day). When the aminotransferase level has fallen to less than twice the upper limit of the reference range (usually after 2–8 weeks), the dose of prednisolone is gradually reduced. Azathioprine (1 mg/kg) is often added at this stage as a 'steroid sparing' agent. Azathioprine cannot be used alone to induce remission, possibly because is seems to act on K and NK stem cells and many months of treatment are required for marked depletion of mature K/NK cells (Pedersen *et al.*, 1984; Pedersen & Beyer, 1986) in contrast to corticosteroids, which have rapid and direct effects on immunoglobulin (including auto-antibody) production – a further clue to the possible importance of ADCC reactions in the mechanisms of hepatocellular damage in AIH (McFarlane & Eddleston, 1990).

Thereafter, the approach depends on the severity of the disease and the patient's response to the initial treatment. Our practice, based almost entirely on management of severe cases, is to titrate the steroid dose against the serum aminotransferase (AST) level until this is completely normal and then to maintain the patient in remission for at least one year on between 0.1 and 0.2 mg/kg/day of prednisolone and 1 mg/kg/day azathioprine. In our experience, even after several years of apparently complete remission, attempts to withdraw all immunosuppressive therapy in such patients are invariably unsuccessful, but it is usually possible to gradually (by 2.5 mg/day per month) withdraw the corticosteroid component, if the dose of azathioprine is first increased from 1 mg to 2 mg/kg/day (Stellon *et al.*, 1988). This approach is probably particularly useful in those patients in whom corticosteroid side-effects are prominent.

Leucopenia and/or thrombocytopenia due to hypersplenism are common features in AIH but may occasionally be related to azathioprine-induced myelosuppression, necessitating discontinuation of the drug. In such cases and in the few others who cannot tolerate the drug, relapse is very likely

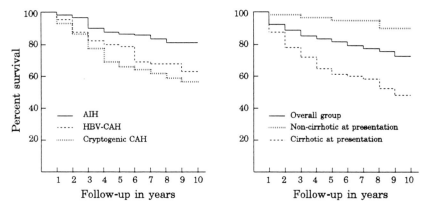

Fig. 14.3. Survival data for chronic active hepatitis. *Left:* according to aetiology; *Right:* according to presence or absence of cirrhosis at presentation (adapted from Keating *et al.*, 1987).

unless steroids are re-introduced before withdrawal of the azathioprine (Stellon *et al.*, 1988). Relapse is also likely in patients maintained on the combination therapy, if the azathioprine is discontinued without a compensatory increase in the steroid dosage (Stellon *et al.*, 1985).

In severe cases (i.e. symptomatic, with histological evidence of bridging necrosis, AST greater than ten-fold elevated, and/or jaundiced), immunosuppressive therapy is clearly associated with markedly improved survival; in asymptomatic patients with milder disease, the benefits of immunosuppressive therapy are less clear cut. After many years, the disease does enter a 'burnt-out' phase, when all treatment can be withdrawn, but patients should still be checked at least at yearly intervals, as relapse can occur at any time over the next decade.

In a large, retrospective analysis of our own experience, in whom all patients received immunosuppressive therapy, the five-year survival in AIH was 85%, compared with 65% in cryptogenic CAH (Keating *et al.*, 1987). This difference is accounted for by the significantly higher frequency of cirrhosis in the cryptogenic group at presentation (Fig. 14.3). Patients with LKM-1 antibody-positive disease are reported to have a worse prognosis, with a 10-year survival of about 75% but, allowing for the high frequency of cirrhosis in this group, the figure is very similar to that for the other non-viral CAH groups (Homberg *et al.*, 1987).

About 10% of patients will never achieve full remission and a smaller proportion become unresponsive, after initially successful treatment. In these situations, remission can occasionally be re-induced by increasing corticosteroid therapy but more often there is progressive liver failure, and early referral to a liver transplant unit is indicated.

Chronic active viral hepatitis types B and D

Hepatitis B virus (HBV) is transmitted parenterally. The majority of healthy adults, exposed to HBV, have an acute hepatitis (which may be asymptomatic) and less than 5% will become chronic carriers of the virus. In contrast, the majority of children infected at birth will become chronic carriers, as will many adults who are immunosuppressed. Males become carriers more frequently than females. 'Vertical transmission' from mother to child is the main mechanism of spread in high incidence areas such as the Far East; the mode of transmission in other high incidence areas such as Southern Africa is not known (Dudley, Scheuer & Sherlock, 1972; Stevens et al., 1975). Some carriers will remain 'healthy', with normal serum aminotransferase activities and minimal histological changes in the liver, while others will develop CAH. It is impossible to define the proportions with these two outcomes, because even those with CAH can remain asymptomatic for long periods, while apparently 'healthy' carriers may develop CAH at some stage.

Clinical features

Aside from the extrahepatic presentations outlined above, the clinical features of HBV-CAH depend on the degree of liver damage and this in turn depends on the stage of the disease. Two main phases are recognised (Hoofnagle et al., 1981): an initial stage of active viral replication which is characterised by high serum levels of hepatitis B 'e' antigen (HBeAg), HBV-DNA and virus-associated DNA polymerase (DNA-P) and with the core antigen (HBcAg) present in the nuclei of infected hepatocytes. After several years there is spontaneous disappearance of serum HBV-DNA and DNA-P, which coincides with seroconversion from HBe antigen to HBe antibody seropositivity. Typically, there is a 'flare' of aminotransferase activity just before seroconversion. In this second phase, hepatic inflammation decreases and biochemical liver tests return toward normal, but the patient usually remains HBsAg (viral surface antigen) seropositive (Brook et al., 1989).

Superinfection with the hepatitis delta virus (HDV), a defective RNA pathogen which is wholly dependent for its replication on obligatory helper functions provided by HBV, may mimic an exacerbation of the underlying chronic HBV infection (Rizzetto, 1990). In such cases, there is an IgM and IgG anti-HDV response, that gives the clue to the superinfection (Di Bisceglei & Negro, 1989). IgA anti-HDV antibodies, may also be detected and these usually indicate underlying CAH attributable to HDV (McFarlane et al., 1991). IgM anti-HDV was also thought to be a marker of underlying CAH (Farci et al., 1986; Buti et al., 1987) but later studies have shown that, whereas this antibody is associated with active viral infection, it does not correlate with histological activity (Lau et al., 1991). Up to 50% of patients with chronic HDV infection are reported to have antibodies (BCLA) reacting with the basal cell layer of rodent fore-stomach and up to 20% may have liver–kidney microsomal antoantibodies (designated LKM-3), which react with a human-specific epitope in microsomes (Negro & Rizzetto, 1993) and thus differ in specificity from the LKM-1 antibodies seen in AIH.

Humoral and cellular mechanisms and immunoregulation

The hepatitis B virus appears not to be inherently cytopathic and, in the normal host, the virus replicates in infected cells and may become integrated into the host genome. Host humoral and cellular immune reactions against the viral surface (HBsAg), envelope (HBenvAg) and core (HBc) proteins are essential for elimination of the virus and for protection against re-infection and it seems that it is the failure or inadequacy of one or more of these host responses that leads to the carrier state (Barnaba & Balsano, 1992). The high frequency of persistent infection associated with vertical transmission of HBV is probably due to the immaturity of the immune system in neonates but the reasons why some adults (other than frankly immunocompromised individuals) become carriers are poorly understood. Mutations by the virus to escape immune surveillance may be a factor and the predilection for males to become carriers suggests that hormonal influences also play a role (Barnaba & Balsano, 1992).

Tissue damage in HBV infections is thought to be due mainly to T cell cytotoxic responses against virus-infected cells, possibly aided by 'non-specific' reactions mediated by cytokines released during the virus-specific inflammatory response (Gudat et al., 1975; Mills, Lee & Perrillo, 1990; Hoofnagle et al., 1982; Mondelli et al., 1982; Gerber & Thung, 1985; Ferrari et al., 1988; Bonino & Brunetto, 1993). It is not at all clear, however, how these events lead to development of CAH in HBV carriers. Since HBV-infected cells are scattered throughout the liver lobule and are not especially concentrated in the periportal areas of the liver lobules (Mills, Lee & Perrillo, 1990; Moreno, Martinez & Carreno, 1993), it seems unlikely that a virus-directed T cell cytotoxic reaction can, alone, account for this histological picture and it is difficult to understand why a 'non-specific' cytokine-mediated response should be particularly targeted against periportal hepatocytes. A possible explanation may relate to the finding that, in addition to the T cell responses directed at viral antigens, patients with HBV-CAH show non-T cell (ADCC) reactions in vitro against normal liver antigens on uninfected hepatocytes (Cochrane et al., 1976; Mieli-Vergani et al., 1982). Most patients with acute hepatitis B have circulating autoantibodies against various normal liver antigens, including the ASGP-R (McFarlane, 1991). These usually disappear during recovery but tend to persist in individuals who do not clear the virus and, as in AIH, a high proportion of those with HBV-CAH have anti-ASGP-R and other antibodies associated with AIH (McFarlane et al., 1986; Treichel et al., 1990; Louzir et al., 1992). In contrast to AIH, however, HBV-infected subjects do not show T cell responses to liver auto-antigens and production of the auto-antibodies cannot therefore be due to liver-auto-antigen-specific T helper (T_H) cell functions. Nor does it appear to be related to a generalised polyclonal B-cell activation by the virus but, rather, to HBV-reactive T_H cells providing help for naturally occurring ASGP-R-auto-reactive B-cells (Vento et al., 1988).

It is less certain that virus-induced auto-reactivity is pathogenetically involved in delta virus infections. HDV seems to be cytopathic for hepatocytes and the various auto-antibodies that have been described in chronic HDV do not correlate with activity of the infection, nor with histological severity of liver damage, in contrast to IgA anti-HDV antibodies (see above).

Extrahepatic manifestations

Myalgia, arthralgia and skin rashes are common in women and vasculitis and/or polyarteritis (Combs et al., 1971; Wands et al., 1975) are also seen but appear much less common than suggested by initial reports. Active viral replication is associated with membranous nephritis, a common cause of nephrotic syndrome in African children with HBV infections (Milner et al., 1988). Most of these complications have been attributed to immune complex formation (Levo et al., 1977; Gorevic et al., 1980; Caporali et al., 1988) but other studies have failed to confirm this (McIntosh, Koss & Gocke, 1976; Dienstag, Wands & Isselbacher 1977; Popp et al., 1984).

Response to treatment

The overall management of patients with HBsAg seropositive CAH is beyond the scope of this chapter and only the two main therapeutic strategies, corticosteroids and alpha-interferon (used individually or in combination), will be reviewed. Large-scale trials have shown that corticosteroids will suppress the inflammatory response in HBV-CAH, but not predictably (Eur. Assn. Study of Liver, 1986), and their use may be deleterious because suppression of the host immune response may delay elimination of the virus, and also because they may enhance viral replication (Schalm et al., 1976; Lam et al., 1981). Following withdrawal of corticosteroids, exacerbation of the condition (with a 'flare' of serum aminotransferase activity) is often seen (Nair *et al.*, 1986; Hanson, Peters & Hoofnagle, 1986; Hoofnagle *et al.*, 1986).

Alpha-interferon is the only well-documented specific therapeutic agent available (Perrillo, 1993). A wide variety of dose regimens, ranging from 3–18 million units, daily, alternate day, or three times weekly over a period of 3–6 months, has been used. The aim is to eradicate viral replication in patients in the early phase of the disease and thereby decrease severity of liver damage. In effect, it seems that interferon treatment, perhaps by augmenting the immune response to HBV, will advance the time at which the 'spontaneous' seroconversion takes place. A small minority will actually lose all evidence of viral infection but, in the majority of cases, successful treatment is characterised by HBeAg/anti-HBe seroconversion and loss of HBV-DNA (Alexander *et al.*, 1987). These changes in viral indices are accompanied by an initial rise in the serum activity of the aminotransferase and a subsequent fall to the reference range together with a marked decrease in histological activity.

Overall, 30–50% of patients respond to alpha-interferon (Perrillo, 1993). Those most likely to do so have moderately elevated serum AST activity, a clear history of acute hepatitis and low levels of circulating HBV-DNA, while the treatment is less successful in patients who acquired the infection at birth and have low pre-treatment aminotransferase levels and marked viraemia (Alexander *et al.*, 1987). This observation has led to several attempts to exploit the 'flare' of disease activity following corticosteroid withdrawal, to enhance the effects of alpha-interferon, by giving the latter after a short course of prednisolone, with variable results (Perrillo *et al.*, 1990; Fevery *et al.*, 1990; Lok *et al.*, 1992).

On a cautionary note, interferon therapy should never be undertaken lightly, particularly in patients with signs of decompensation of their liver disease. Apart from the immediate side effects of fatigue, fever, rigors, myalgia, arthralgia, and myelosuppression, which occur with varying severity and duration in most patients, there is the potentially hazardous risk of unmasking previously unsuspected anto-immune diseases, or inducing these *de novo*, and careful monitoring is essential (Vento *et al.*, 1990; Conlon *et al.*, 1990; Roonbloom, Alm & Oberg, 1991; Pateron *et al.*, 1993).

Chronic active viral hepatitis type C

The development of an acute viral-type hepatitis after transfusion with blood that is negative for markers of the hepatitis A and B viruses has been recognised as 'Non-A, Non-B, (NANB) hepatitis' (Koretz, Suffin & Gitnick, 1976; Koretz *et al.*, 1985). In nearly 50% of cases the illness progressed to a chronic phase, in which the liver histology revealed a typical picture of CAH, except that there was a more prominent lobular component to the inflammation and cholangiolytic features were more frequently seen than in auto-immune CAH (Scheuer, 1987).

With the identification of the hepatitis C virus (HCV) and development of a serological test for anti-HCV antibodies in 1989 (Choo *et al.*, 1989; Kuo *et al.*, 1989), it became apparent that many subjects with what was previously classified as 'cryptogenic liver disease', in fact had chronic HCV infections. Only a minority gave a history of blood transfusion, or of acute hepatitis and indeed the source of infection, in the majority of cases classified as 'community acquired', remains unknown (Alter, 1991). In contrast to hepatitis B, perinatal and sexual transmission rates seem to be very low (Alter, 1991; Esteban, 1993).

The situation has been complicated by problems of false-positivity with the early tests for HCV (McFarlane *et al.*, 1990*b*; Ikeda *et al.*, 1990; Nicholson *et al.*, 1991), but even after the development of more specific tests for anti-HCV (Hosein *et al.*, 1991; Van der Poel *et al.*, 1991; Chien *et al.*, 1992; Yatsuhashi *et al.*, 1992) and to detect viraemia by measurement of circulating HCV-RNA using the polymerase chain reaction (PCR) technique (Garson *et al.*, 1990; Ulrich *et al.*, 1990; Hu, Yu & Vierling, 1993), there is still very little known about the natural history of HCV infections. It is clear, however, that there is very marked variation in severity – ranging from slowly resolving, through mild, stable, disease in the majority of patients, to a rapidly progressive disorder in some (Alter *et al.*, 1992).

The liver morphology of chronic hepatitis C is perhaps the one area that is becoming more clearly defined. In addition to the lobular and biliary changes noted above, most authorities now agree that well-organised lymphoid aggregates, particularly in the portal tracts, are a prominent feature of the disease (Moreno, Martinez & Carreno, 1993; Scheuer *et al.*, 1992; Bach, Thung & Schaffner, 1992). Indeed, although periportal inflammation and piecemeal necrosis of hepatocytes (the hallmark of CAH) is often seen, this tends to be significantly less marked than in CAH of other aetiologies and it must be questioned whether the morphological changes in chronic HCV do constitute part of the spectrum of CAH.

Humoral and cellular mechanisms and immunoregulation

Even less is currently known about the humoral and cellular processes involved in the host immune response to the virus, or the mechanisms of tissue damage, than about the natural history of HCV infections. In contrast to most other viral infections (with the notable exception of HIV), in which the appearance of antibodies to the virus is usually associated with clearance of the infection and, often, protection against re-infection, the majority of patients with anti-HCV antibodies have concurrent viraemia. These antibodies variously recognise a range of peptides corresponding to different regions of the viral genome, but the pattern and timing of the different antibody responses varies widely between individual patients (Giuberti *et al.*, 1992; Puoti *et al.*, 1992). Some patients may have persistent infection (HCV-RNA seropositive) without anti-HCV (Alter *et al.*, 1992), or with normal serum aminotransferases (Alberti *et al.*, 1992; McGuinness *et al.*, 1993) and even, reportedly, without liver disease (Brillianti *et al.*, 1993). Interpretation is complicated by the knowledge that there is considerable genomic variation between different HCV isolates, suggesting a high level of viral mutation (Brechot & Kremsdorf, 1993).

One of the consequences of widespread screening of patients, with chronic liver disease for anti-HCV antibodies, was the finding of positive results in patients with disorders which had not previously been thought to be virus-mediated. A particular case in point was the observation that between 40% and 88% of patients with AIH in Spain and Italy apparently had chronic HCV, on the basis of anti-HCV seropositivity (Lenzi *et al.*, 1990; Esteban *et al.*, 1989). There was some initial confusion because of the problem of false-positivity with the earlier anti-HCV tests, but it now seems that many patients with AIH, from areas where HCV is prevalent do have chronic HCV infections and this has led to the suggestion that the virus may induce AIH (Lenzi *et al.*, 1991; Magrin *et al.*, 1991; Todros *et al.*, 1991; Garson *et al.*, 1991). Such patients tend to be older and more often male than those without evidence of HCV (Lunel *et al.*, 1991). The highest frequencies are seen among patients with LKM antibodies (Lenzi *et al.*, 1991) but recent evidence suggests that, in many cases, these are not reacting with the same epitope as that recognised by the LKM-1 antibodies characteristic of AIH (Ma *et al.*, 1993).

It is not at all clear whether these are patients in whom the virus has triggered AIH or are cases of AIH with superimposed HCV infections. Additional evidence that HCV may induce anto-immune disease comes from the finding that a high proportion have circulating antibodies against a naturally occurring pentadecapeptide, GOR (Mishiro, Hoshi & Takeda, 1990). This peptide has, however, been shown to share partial homology with HCV at both the amino acid and genomic sequence levels (Hosein, Fang & Wang, 1992) and anti-GOR therefore seems to be another anti-HCV antibody, rather than a true auto-antibody (Mehta *et al.*, 1992; McFarlane *et al.*, 1993). Findings in our laboratories, that auto-antibodies are very rare in Italian patients presenting with acute HCV infections, suggest that the virus is not inherently anto-inductive (McFarlane *et al.*, 1993) and this is supported by studies in AIH patients in the USA (Czaja *et al.*, 1993*b*). On the other hand, a study in France has found a high frequency of auto-antibodies (mainly at low titres) in a high proportion of patients with chronic hepatitis C (Abuaf *et al.*, 1993) and another recent report documents thyroid auto-antibodies in nearly a third of patients with apparently primary HCV infections, 14% of whom had overt auto-immune thyroid disease (Tran et al., 1993).

Extrahepatic manifestations

The extrahepatic manifestations of chronic hepatitis C are very similar to those seen in chronic hepatitis B, but symptoms of cryoglobulinaemia (arthritis, vasculitis, purpura, peripheral neuropathy, glomerulonephropathy and Raynaud's phenomenon) appear to occur much more frequently. Indeed, there has recently been a flood of reports of a high frequency of HCV infections in patients with essential mixed cryoglobulinaemia (EMC) (Phillips & Dougherty, 1991; McFarlane, 1992; Agnello, Chung & Kaplan, 1992; Pechere-Bertschi et al., 1992; Misiani et al., 1992; Relman, 1992; Marcellin et al., 1993), glomerulonephritis (Johnson et al., 1993), polyarteritis nodosa (Cacoub, Lunel-Fabiani & Du, 1992), Sjogren's syndrome (Haddad et al., 1992), and even porphyria cutanea tarda (Fargion et al., 1992; Herrero, Arroya & Bruguero, 1993). Some of the later studies have demonstrated anti-HCV antibodies and HCV-RNA in cryoprecipitates from the patients, suggesting that immune complexes containing viral particles are a key factor.

Almost all of these studies have been undertaken in patients presenting with symptomatic EMC in rheumatology, nephrology, dermatology and other specialist clinics but there have been no large-scale studies to date of the incidence of this complication in patients who present with chronic HCV infections. While cryoglobulinaemia in liver disease has long been recognized (Florin-Christensen, Roux & Aran, 1974; Jori et al., 1977; Garcia-Bragado et al., 1984; Zarski et al., 1984), the underlying mechanisms are not well understood. Thus, as with the association between HCV and AIH, it is still uncertain whether it is the virus or the liver disease that is the cause of the EMC or whether, since most of the reports are from areas where the virus is prevalent, these are cases of primary EMC with superimposed HCV infections. In this regard, it is interesting to note that the cryoglobulinaemia seems to disappear with response of the liver disease to interferon therapy (Marcellin et al., 1993; Johnson et al., 1993; Knox, Hillyer & Kaplan, 1991).

Response to treatment

Treatment of HCV is still in its infancy. Once again the only effective agent is alpha-interferon, but the monitoring of response is particularly difficult, and the physician has to rely on the inaccurate parameter of the aminotransferase level. Carefully controlled clinical trials show that 30–50% of patients normalise serum aminotransferase levels and that this is associated with a

reduction of hepatic inflammation on biopsy (Davis, 1990) but it appears
that the disease recurs in the majority of patients when treatment is stopped.
Different regimens under investigation may prove to be more effective at
inducing long-term remission (Alberti et al., 1993; Carreño, Marriott &
Quiroga, 1993). However, as with interferon therapy in HBV-CAH
(above), caution should be exercised – particularly until the association
between HCV and auto-immunity is clarified.

Chronic active hepatitis in other disorders

In most cases, the other disorders, in which the histological features of CAH
can be seen (Table 14.1), can be distinguished on the basis of specific
morphological findings and clinical and serological parameters. Diagnoses,
particularly in those who are seronegative for all of the viral markers, may,
however, be complicated by features that overlap with those of AIH.
Patients presenting with anti-mitochondrial antibodies (AMA) without
biliary changes on liver biopsy or, conversely, without AMA but with ANA
and histological features of primary biliary cirrhosis (PBC), form part of one
well-recognised overlap group.
    In those with AMA it may be possible to differentiate on the basis of the
sub-type of the auto-antibody. Of the nine major sub-types (M1–M9) of
AMA that have been described (see Chapter 15), the M2 antibody, which
reacts against the E2 subunit of the pyruvate dehydrogenase complex (PDC-
E2), is specific for PBC (Fussey et al., 1988; Van der Water et al., 1988;
Briand et al., 1992). The M4 sub-type is said to react with sulphite oxidase
and reportedly identifies patients with the PBC/AIH overlap syndrome who
have a poor prognosis, while the M9 antibody is said to recognise glycogen
phosphorylase and to identify PBC patients with benign disease (Berg &
Klein, 1990; Klein & Berg, 1990, 1991). Two later independent studies, in
which no evidence for specific reactivity with these antigens or disease-
specific associations with the M4 and M9 antibodies could be found, dispute
this (Davis et al., 1992; Palmer et al., 1993).
    In patients with both CAH and biliary lesions on liver biopsy, who present
without AMA but have circulating ANA, SMA or other auto-antibodies,
the diagnosis can be particularly difficult (Rabinovitz et al., 1992). In the
absence of markers of hepatitis virus infections, the differential diagnosis is
of AIH from PBC and primary sclerosing cholangitis (PSC). There is an
increasing trend towards defining this group of cases under the general
headings of autoimmune cholangitis or autoimmune cholangiopathy, partly
because of the overlapping features but also because some seem to respond
to corticosteroid therapy (Ben-Ari, Dhillon & Sherlock, 1993). Endoscopic

retrograde cholangiopancreatography (ERCP) is recommended, especially in children (Mieli-Vergani et al., 1989), to exclude PSC.

The diagnosis of Wilson's disease is classically based on the finding of low serum copper and ceruloplasmin concentrations, high liver and urinary copper concentrations, and ocular Kaiser-Fleischer rings (Marsden, 1987; Sternlieb, 1990). Some of these abnormalities may be absent in children with this disorder and other patients who present with histological features of CAH and auto-antibodies suggestive of AIH (Da Costa et al., 1992). Conversely, similar abnormalities in copper parameters are occasionally seen in patients with AIH (Hodges et al., 1991; Ilan et al., 1991). Early diagnosis is essential because specific treatment can prevent further liver injury in both conditions and the development of neurological complications in Wilson's disease. It also allows for early liver transplantation in those with very severe liver damage. Fortunately, the distinction can be made fairly easily by measuring the 24-hour urinary copper excretion after D-penicillamine challenge (Da Costa et al., 1992).

The morphological features of alcoholic liver disease are well recognised: fatty infiltration, an inflammatory infiltrate composed predominantly of polymorphonuclear leucocytes, swelling and degeneration of perivenular hepatocytes, and Mallory's hyaline. However, lymphocytic infiltration and piecemeal necrosis of periportal hepatocytes is also often seen and ANA, SMA and other auto-antibodies associated with AIH occur in 20–40% of cases (Johnson & Williams, 1986; Lieber, 1988; Ishak, Zimmerman & Ray, 1991). Also, as in AIH, some patients respond to corticosteroid therapy (Hofer & McMahon, 1991). At the present time, it is almost impossible to determine whether such cases are patients with AIH who consume excessive amounts of alcohol or patients with alcoholic liver disease with auto-antibodies.

The drugs that have been implicated in idiosyncratic reactions associated with a histological picture of CAH with clinical and immunological features of AIH include a very broad spectrum of therapeutic agents, a comprehensive discussion of which is beyond the scope of this chapter. Suffice it to say that alpha-methyldopa, oxyphenisatin, isoniazid, nitrofurantoin, tienilic acid, diclofenac and other non-steroidal anti-inflammatory agents, and some anti-thyroid drugs are perhaps the best documented (Hofer & McMahon, 1991; Ludwig, 1979; Zimmerman & Maddrey, 1987; Johnson & McFarlane, 1989; Scully, Clarke & Barr, 1993). That some of these drugs are used to treat conditions which may themselves be part of the spectrum of extrahepatic manifestations of AIH (see above), complicates diagnosis of these idiosyncratic reactions. However, the hepatic abnormalities usually resolve upon discontinuation of the drug.

References

A Trial Group of the European Association for the Study of the Liver: steroids in chronic B hepatitis. (1986). A randomized, double-blind, multinational trial on the effect of low-dose long term treatment on survival. *Liver*, **6**, 227–32.

Abuaf, N., Lunel, F., Giral. P. *et al.* (1993). Non-organ specific autoantibodies associated with chronic C virus hepatitis. *Journal of Hepatology*, **18**, 359–64.

Agnello, V., Chung, R. T. & Kaplan, L. M. (1992). A role for hepatitis C virus infection in type II cryoglobulinemia. *New England Journal of Medicine*, **327**, 1490–5.

Alberti, A., Morsica, G., Chemello, L., Cavelletto, D., Noventa, P., Pontisso, P. & Rual, A. (1992). Hepatitis C viraemia and liver disease in symptom-free individuals with anti-HCV. *Lancet*, **340**, 697–8.

Alberti, A., Chemello, L., Bonetti, P. *et al.* (1993). Treatment with interferon(s) of community-acquired chronic hepatitis and cirrhosis type C. *Journal of Hepatology*, **17**(Suppl. 3), S123–6.

Alexander, G. J. M., Brahm, J., Fagan, E. A. *et al.* (1987). Loss of HBsAg with interferon therapy in chronic hepatitis virus infection. *Lancet*, **ii**, 66–8.

Alter, M. J. (1991). Inapparent transmission of hepatitis C: footprints in the sand. *Hepatology*, **14**, 389–91.

Alter, M. J., Margolis, H. S., Krawczynski, K. *et al.* (1992), for the Sentinel Counties Chronic Non-A, Non-B Hepatitis Study Team. The natural history of community-acquired hepatitis C in the United States. *New England Journal of Medicine*, **327**, 1899–905.

Amberg, S. (1942) Hyperproteinaemia associated with severe liver damage. *Proceedings of the Staff Meeting Mayo Clinic*, **17**, 360–2.

Aronson, A. R. & Montgomery, M. M. (1959). Chronic liver disease with a 'lupus erythematosus-like syndrome'. *Archives of Internal Medicine*, **104**, 544–52.

Bach, N., Thung, S. N. & Schaffner, F. (1992). The histological features of chronic hepatitis C and autoimmune chronic hepatitis: a competitive analysis. *Hepatology*, **15**, 572–7.

Barnaba, V. & Balsano, F. (1992). Immunologic and molecular basis of viral persistence: The hepatitis B virus model. *Journal of Hepatology*, **14**, 391–400.

Bartholomew, L. G., Cain, J. C., Baggenstoss, A. H. & Hagedorn, A. B. (1960). Further observations on hepatitis in young women with positive clot tests for lupus erythematosus. *Gastroenterology*, **39**, 730–6.

Bartholomew, L. G., Hagedorn, A. B., Cain, J. C. & Baggenstoss, A. H. (1958). Hepatitis and cirrhosis in women with positive clot tests for lupus erythematosus. *New England Journal of Medicine*, **259**, 947–56.

Beaune, P., Dansette, P. M., Mansuy, D. *et al.* (1987). Human anti-endoplasmic reticulum autoantibodies appearing in a drug-induced hepatitis are directed against a human liver cytochrome P-450 that hydroxylates the drug. *Proceedings of the National Academy of Sciences, USA*, **84**, 551–5.

Ben-Ari, Z., Dhillon, A. P. & Sherlock, S. (1993). Autoimmune cholangiopathy: part of the spectrum of autoimmune chronic active hepatitis. *Hepatology*, **18**, 10–15.

Berg, P. A. & Klein, R. (1990). Autoantibodies in primary biliary cirrhosis. *Springer Seminars in Immunopathology*, **12**, 85–99.

Bonino, F. & Brunetto, M. R. (1993). Hepatitis B virus heterogeneity, one of many factors influencing the severity of hepatitis B. *Journal of Hepatology*, **18**, 5–8.

Brechot, C. & Kremsdorf, D. (1993). Genetic variation of the hepatitis C virus (HCV) genome: random events of a clinically relevant issue? *Journal of Hepatology*, **17**, 265–8.

Briand, J. P., André, C., Tuaillon, N., Herve, L., Neimark, J. & Muller, S. (1992). Multiple autoepitope presentation for specific detection of antibodies in primary biliary cirrhosis. *Hepatology*, **16**, 1395–403.

Brillianti, S., Foli, M., Gaiani, S., Masci, C., Miglioli, M. & Barbara, L. (1993). Persistent hepatitis C viraemia without liver disease. *Lancet*, **341**, 464–5.

Brook, M. G., Petrovic, L., McDonald, J. A., Scheuer, P. J. & Thomas, H. C. (1989). Evidence of histological improvement following anti-viral treatment in chronic hepatitis B virus carriers and identification of histological features that predict response. *Journal of Hepatology*, **8**, 218–25.

Buti, M., Esteban, R., Esteban, J. F., Allende, H., Jardi, R. & Guardia, J. (1987). Anti-HD IgM as a marker of chronic delta infection. *Journal of Hepatology*, **4**, 62–5.

Cacoub, P., Lunel-Fabiani, F. & Du, L. T. H. (1992). Polyarteritis nodosa and hepatitis C virus infection. *Annals of Internal Medicine*, **7**, 605.

Caporali, R., Longhi, M., Zorzoli, I. *et al.* (1988). Hepatitis B virus markers in monoclonal (Type I and II) polyclonal (Type III) cryoglobulinemia. *Haematologica*, **73**, 375–8.

Carreño, V., Marriott, E. & Quiroga, J. A. (1993). Other approaches to the treatment of chronic viral hepatitis. *Journal of Hepatology*, **17**(Suppl. 3), S127–9.

Chien, D. Y., Choo, Q. L., Tabrizi, A. *et al.* (1992). Diagnosis of hepatitis C virus (HCV) infection using an immunodominant chimeric polyprotein to capture circulating antibodies: Re-evaluation of the role of HCV in liver disease. *Proceedings of the National Academy of Sciences, USA*, **89**, 10011–15.

Choo, Q.-L., Kuo, G., Weiner, A. J. *et al.* (1989). Isolation of a cDNA clone derived from a blood-borne non-A, non-B hepatitis genome. *Science*, **244**, 359–61.

Cochrane, M. A. G., Moussouros, A., Thomson, A. D. *et al.* (1976). Antibody-dependent cell-mediated (K-cell) cytotoxicity against isolated hepatocytes in chronic active hepatitis. *Lancet*, **i**, 441–4.

Combs, B., Stasny, P., Shorey, J. *et al.* (1971). Glomerolonephritis with deposition of Australia antigen–antibody complexes in glomerular basement membrane. *Lancet*, **i**, 234–7.

Conlon, K. C., Urba, W. J., Smith, J. W., Steis, R. G., Longo, D. L. & Clark, J. W. (1990). Exacerbation of symptoms of autoimmune disease in patients receiving alpha-interferon therapy. *Cancer*, **65**, 2237–42.

Crivelli, Q., Lavarini, C., Chiaberge, E. *et al.* (1983). Microsomal autoantibodies in chronic infection with the HBsAg associated delta agent. *Clinical Experimental Immunology*, **54**, 232–8.

Cullinan, E. R. (1936). Idiopathic jaundice (often recurrent) associated with subacute necrosis of the liver. *St. Bartholomew Hospital Reports*, **69**, 55–142.

Czaja, A. J., Hay, J. E. & Rakela, J. (1990). Clinical features and prognostic implications of severe corticosteroid-treated cryptogenic chronic active hepatitis. *Mayo Clinic Proceedings*, **65**, 23–30.

Czaja, A. J., Carpenter, H. A., Santrach, P. J., Moore, S. B. & Homburger, H. A. (1993a). The nature and prognosis of severe cryptogenic chronic active hepatitis. *Gastroenterology*, **104**, 1755–61.

Czaja, A. J., Carpenter, H. A., Santrach, P. J., Moore, S. B., Taswell, H. F. & Homburger, H. A. (1993b). Evidence against hepatitis viruses as important causes of severe autoimmune hepatitis in the United States. *Journal of Hepatology*, **18**, 342–52.

Da Costa, C. D., Baldwin, D., Portmann, B., Lolin, Y., Mowat, A. P. & Mieli-Vergani, G. (1992). Value of urinary copper excretion after penicillamine challenge in the diagnosis of Wilson's disease. *Hepatology*, **15**, 609–15.

Daniels, C. K., Smith, K. M. & Schmucker, D. L. (1987). Asialoorosomucoid hepatobiliary transport is unaltered by the loss of liver asialoglycoprotein receptors in aged rats. *Proceedings of the Society of Experimental and Biological Medicine*, **186**, 246–50.

Davis, G. L. (1990). Recombinant α-interferon treatment of non-A, non-B (type C) hepatitis: review of studies and recommendations for treatment. *Journal of Hepatology*, **11**, s72–7.

Davis, P. A., Leung, P., Manns, M. *et al.* (1992). M4 and M9 antibodies in the overlap syndrome of primary biliary cirrhosis and chronic active hepatitis: epitopes of epiphenomena? *Hepatology*, **16**, 1128–36.

Di Bisceglie, A. M. & Negro, F. (1989). Diagnosis of hepatitis delta infection. *Hepatology*, **10**, 1014–16.

Diederichsen, H. & Riisom, K. (1980). Anti-actin antibodies revealed by counter-immunoelectrophoresis. *Journal of Clinical Pathology*, **33**, 876–9.

Dienstag, J. L., Wands, J. R. & Isselbacher, K. J. (1977). Hepatitis B and essential mixed cryoglobulinemia. *New England Journal of Medicine*, **297**, 946–7.

Dighiero, G., Lymberi, P., Monot, C. & Abuaf, N. (1990). Sera with high levels of anti-smooth muscle and anti-mitochondrial antibodies frequently bind to cytoskeletal proteins. *Clinical and Experimental Immunology*, **82**, 52–6.

Donaldson, P. T., Doherty, D. G., Hayllar, K. M., McFarlane, I. G., Johnson, P. J. & Williams, R. (1991). Susceptibility to autoimmune chronic active hepatitis: human leukocyte antigens DR4 and AI-B8-DR3 are independent risk factors. *Hepatology*, **13**, 701–6.

Doniach, D., Roitt, I. M., Walker, J. G. & Sherlock, S. (1966). Tissue antibodies in primary biliary cirrhosis, active chronic (lupoid) hepatitis, cryptogenic cirrhosis and other liver diseases and their clinical implications. *Clinical and Experimental Immunology*, **1**, 237–62.

Dudley, F. J., Scheuer, P. J. & Sherlock, S. (1972) Natural history of hepatitis-associated antigen-positive chronic liver disease. *Lancet*, **ii**, 1388–93.

Esteban, J. I., Esteban, R., Viladomiu, L. *et al.* (1989). Hepatitis C virus antibodies among risk groups in Spain. *Lancet*, **ii**, 294–7.

Esteban, R. (1993). Epidemiology of hepatitis C virus infection. *Journal of Hepatology*, **17**(Suppl. 3), S67–S71.

Farci, P., Gerin, J. L., Aragona, M., *et al.* (1986). Diagnostic and prognostic significance of the IgM antibody to the hepatitis delta virus. *Journal of the American Medical Association*, **255**, 1443–6.

Fargion, S., Piperno, A., Cappellini, M. D. *et al.* (1992). Hepatitis C virus and porphyria cutanea tarda: evidence of a strong association. *Hepatology*, **16**, 1322–6.

Ferrari, C., Penna, A., Degliantoni, A. *et al.* (1988). Cellular immune response to hepatitis B virus antigens. An overview. *Journal of Hepatology*, **7**, 21–33.

Fevery, J., Elewaut, A., Michielsen, P. *et al.* (1990). Efficacy of interferon alfa-2b with or without prednisone withdrawal in the treatment of chronic viral hepatitis B. A prospective double-blind Belgian–Dutch study. *Journal of Hepatology*, **11**, S108–12.

Florin-Christensen, A., Roux, M. E. B. & Aran, R. M. (1974). Cryoglobulins in acute and chronic liver disease. *Clinical and Experimental Immunology*, **16**, 595–605.

Fussey, S. P. M., Guest, J. R., James, O. F. W., Bassendine, M. F. & Yeaman, S. J. (1988). Identification and analysis of the major M2 autoantigen in primary biliary cirrhosis. *Proceedings of the National Academy of Sciences, USA*, **85**, 8654–8.

Gabbiani, G., Ryan, G. B., Lamelin, J. P. *et al.* (1973). Human smooth muscle autoantibody. Its identification as antiactin antibody and a study of its binding to non-muscular cells. *American Journal of Pathology*, **72**, 473–88.

Galbraith, R. M., Eddleston, A. L. W. F., Smith, M. G. M. *et al.* (1974). Histocompatibility antigens in active chronic hepatitis and primary biliary cirrhosis. *British Medical Journal*, **3**, 604–5.

Garcia-Bragado, F., Biosca, M., Villar, M., De La Figuera, M., Rodrigo, M. J. & Vilardell, M. (1984). Maladies hépatiques et cryoglobulinémie mixte. *Gastroenterological Clinical Biology*, **9**, 456–7.

Garson, J. A., Tedder, R. S., Briggs, M. *et al.* (1990). Detection of hepatitis C viral sequences in blood donations by 'nested' polymerase chain reaction and prediction of infectivity. *Lancet*, **335**, 1419–22.

Garson, J. A., Lenzi, M., Ring, C., *et al.* (1991). Hepatitis C viraemia in adults with Type 2 autoimmune hepatitis. *Journal of Medical Virology*, **34**, 223–6.

Geall, M. G., Schoenfield, L. J. & Summerskill, W. H. J. (1968). Classification and treatment of chronic active liver disease. *Gastroenterology*, **55**, 724–9.

Gerber, M. A. & Thung, S. N. (1985). Biology of disease. Molecular and cellular pathology of hepatitis B. *Laboratory Investigations*, **52**, 572–90.

Giuberti, T., Ferrari, C., Marchelli, S. *et al.* (1992). Long-term follow-up of anti-hepatic C virus antibodies in patients with acute non-A non-B hepatitis and different outcome of liver disease. *Liver*, **12**, 94–9.

Golding, P. L., Smith, M. & Williams, R. (1973). Multisystem involvement in chronic liver disease. *American Journal of Medicine*, **55**, 772–82.

Gorevic, P. D., Kassab, H. J., Levo, Y. *et al.* (1980). Mixed cryoglobulinemia: clinical aspects and long-term follow-up of 40 patients. *American Journal of Medicine*, **69**, 287–308.

Gudat, F., Bianchi, L., Sonnabend, W. *et al.* (1975). Pattern of core and surface expression in liver tissue reflects state of specific immune response in hepatitis B. *Laboratory Investigations*, **32**, 1–9.

Gurian, L. E., Rogoff, T. M., Ware, A. J. *et al.* (1985). The immunologic diagnosis of chronic active 'autoimmune' hepatitis: distinction from systemic lupus erythematosus. *Hepatology*, **5**, 397–402.

Haddad, J., Deny, P., Munz-Gotheil, C. *et al.* (1992). Lymphocytic sialadenitis of Sjogren's syndrome associated with chronic hepatitis C virus liver disease. *Lancet*, **339**, 321–3.

Hamlyn, A. N. & Berg, P. A. (1980). Haemagglutinating anti-actin antibodies in acute and chronic liver disease. *Gut*, **21**, 311–17.

Hanson, R. G., Peters, M. G. & Hoofnagle, J. H. (1986). Effects of immunosuppressive therapy with prednisolone on B and T lymphocyte function in patients with chronic type B hepatitis. *Hepatology*, **6**, 173–9.

Hay, J. E., Czaja, A. J., Rakela, J. & Ludwig, J. (1989). The nature of unexplained chronic aminotransferase elevations of a mild to moderate degree in asymptomatic patients. *Hepatology*, **9**, 193–7.

Herrero, C., Arroyo, V. & Bruguera, M. (1993). Is hepatitis C virus infection a trigger of porphyria cutanea tarda? *Lancet*, **341**, 788–9.

Hodges, S., Lobo-Yeo, A., Donaldson, P., Tanner, M. S. & Vergani, D. (1991). Autoimmune chronic active hepatitis in a family. *Gut*, **32**, 299–302.

Hofer, T. & McMahon, L. (1991). Corticosteroids and alcoholic hepatitis. *Hepatology*, **13**, 199–201.

Homberg, J. C., Andre, C. & Abuaf, N. (1984). A new anti-liver -kidney microsome antibody (LKM-2) in tienilic acid induced hepatitis. *Clinical Experimental Immunology*, **55**, 561–70.

Homberg, J.-C., Abauf, N., Bernard, O. *et al.* (1987). Chronic active hepatitis associated with antiliver/kidney microsome antibody type 1: a second type of 'autoimmune' hepatitis. *Hepatology*, **7**, 1333–9.

Hoofnagle, J. H., Dusheiko, G. M., Seef, L. B., Jones, E. A., Waggoner, J. G. & Bales, Z. B. (1981). Seroconversion from hepatitis B e antigen to antibody in chronic type B hepatitis. *Annals of Internal Medicine*, **94**, 744–8.

Hoofnagle, J. H., Dushieko, G. M., Schafer, D. F. *et al.* (1982). Reactivation of chronic hepatitis B virus infection by cancer chemotherapy. *Annals of Internal Medicine*, **96**, 447–9.

Hoofnagle, J. H., Davis, G. L., Pappas, C. *et al.* (1986). A short course of prednisolone in chronic type B hepatitis: report of a randomized, double-blind, placebo-controlled trial. *Annals of Internal Medicine*, **104**, 12–17.

Hosein, B., Fang, C. T., Popovsky, M. A. *et al.* (1991). Improved serodiagnosis of hepatitis C virus infection with synthetic peptide antigen from capsid protein. *Proceedings of the National Academy of Sciences, USA*, **88**, 3647–51.

Hosein, B., Fang, X. & Wang, C. Y. (1992). Anti-HCV, anti-GOR, and autoimmunity. *Lancet*, **339**, 871 (letter).

Hu, K.-Q., Yu, C.-H. & Vierling, J. M. (1993). One-step RNA polymerase chain reaction for detection of hepatitis C virus RNA. *Hepatology*, **18**, 270–4.

Ikeda, Y., Toda, G., Hashimoto, N. *et al.* (1990). Antibody to superoxide dismutase, autoimmune hepatitis, and antibody tests for hepatitis C virus. *Lancet*, **335**, 1345–6.

Ilan, Y., Hillman, M., Oren, R., Galun, E. & Shalit, M. (1991). Undetectable caeruloplasmin values in a patient with autoimmune chronic active hepatitis. *Gut*, **32**, 549–50.

Ishak, K. G., Zimmerman, H. J. & Ray, M. B. (1991). Alcoholic liver disease: pathologic pathogenetic and clinical aspects. *Alcoholism Clinical and Experimental Research*, **15**, 45–66.

Johnson, P. J. & McFarlane, I. G. (1989). *The Laboratory Investigation of Liver Disease*. pp. 179–204. London: Ballière Tindall.

Johnson, P. J., McFarlane, I. G., McFarlane, B. M. & Williams, R. (1990). Auto-immune features in patients with idiopathic chronic active hepatitis who are seronegative for conventional autoantibodies. *Journal of Gastroenterology and Hepatology*, **5**, 244–51.

Johnson, P. J. & McFarlane, I. G. (1993). Meeting report: International Autoimmune Hepatitis Group. *Hepatology*, **18**, 998–1005.

Johnson, R. D. & Williams, R. (1986). State of the art: Immune responses in alcoholic liver disease. *Alcoholism and Clinical Experimental Research*, **10**, 471–86.

Johnson, R. J., Gretch, D. R., Yamabe, H. *et al.* (1993). Membranoproliferative glomerulo-nephritis associated with hepatitis C virus infection. *New England Journal of Medicine*, **328**, 465–70.

Jori, G. P., Buonanno, G., D'Onofrio, F., Tirelli, A., Gonnela, F. & Gentile, S. (1977). Incidence and immunochemical features of serum cryoglobulin in chronic liver diseases. *Gut*, **18**, 245–9.

Joske, R. A. & King, W. E. (1955). The 'L.E.-cell' phenomenon in active chronic viral hepatitis. *Lancet*, **ii**, 477–9.

Keating, J. J., O'Brien, C. J., Stellon, A. J. *et al.* (1987). Influence of aetiology, clinical and histological features on survival in chronic active hepatitis: an analysis of 204 patients. *Quarterly Journal of Medicine*, **62**, 59–66.

Kenny, R. P., Czaja, A. J., Ludwig, J. & Dickson, E. R. (1986). Frequency and significance of antimitochondrial antibodies in severe chronic active hepatitis. *Digest Disease Science*, **31**, 705–11.

Klein, R. & Berg, P. A. (1990). Anti-M9 antibodies in sera from patients with primary biliary cirrhosis recognise an epitope of glycogen phosphorylase. *Clinical Experimental Immunology*, **81**, 65–7.

Klein, R. & Berg, P. A. (1991). Anti-M4 antibodies in primary biliary cirrhosis react with sulphite oxidase, an enzyme of the mitochondrial inter-membrane space. *Clinical and Experimental Immunology*, **84**, 445–8.

Knox, T. A., Hillyer, C. D. & Kaplan, M. M. (1991). Mixed cryoglobulinemia responsive to interferon-α. *American Journal of Medicine*, **91**, 554–5.

Koretz, R. L., Suffin, S. C. & Gitnick, G. L. (1976). Post transfusion chronic liver disease. *Gastroenterology*, **71**, 797–803.

Koretz, R. L., Stone, O., Moussa, M. & Gitnick, G. L. (1985). Non-A, Non-B post-transfusion hepatitis—A decade later. *Gastroenterology*, **88**, 1251–4.

Kuo, G., Choo, O.-L., Alter, H. J. *et al.* (1989). An assay for circulating antibodies to a major etiologic virus of human non-A, non-B hepatitis. *Science*, **244**, 362–4.

Lam, K. C., Lai, C. L., Ng, T. P. *et al.* (1981). Deleterious effect of prednisone in HBsAg positive chronic active hepatitis. *New England Journal of Medicine*, **304**, 380–6.

Lau, J. Y. N., Smith, H. M., Chaggar, K. *et al.* (1991). Significance of IgM anti-hepatitis delta virus (HDV) in chronic HDV infection. *Journal of Medical Virology*, **33**, 273–6.

Lenzi, M., Ballardini, G., Fusconi, M. *et al.* (1990). Type 2 autoimmune hepatitis and hepatitis C virus infection. *Lancet*, **335**, 258–9.

Lenzi, M., Johnson, P. J., McFarlane, I. G. *et al.* (1991). Antibodies to hepatitic C virus in autoimmune liver disease: evidence for geographical heterogeneity. *Lancet*, **338**, 277–80.

Levo, Y., Gorevic, P. D., Kassab, H. J., Zucker-Franklin, D. & Franklin, E. C. (1977). Association between hepatitis B virus and essential mixed cryoglobulinemia. *New England Journal of Medicine*, **296**, 1501–4.

Lidman, K., Biberfeld, G., Fagraeus, A. *et al.* (1976). Anti-actin specificity of human smooth muscle antibodies in chronic active hepatitis. *Clinical and Experimental Immunology*, **24**, 266–72.

Lieber, C. S. (1988). Biochemical and molecular basis of alcohol-induced injury to liver and other tissues. *New England Journal of Medicine*, **319**, 1639–50.

Loeper, J., Descatoire, V., Maurice M. *et al.* (1993). Cytochromes P-450 in human hepatocyte plasma membrane: recognition by several autoantibodies. *Gastroenterology*, **104**, 203–16.

Lohr, H., Treichel, U., Poralla, T., Manns, M. Meyer zum Buschenfelde, K. H. & Fleischer, B. (1990). The human hepatic asialoglycoprotein receptor is a target antigen for liver-infiltrating T cells in autoimmune chronic active hepatitis and primary biliary cirrhosis. *Hepatology*, **12**, 1314–20.

Lok, A. S. F., Wu, P. C., Lai, C. L. *et al.* (1992). A controlled trial of interferon with or without prednisone priming for chronic hepatitis B. *Gastroenterology*, **102**, 2091–7.

Louzir, H., Ternynck, T., Gorgi, Y., Tahar, S., Ayed, K. & Avrameas, S. (1992). Autoantibodies and circulating immune complexes in sera from patients with hepatitis B virus-related chronic liver disease. *Clinical Immunology and Immunopathology*, **62**, 160–7.

Ludwig, J. (1979). Drug effects on the liver: a tabular compilation of drugs and drug-related hepatic diseases. *Digest Disease Science*, **24**, 785–91.

Ludwig, J. (1992). *Practical Liver Biopsy Interpretation*. pp. 9–19. Chicago: ASCP Press.

Lunel, E., Homberg, J. C., Grippon, P. *et al.* (1991). Type 2 autoimmune hepatitis and hepatitis C virus: A study of 83 patients. *Journal of Hepatology*, **13**(Suppl. 2): s47.

Ma, Y., Peakman, M., Lenzi, M. *et al.* (1993). Case against subclassification of type II autoimmune chronic active hepatitis. *Lancet*, **341**, 60 (letter).

McFarlane, I. G. (1991). Autoimmunity and hepatotropic viruses. *Seminars in Liver Diseases*, **11**, 221–3.

McFarlane, I. G. (1992). Editorial review: Immunological abnormalities and hepatotropic viral infections. *Clinical and Experimental Immunology*, **87**, 337–9.

McFarlane, I. G. (1993). Clinical spectrum and heterogeneity of autoimmune hepatitis: an overview. In *Falk Symposium 70 – Immunology and the Liver*, ed. K. H. Meyer zum Buschenfelde, J. H. Hoofnagle & M. Manns, pp. 179–192. Kluwer Academic Press

McFarlane, I. G. & Eddleston, A. L. W. F. (1990). Chronic active hepatitis. In *Immunology and Immunopathology of the Liver and Gastrointestinal Tract*, ed. S. R. Targan & F. Shanahan, pp. 281–304. New York: Igaku-Shoin.

McFarlane, I. G. & Williams, R. (1985). Liver membrane antibodies. *Journal of Hepatology*, **1**, 313–19.

McFarlane, B. M., McSorley, C. G., Vergani, D., McFarlane, I. G. & Williams, R. (1986). Serum autoantibodies reacting with the hepatic asialoglycoprotein receptor protein (hepatic lectin) in acute and chronic liver disorders. *Journal of Hepatology*, **3**, 196–205.

McFarlane, B. M., Sipos, J., Gove, C. D. *et al.* (1990*a*). Antibodies against the hepatic asialoglycoprotein receptor perfused *in situ* preferentially attach to periportal liver cells in the rat. *Hepatology*, **11**, 408–415.

McFarlane, I. G., Smith, H. M., Johnson, P. J., Bray, G. P., Vergani, D. & Williams, R. (1990*b*). Hepatitic C virus antibodies in chronic active hepatitis: pathogenetic factors of false-positive result? *Lancet*, **335**, 754–7.

McFarlane, B. M., Bridger, C., Tibbs, C. J. *et al.* (1994). Virus-induced autoimmunity in hepatitis C virus infections: a rare event. *Journal of Medical Virology*, **42**, 66–72.

McFarlane, I. G., Chaggar, K., Davies, S. E., Smith, H. M., Alexander, G. J. M. & Williams, R. (1991). IgA class antibodies to hepatitis delta virus antigen in acute and chronic hepatitis delta virus infections. *Hepatology*, **14**, 980–4.

McFarlane, I. G., Farrant, J. M. & Eddleston, A. L. W. F. (1993). Autoimmune liver disease. In *Clinical Aspects of Immunology*, ed. P. J. Lachmann, K. Peters, F. S. Rosen & M. J. Walport, 5th edn. pp. 1969–1985. Oxford: Blackwell.

McGuinness, P. H., Bishop, G. A., Lien, A., Wiley, B., Parsons, C. & McCaughan, G. W. (1993). Detection of serum hepatitis C virus RNA in HCV antibody-positive volunteer blood donors. *Hepatology*, **18**, 485–90.

McIntosh, R. M., Koss, M. N. & Gocke, D. J. (1976). The nature and incidence of cryoproteins in hepatitis B antigen (HBsAg) positive patients. *Quarterly Journal of Medicine*, **45**, 23–8.

Mackay, I. R., Taft, L. I. & Cowling, D. C. (1956). Lupoid hepatitis. *Lancet*, **ii**, 1323–6.

Mackay, I. R., Taft, L. I. & Cowling, D. C. (1959). Lupoid hepatitis and the hepatic lesions of systemic lupus erythematosus. *Lancet*, **i**, 65–9.

Mackay, I. R. & Wood, I. J. (1962). Lupoid hepatitis: a comparison of 22 cases with other types of liver disease. *Quarterly Journal of Medicine*, **31**, 485–507.

Mackay, I. R. & Tait, D. B. (1980). HLA associations with autoimmune type chronic active hepatitis: identification of B8-DRw3 haplotype by family studies. *Gastroenterology*, **79**, 95–9.

Magrin, S., Craxi, A., Fiorentino, G. *et al.* (1991). Is autoimmune chronic active hepatitis a HCV-related disease? *Journal of Hepatology*, **13**, 56–60.

Manns, M. P. (1991). Cytoplasmic autoantigens in autoimmune hepatitis: molecular analysis and clinical relevance. *Seminars in Liver Diseases*, **11**, 205–14.

Manns, M., Gerken, G., Kyriatsoulis, A., Staritz, M. & Meyer zum Buschenfelde, K.-H. (1987). Characterisation of a new subgroup of autoimmune chronic active hepatitis by autoantibodies against a soluble liver antigen. *Lancet*, **i**, 292–4.

Manns, M., Johnson, E. F., Griffin K. J. *et al.* (1989). Major antigen of liver kidney microsomal autoantibodies in idiopathic autoimmune hepatitis is cytochrome P450db1. *Journal of Clinical Investigation*, **83**, 1066–72.

Manns, M. P., Griffin, K. J., Sullivan, K. F. & Johnson, E. F. (1991). LKM-1 autoantibodies recognize a short inner sequence in P450IID6, a cytochrome P450 monooxygenase. *Journal of Clinical Investigation*, **88**, 1370–8.

Marcellin, P., Descamps, V., Martinot-Peignoux, M. *et al.* (1993). Cryoglobulinemia with vasculitis associated with hepatitis C virus infection. *Gastroenterology*, **104**, 272–7.

Marsden, C. D. (1987). Wilson's disease. *Quarterly Journal of Medicine*, **65**, 959–66.

Mehta, S., Mishiro, S., Sekiguchi, K. *et al.* (1992). Immune response to GOR, a marker for non-A, non-B hepatitis and its correlation with hepatitic C virus infection. *Journal of Clinical Immunology*, **12**, 178–84.

Mieli-Vergani, G., Vergani, D, Portmann, B. *et al.* (1982). Lymphocyte cytotoxicity to autologous hepatocytes in HBsAg-positive chronic liver disease. *Gut*, **23**, 1029–36.

Mieli-Vergani, G., Lobo-Yeo, A., McFarlane, B. M., McFarlane, I. G., Mowat, A. T. & Vergani, D. (1989). Different immune mechanisms leading to autoimmunity in primary sclerosing cholangitis and autoimmune chronic active hepatitis of childhood. *Hepatology*, 9, 198–203.

Mieli-Vergani, G., Civeira, M. P. & Vergani, D. (1992). Immunology and the liver. In *Hepatobiliary Diseases*, ed. J. Prieto, J. Rodes & D. A. Schafritz, pp. 95–116. New York: Springer-Verlag.

Milner, L. S., Dusheiko, G. M., Jacobs, D. *et al.* (1988). Biochemical and serological characteristics of children with membranous nephropathy due to hepatitis B virus infection: correlation with hepatitis Be antigen, hepatitis B DNA and hepatitis D. *Nephron*, 49, 184–9.

Mills, C. T., Lee, E. & Perrillo, R. (1990). Relationship between histology, aminotransferase levels, and viral replication in chronic hepatitis B. *Gastroenterology*, 99, 519–24.

Mishiro, S., Hoshi, Y. & Takeda, K. (1990). Non-A, non-B hepatitis specific antibodies directed at host-derived epitope: implications for an autoimmune process. *Lancet*, 336, 1400–3.

Misiani, R., Bellavita, P., Fenili, D. *et al.* (1992). Hepatitis C virus infection in patients with essential mixed cryoglobulinemia. *Annals of Internal Medicine*, 117, 573–7.

Mondelli, M., Mieli-Vergani, G., Alberti, A. *et al.* (1982). Specificity of T-lymphocyte cytotoxicity to autologous hepatocytes in chronic hepatitis B virus infection: evidence that T cells are directed against HBV core antigen expressed on hepatocytes. *Journal of Immunology*, 129, 2773–8.

Moreno, A., Martinez, C. J. & Carreno, V. (1993). Liver biopsy and the etiologic diagnosis of chronic hepatitis. *Journal of Hepatology*, 17(Suppl. 3), S112–15.

Nair, P. V., Tong, M. J., Stevenson, D., Roskanp, D. & Boone, C. (1986). A pilot study on the effects of prednisone withdrawal on serum hepatitis B virus DNA and HBeAg in chronic active hepatitis B. *Hepatology*, 6, 1319–24.

Negro, F. & Rizzetto, M. (1993). Pathobiology of hepatitis delta virus. *Journal of Hepatology*, 17, (Suppl. 3), S149–53.

Nicholson, S., Leslie, D. E., Efandis, T. *et al.* (1991). Hepatitis C antibody testing: Problems associated with non-specific binding. *Journal of Virology Methods*, 33, 311–17.

Nishioka, M. (1993). Nuclear antigens in autoimmune hepatitis. In *Falk Symposium 70 – Immunology and the Liver,* ed. K. H. Meyer zum Buschenfelde, J. H. Hoofnagle & M. Manns, pp. 193–205. Kluwer Academic Press.

O'Brien, C. J., Vento, S., Donaldson, P. T. *et al.* (1986). Cell-mediated immunity and suppressor-T-cell defects to liver-derived antigens in families of patients with autoimmune chronic active hepatitis. *Lancet*, i, 350–3.

Opelz, G., Vogten, A. J., Summerskill, W. H., Schalm, S. W. & Terasaki, P. I. (1977). HLA determinants in chronic active liver disease: possible relation of HLA-Dw3 to prognosis. *Tissue Antigens*, 9, 36–40.

Palmer, J. M., Yeaman, S. J., Bassendine, M. F. & James, O. F. W. (1993). M4 and M9 autoantigens in primary biliary cirrhosis – a negative study. *Journal of Hepatology*, 18, 251–4.

Pateron, D., Hartmann, D. J., Duclos-Vallée, J. C., Jouanolle, H. & Beaugrand, M. (1993). Latent autoimmune thyroid disease in patients with chronic HCV hepatitis. *Journal of Hepatology*, 17, 417–19.

Pechere-Bertschi, A., Perrin, L., De Saussure, P., Widmann, J. J., Giostra, E. & Schifferli, J. A. (1992). Hepatitis C: a possible etiology for cryoglobulinemia type II. *Clinical and Experimental Immunology*, 89, 419–22.

Pedersen, B. K., Beyer, J. M., Rasmussen, A. *et al.* (1984). Azathioprine as single drug in the treatment of rheumatoid arthritis induces complete suppression of natural killer cell activity. *Acta Pathologica Microbiologica Immunologica Scandinavica* (C) 92, 221–5.

Pedersen, B. K. & Beyer, J. M. (1986). A longitudinal study of the influence of azathioprine on natural killer cell activity. *Allergy*, **41**, 286–9.

Perrillo, R. P. (1993). Interferon in the management of chronic hepatitis B. *Digest Disease Science*, **38**, 577–93.

Perrillo, R. P., Schiff, E. R., Davis, G. L. *et al.* (1990). A randomized, controlled trial of interferon alfa-2b alone and after prednisone withdrawal, in the treatment of chronic hepatitis B. *New England Journal of Medicine*, **232**, 295–301.

Phillips, P. E. & Dougherty, R. M. (1991). Editorial: Hepatitis C and mixed cryoglobulinemia. *Clinical and Experimental Rheumatology*, **9**, 551–5.

Popp. J. W., Dienstag, J. L., Wands, J. R. & Bloch, K. J. (1984). Essential mixed cryoglobulinemia without evidence for hepatitis B virus infection. *Annals of Internal Medicine*, **92**, 379–83.

Poralla, T., Treichel, U., Lohr, H. & Fleischer, B. (1991). The asialoglycoprotein receptor as target structure in autoimmune liver diseases. *Seminars in Liver Disease*, **11**, 215–22.

Puoti, M., Zonaro, A., Ravagii, A. *et al.* (1992). Hepatitis C virus RNA and antibody response in the clinical course of hepatitis C virus infection. *Hepatology*, **16**, 877–81.

Rabinovitz, M., Demetris, A. J., Bou-Abboud, C. F. & Van Thiel, D. H. (1992). Simultaneous occurrence of primary sclerosing cholangitis and autoimmune chronic active hepatitis in a patient with ulcerative colitis. *Digest Disease Science*, **37**, 1606–11.

Relman, A. S. (1992). Cryoglobulinemia and hepatitis C virus. *New England Journal of Medicine*, **327**, 1521–2.

Rizzetto, M. (1990). Hepatitis delta: the virus and the disease. *Journal of Hepatology*, **11**, s145–8.

Rizzetto, M., Swana, G. & Doniach, D. (1973). Microsomal antibodies in active chronic hepatitis and other disorders. *Clinical and Experimental Immunology*, **15**, 331–44.

Roonbloom, L. E., Alm, G. V. & Oberg, K. E. (1991). Autoimmunity after alpha-interferon therapy for malignant carcinoid tumours. *Annals of Internal Medicine*, **115**, 178–83.

Schalm, S. W., Summerskill, W. J. H., Gitnick, G. L. *et al.* (1976). Contrasting features and responses to treatment for severe chronic active liver disease with and without hepatitis B s antigen. *Gut*, **17**, 781–786.

Scheuer, P. J. (1987). Viral hepatitis. In *Pathology of the Liver*, ed. R. N. M. McSween, P. P. Anthony & P. J. Scheuer, pp. 202–3. Edinburgh: Churchill Livingstone.

Scheuer, P. J., Ashrafzadeh, P., Sherlock, S., Brown, D. & Dusheiko, G. M. (1992). The pathology of hepatitis C. *Hepatology*, **15**, 567–71.

Scully, L. J., Clarke, D. & Barr, R. J. (1993). Diclofenac induced hepatitis. Three cases with features of autoimmune chronic active hepatitis. *Digest Disease Science*, **38**, 744–51.

Seki, T., Kiyosawa, K., Inoko, H. & Ota, M. (1990). Association of autoimmune hepatitis with HLA-Bw54 and DR4 in Japanese patients. *Hepatology*, **12**, 1300–4.

Stechemesser, E., Klein, R. & Berg, P. A. (1993). Characterization and clinical relevance of liver-pancreas antibodies in autoimmune hepatitis. *Hepatology*, **18**, 1–9.

Stellon, A. J., Hegarty, J. E., Portmann, B. & Williams, R. (1985). Randomised controlled trial of azathioprine withdrawal in autoimmune chronic active hepatitis. *Lancet*, **i**, 668–70.

Stellon, A. J., Keating, J. J., Johnson, P. J., McFarlane, I. G. & Williams, R. (1988). Maintenance of remission in autoimmune chronic active hepatitis with azathioprine after corticosteroid withdrawal. *Hepatology*, **8**, 781–4.

Sternlieb, I. (1990). Perspective in Wilson's disease. *Hepatology*, **12**, 1234–9.

Stevens, C. E., Beasley, R. P., Tsui, J. & Lee, W. C. (1975). Vertical transmission of hepatitis B antigen in Taiwan. *New England Journal Medicine*, **292**, 771–5.

Swanson, N. R., Reed, W. D., Yarred, L. J., Shilkin, K. B. & Joske, R. A. (1990). Autoantibodies to isolated human hepatocyte plasma membranes in chronic active hepatitis. II. Specificity of antibodies. *Hepatology*, **11**, 613–21.

Toda, G., Ikeda, Y., Kashiwagi, M., Iwamori, M. & Oka, H. (1990). Hepatocyte plasma membrane glycosphingolipid reactive with sera from patients with autoimmune chronic active hepatitis: its identification as sulfatide. *Hepatology*, **12**, 664–70.

Todros, L., Touscoz, G., D'Urso, N. *et al.* (1991). Hepatitis C virus-related chronic liver disease with autoantibodies to liver-kidney microsomes (LKM). *Journal of Hepatology*, **13**, 128–31.

Tran, A., Quaranta, J.-F., Benzaken, S. *et al.* (1993). High prevalence of thyroid autoantibodies in a prospective series of patients with chronic hepatitis C before interferon therapy. *Hepatology*, **18**, 253–7.

Treichel, U., Poralla, T., Hess, G., Manns, M. & Meyer zum Buschenfelde, K.-H. (1990). Autoantibodies to human asialoglycoprotein receptor in autoimmune-type chronic hepatitis. *Hepatology*, **11**, 606–12.

Ulrich, P. P., Romeo, J. M., Lane, P. K. *et al.* (1990). Detection, semiquantitation, and genetic variation in hepatitis C virus sequences amplified from the plasma of blood donors with elevated alanine aminotransferase. *Journal of Clinical Investigation*, **86**, 1609–14.

Van der Poel, C. L., Cuypers, H. T. M., Reesink, H. W. *et al.* (1991). Confirmation of hepatitis C virus infection by new four-antigen recombinant immunoblot assay. *Lancet*, **337**, 317–9.

Van der Water, J., Gershwin, M. E., Leung, P., Ansari, A. & Coppel, R. L. (1988). The autoepitope of the 74 kD mitochondrial autoantigen of primary biliary cirrhosis corresponds to the functional site of dihydrolipoamide acetyltransferase. *Journal of Experimental Medicine*, **167**, 1791–9.

Vento, S., O'Brien, C. J., McFarlane, B. M., McFarlane, I. G., Eddleston, A. L. W. F. & Williams, R. (1986). T-lymphocyte sensitization to hepatocyte antigens in autoimmune chronic active hepatitis and primary biliary cirrhosis. Evidence for different underlying mechanisms and different antigenic determinants as targets. *Gastroenterology*, **91**, 810–17.

Vento, S., O'Brien, C. J., McFarlane, I. G., Williams, R. & Eddleston, A. L. W. F. (1987). T-cell inducers of suppressor lymphocytes control liver-directed autoreactivity. *Lancet*, **i**, 886–8.

Vento, S., McFarlane, B. M., Garofano-Vento, T. *et al.* (1988). Serial study of liver-directed autoantibodies and autoreactive T-lymphocytes in acute viral hepatitis B. *Journal of Autoimmunity*, **1**, 229–307.

Vento, S., Di Perri, G., Garofano, T. *et al.* (1990). Hazards of interferon therapy for HBV-seronegative chronic hepatitis. *Lancet*, **ii**, 926 (letter).

Vergani, D. & Mieli-Vergani, G. (1993). Editorial review. Type II autoimmune hepatitis: the conundrum of cytochrome P450IID6. *Clinical and Experimental Immunology*, **92**, 367–8.

Waldenstrom, J. (1950). Leber, blutproteine und Nahrungseiweiss. *Deutsch Gesellschaft Z Verdau Stoffwechselkr*, **15**, 113–9.

Wands, J. R., Mann, E., Alpert, E. & Isselbacher, K. J. (1975). The pathogenesis of arthritis associated with hepatitis B surface antigen-positive hepatitis. *Journal of Clinical Investigation*, **55**, 930–5.

Wen, L., Peakman, M., Lobo-Yeo, McFarlane, B. M., Mowat, A. P., Mieli-Vergani, G. & Vergani, D. (1990). T-cell-directed hepatocyte damage in autoimmune chronic active hepatitis. *Lancet*, **336**, 1527–30.

Whittingham, S., Irwin, J., Mackay, I. R. & Smalley, M. (1966). Smooth muscle autoantibody in 'autoimmune' hepatitis. *Gastroenterology*, **51**, 499–505.

Whittingham, S., Mackay, I. R. & Irwin, J. (1966). Autoimmune hepatitis: immunofluorescence reactions with cytoplasm of smooth muscle and glomerular cells. *Lancet*, **i**, 1333–5.

Worman, H. J. & Courvalin, J.-C. (1991). Autoantibodies against nuclear envelope proteins in liver disease. *Hepatology*, **14**, 1269–79.

Yamamoto, A. M., Mura, C., De Lemos-Chiarandini, C., Krishnamoorthy, R. & Alvarez, F. (1993). Cytochrome P450IID6 recognized by LKM-1 antibody is not exposed on the surface of hepatocytes. *Clinical and Experimental Immunology*, **92**, 381–90.

Yatsuhashi, H., Inoue, O., Koga, M. *et al.* (1992). Comparison of hepatitis C virus markers in patients with NANB hepatitis. *Journal Virology Methods*, **37**, 13–21.

Zarski, J. P., Rougier, D., Aubert, H. *et al.* (1984). Association cryoglobuline et maladie hépatique: fréquence, nature et caractères immuno-chiminiques de la cryoglobulinémie. *Gastroenterology and Clinical Biology*, **8**, 845–50.

Zimmerman, H. J. & Maddrey, W. C. (1987). Toxic and drug-induced hepatitis. In *Diseases of the Liver*, 6th edn. ed. L. Schiff & E. R. Schiff, pp. 591–668. Philadelphia: JB Lippincott.

–15–
Primary biliary cirrhosis

M. H. DAVIES and J. M. NEUBERGER

Foreword

It would be improper to proceed with a chapter on primary biliary cirrhosis, without first reflecting upon a great contribution to the knowledge and understanding of the disease made by the late David R. Triger. Unfortunately, his premature and untimely death prevented him from writing this chapter. David Triger had a lifelong zest for the disease, its pathophysiology, clinical management and provided novel observations concerning its epidemiology.

Introduction

Primary biliary cirrhosis (PBC) is a disease of unknown aetiology associated with a variety of immunological disturbances which suggest a breakdown of immune tolerance. It is characterised by chronic infiltration in the liver and destruction of intrahepatic bile ducts and usually leads to cholestasis, portal hypertension, cirrhosis and death due to liver failure.

Incidence and geography

The disease has been reported from most parts of the world and appears to affect all ethnic populations studied. A study of the prevalence, incidence and death rates in various countries is presently being carried out under the direction of the International Association for the Study of the Liver. Provisional data suggest a marked variation across the world, which probably cannot be adequately explained by differences in clinical practice and diagnostic accuracy alone.

Many series have described incidence and prevalence of PBC in predominantly Caucasian populations. In the UK the incidence is reported to be 5–10/million/year and prevalence of approximately 25–50/million (Triger, 1980; Hamlyn, Macklon & James, 1983).

Familial clustering of PBC occurs and it has been reported in sisters, twins, and mothers and daughters. An association between HLA and PBC has been sought. There appears to be no class I association, although a number of class II associations have been reported. Early studies in Japan (Miyamori et al., 1983) and Spain (Hamlyn, Adams & Sherlock, 1980) suggested associations with DR2 and DR3 respectively, although subsequent studies failed to confirm this. Two subsequent reports have noted association with DR8 and DR5 (Gores et al., 1987; Manns et al., 1991). There is also association with the class three haplotype C4 B2. Most recently the association with DR8 has been supported from data resulting from restriction-fragment-length polymorphism HLA genotyping (Underhill et al., 1992).

Marked geographical clustering has been noted in one study (Triger, 1980). The point prevalence was 54 per million, but inhabitants whose water supply was from one particular reservoir were 10 times more likely to have the disease than people served from other reservoirs. Another study has suggested a predominance of cases arising within urban dwellers (Goudie et al., 1987) and a study from Sweden reported a statistically significant difference in incidence in the most Northerly population studied.

Clinical features

Ninety per cent of patients with PBC are female (Sherlock & Scheuer, 1973; Christensen et al., 1980) and the disease is usually diagnosed between the ages of 40 and 60 years. The disease usually presents in one of four ways.

In the classical presentation of PBC, clinical features are typically gradual in onset, often with pruritus as the earliest symptom (Sherlock & Scheuer, 1973; Ahrens et al., 1950; Long, Scheuer & Sherlock, 1977; Tornay, 1980; James, Macklon & Watson, 1981). This is followed by constitutional disturbance, fatigue, lethargy and general malaise (Long, Scheuer & Sherlock, 1977). Jaundice with features of cholestasis tends to occur late, but occasionally is the presenting feature (Sherlock & Scheuer, 1973; Ahrens et al., 1950; Long, Scheuer & Sherlock, 1977; Tornay, 1980; James, Macklon & Watson, 1981). As the disease progresses, features of portal hypertension may develop with ascites and gastrointestinal bleeds from oesophageal varices. Skin changes often include pigmentation and excoriations from chronic pruritus. Other cutaneous stigmata typical of chronic liver disease are relatively infrequent. Xanthelasmata are common, but xanthomata, which may cause neuropathy, are rare. Hepatosplenomegaly is frequent and may cause dragging abdominal discomfort. As disease progresses, cirrhosis may develop with features of hepatocellular failure, manifest by progressive muscle wasting and encephalopathy.

The increased utilisation of automated laboratory equipment has resulted in an increasing number of asymptomatic patients being identified by routine serum biochemical or immunological screening.

In a small proportion of patients complications of portal hypertension may be the presenting feature (James, Macklon & Watson, 1981). This can develop in the absence of other features of advanced liver disease, especially if the patient is pre-cirrhotic. Such patients therefore, may present with variceal bleeding or ascites, with relatively well preserved biochemical and synthetic liver function tests.

Patients may present with an associated auto-immune disease and be identified during investigation.

Overlap syndromes

A degree of histological overlap exists between primary biliary cirrhosis and a number of other conditions. A loss of small and intermediate-sized bile ducts may occur in primary sclerosing cholangitis, antibiotic-associated hepatotoxicity, graft versus host disease, liver allograft rejection, non Hodgkin's lymphoma, sarcoidosis and an apparent adult idiopathic form. Some cases of PBC or PBC-like syndromes have occurred following drug-induced reactions, with precipitants including chlorpromazine, benoxaprofen and imipramine. An overlap between PBC and auto-immune chronic active hepatitis may occur, making differentiation between the two difficult in some. In addition to the development of a vanishing bile duct syndrome in sarcoidosis, other similarities, such as hepatic granulomas occasionally make differentiation between the two conditions difficult.

In addition to these specific syndromes, a small minority of patients with PBC are consistently negative for mitochondrial antibody (AMA negative PBC) (see later).

Prognosis

The course of the disease is highly variable. In an early series (Ahrens *et al.*, 1950) 17 patients were described, of whom 6 died within 7 years of the diagnosis. Other early series reported similar survival data, but the majority of these series predominantly reviewed patients who already had advanced disease at presentation.

Symptomatic disease

James, Macklon & Watson in 1981 reported 11 deaths from 48 cases of PBC. Nine of these deaths were attributed to liver disease during a mean follow-up of 4.1 years. The mortality rate was markedly higher than standardised mortality matched for age and sex. Another series described median survival of 10 years following onset of symptoms in 243 patients over a 12 year period (Moll *et al.*, 1983). More recently Mitchison reported median survival from diagnoses of 78 months and 61 months in symptomatic patients from a regional liver unit and tertiary referral centre respectively (Mitchison *et al.*, 1990).

Asymptomatic disease

Asymptomatic disease is defined in the presence of a positive anti-mitochondrial antibody titre greater than 1/40, with liver histology consistent with primary biliary cirrhosis (which is almost invariably present). Biochemistry is not necessarily deranged.

A series of patients with asymptomatic disease was first described in 1973 (Fox, Scheuer & Sherlock, 1973). Four patients all presented for reasons unrelated to the liver, but were found to have elevated serum alkaline phosphatase. In each case, liver biopsy showed histological features considered diagnostic of PBC. The prognosis of these asymptomatic patients is uncertain. In an early series of 20 patients, 10 remained symptom-free during 2–10 years follow-up (Long, Scheuer & Sherlock, 1977). Two of these died during the study period, but death was not related to liver disease. The other 10 patients developed symptoms of liver disease over a mean period of 2.2 years. Three of these died from liver failure and 7 remained alive at the end of follow-up. The prognosis of such patients was reported in another series (Sherlock, 1984). Many individuals were found to remain asymptomatic for over 10 years, whereas others progressed rapidly to portal hypertension, cirrhosis, hepatocellular failure and death.

Subsequently numerous studies have examined the prognosis of patients with asymptomatic PBC (Roll *et al.*, 1983; Kapelman & Schaffner, 1981; Balasubramaniam *et al.*, 1990; Beswick, Klatskin & Boyer, 1985; Hanik, Eriksson & Lindgren, 1984), but in many the sample size was small, follow-up short and patient populations studied have varied considerably. Conclusions vary, but overall results indicate that a number of patients followed up with asymptomatic PBC will remain well for many years, with no evidence of histological progression, whilst others go on to develop progressive disease. Currently there is no way of predicting which course a patient will follow.

Anti-mitochondrial antibody (AMA) negative PBC

A small proportion of patients with PBC are repeatedly seronegative for AMA. Despite this, histological examination, cholangiography and IgM rises are well consistent with a diagnosis of PBC. They usually have antinuclear antibody (ANA), and higher serum immunoglobulin levels. The proportion of patients with AMA negative PBC is low – of the order of 5% and anecdotal evidence suggests their course is similar to their AMA positive counterparts and they have an unpredictable response to corticosteroid therapy. Whether anti-mitochondrial antibody negative PBC represents a distinct disease entity – an alternative auto-immune cholangitis is unknown.

Prognosis

The ability to predict prognosis is of value in any disease, but in liver disease, this is of particular value since the advent of liver transplantation (see later). In 1979, Shapiro reported serum bilirubin to be an important prognostic factor in PBC (Shapiro, Smith & Schaffner, 1979), and this has been confirmed in subsequent studies (Christensen et al., 1980, 1985; Roll et al., 1983; Dickson et al., 1989). Portal granulomata present in liver biopsy material has been found to be associated with a favourable prognosis by some (Beswick, Klatskin & Boyer, 1985; Lee et al., 1981), although not all agree (Portmann et al., 1985).

Subsequently a number of prognostic models have been developed for patients with PBC.

Prognostic models

Several prognostic models have been developed for predicting survival in non-transplanted individuals with PBC, using the Cox proportional hazards multivariate regression analysis. The prognostic models have been developed in an attempt to predict likely course of disease. The models, however, have limitations; while they identify prognostic factors and provide valuable information regarding population survival, they are of limited value when applied to an individual, because:

- Confidence limits are wide.
- Reapplication is inappropriate unless time-dependent models are used.
- Prognostic factors for end-stage patients may be different to those patients with early disease.
- No account is taken of symptomatic disease.
- Studies are retrospective and cannot take account of new developments.

In the Yale model, Roll reported elevated bilirubin, old age and hepato-megaly to be independently associated with adverse prognosis, whereas portal fibrosis without bridging fibrosis or cirrhosis was associated with a better prognosis (Roll *et al.*, 1983). Serum bilirubin was the most significant variable in this model.

The European model was based on a multicentre trial with azathioprine (Christensen *et al.*, 1985). Serum bilirubin was the most significant of six independent variables which included old age, cirrhosis, low serum albumin and central cholestasis, all indicating poor prognosis.

The Mayo model is the most recent. This includes patient's age, serum bilirubin and albumin, prothrombin time and severity of oedema (Dickson *et al.*, 1989). When applied subsequently to separate databases of 141 and 35 non-Mayo patients it was found to predict survival accurately (Grambsch *et al.*, 1989). When applied to Mayo clinic patients, accuracy was independent of histological stage of disease (Grambsch *et al.*, 1989). Results obtained from the three models correlate well.

Pathology

Macroscopic

In end-stage PBC the liver is enlarged, bile stained with a nodular surface. The extra hepatic biliary system is normal. Enlarged fleshy lymph nodes are present at the porta hepatis and along the common bile duct (Hübscher & Harrison, 1989).

Microscopic

The histological changes associated with PBC are patchy, especially in the early stages. Histological diagnosis can be difficult if characteristic bile duct lesions are absent from a small needle biopsy specimen (Scheuer, 1968). Features of early disease include a mixed portal inflammatory infiltrate and the presence of granulomata. Later there is loss of bile ducts, marginal ductular proliferation, the development of biliary piecemeal necrosis and progression to fibrosis and cirrhosis.

Bile duct lesions

Early bile ducts lesions involve small to medium-sized bile ducts of 40 μm to 75 μm in diameter (MacSween, 1986). A chronic inflammatory cell infiltrate surrounds bile ducts with minimal periportal inflammation and little paren-chymal involvement. The biliary epithelium may be hyperplastic or necrotic

(Scheuer 1968; MacSween, 1986; Portmann & MacSween, 1987). Other features include focal disruption of the basement membrane, ulceration of the epithelium and rupture of the duct. The portal infiltrate consists of lymphocytes, plasma cells and occasional eosinophils but neutrophils are virtually absent. Smaller portal tracts are normal or diffusely infiltrated with mononuclear cells. Limiting plates may remain intact.

Lymphocyte aggregates, sometimes with a germinal centre are seen around or adjacent to the ducts. Intense histiocytic granuloma formation may occur, sometimes with foamy giant cells. Remnants of bile duct epithelium may be seen within these inflammatory aggregates, but eventually disappear. Lymphoid aggregates may persist as 'tombstone' markers of the departed duct – the histological hallmark of primary biliary cirrhosis which are virtually pathognomonic (MacSween, 1986).

Later in the course of the disease characteristic periductal lesions regress and diminish in number. A study incorporating computer assisted three-dimensional reconstruction from tissue sections showed 'amputation' of bile ducts of sizes ranging from $<40\,\mu$m to $>80\,\mu$m (Yamada, Howe & Sheuer, 1987). Irregular bile ductular proliferation develops in the marginal zones of portal tracts. These neoductules are smaller than those seen in large duct obstruction and their lumens tend to be poorly defined.

Parenchymal changes

Changes within the liver parenchyma are characteristically mild (Portmann & MacSween, 1987), but include periportal cholestasis, epithelioid granulomata, focal Kupffer cell hyperplasia and intrasinusoidal accumulation of lymphocytes and other mononuclear cells. Periportal hepatocytes may become ballooned. There is accumulation of copper-associated protein and Mallory's hyaline may be present – all features of chronic cholestatis.

Portal fibrosis/cirrhosis

Portal tracts show irregular expansion, chronic inflammation and destruction of the limiting plate. Irregular fibrous septa often bridge between portal tracts with biliary piecemeal necrosis and cholestasis. The final stage involves extension of fibrous septa to the perivenular zone producing a true micronodular cirrhosis.

Staging

A number of staging systems have been devised, each grading disease from stage 1 to 4. Unfortunately, interpretation of the histological stage is difficult in view of the patchy nature of PBC. Changes are focal and considerable overlap between the stages will occur within the same liver. A biopsy from one area may show stage 1 disease, yet a second needle biopsy might show cirrhosis, stage 4. It is not surprising that correlation between clinical condition and histological state is poor (MacSween, 1986).

Associated auto-immune disease

Primary biliary cirrhosis is associated with a number of non-hepatic auto-immune diseases. Associations with scleroderma (Rudzki, Ishak & Zimmerman, 1975), Sjögren's syndrome (Alarcón-Segovia et al., 1973), arthropathy (Sherlock & Scheuer, 1973) and vitiligo are well recognised. Between 72% and 100% of patients have kerato-conjunctivitis sicca or xerostomia on specific testing (Alarcón-Segovia et al., 1973; Giovaninni et al., 1985) and many have CREST syndrome (calcinosis, Raynaud's, (o)esophageal dysfunction, sclerodactyly and telangiectasia). Arthropathy is frequent and has various causes including rheumatoid arthritis, psoriatic arthritis, chondro-calcinosis, hypertrophic osteodystrophy and avascular necrosis. The prevalence of frank arthritis varies between 5 and 24% in different series (Clarke et al., 1978; Crowe et al., 1980). Hypothyroidism is reported in approximately 20% of cases (James, Macklon & Watson, 1981; Elta et al., 1983; Crowe et al., 1980). A study of auto-immune associations in 113 patients participating in a trial of D-penicillamine revealed at least one association in 84% and two or more associations in 41% (Culp et al., 1982). Renal tubular acidosis is frequently present on formal testing, although it is not usually symptomatic (Parés et al., 1980). Some patients have active glomerulonephritis. An association with coeliac disease has also been reported (Logan et al., 1978). It is advisable to obtain duodenal biopsies in patients, especially if the serum albumin appears inappropriately low for the stage of the disease.

Other markers of possible interference in immune tolerance is the increased rate of certain tumours. The prevalence of hepatocellular (Melia et al., 1984; Nakanuma et al., 1990), and breast carcinoma (Wolke et al., 1984; Goudie et al., 1985), are increased compared with a control population.

Immunological abnormalities

Humoral

Numerous abnormalities of the humoral immune system have been described in patients with PBC, including high levels of immune complexes (Sandilands et al., 1980), elevated serum IgM and IgG (Riggione, Stokes & Thompson, 1983; Mitchison et al., 1986; Zhang et al., 1992), complement activation (Lindgren, Laurell & Eriksson, 1984), elevated serum levels of

β2-microglobulin (Nyberg, Lööf & Hällgren, 1985) and the presence of increased levels of auto-antibodies in the serum.

Alterations in complement metabolism have been reported in patients with PBC, consisting of increased fractional catabolism of C1q. However, these were not specific to PBC, since they occurred also in hepatitis B viral liver disease (Potter *et al.*, 1980). Circulating immune complexes are present in patients with PBC (Sandilands *et al.*, 1980), but their exact composition remains unclear, although some contain AMA.

Auto-antibodies

Anti-mitochondrial antibodies

Anti-mitochondrial antibodies were first described by Walker *et al.* (1965) using immunofluorescence and subsequently by Berg using complement fixation (Berg, Doniach & Roitt, 1967). Several types of AMA have been described, some of which are specific for PBC. These AMA subtypes (M1–M9) differ in their immunofluorescence pattern on tissue sections. Further studies demonstrated complement fixation by serum from PBC patients with a trypsin-sensitive antigen of the inner mitochondrial membrane. The antigen co-purified with the F1 complex of the H^+-ATPase, but further studies using immunoblotting techniques failed to demonstrate reactivity of anti-M2 antibodies with any of the major subunits of F1-ATPase.

Other studies have identified anti-M2 exclusively in sera from patients with PBC (Berg *et al.*, 1982; Berg, Klein & Lindenborn-Fotinos, 1985). Four of the AMAs, anti-M2, -M4, -M8 and -M9 are associated with PBC. Anti M4 was found preferentially in patients with mixed histological features of PBC and auto-immune chronic active hepatitis (Berg *et al.*, 1980; Klöppel, Kirchhof & Berg, 1982). The others, anti-M1, -M3, -M5, -M6 and -M7 are mainly associated with non-hepatic disorders.

An association between urinary tract infection (UTI) and PBC has been reported (Burroughs *et al.*, 1984), with an increased incidence of UTI in patients with PBC compared with age and sex matched controls with other forms of chronic liver disease. There is also a high incidence of the rough-form mutants of *Escherichia coli* in the urine of patients with PBC. In a subsequent study (Butler *et al.*, 1993), patients with recurrent UTI, but no history of liver or other auto-immune disease were studied, for the presence of rough mutants and anti-mitochondrial antibody. Of patients with recurrent UTI receiving prophylactic antibiotics, 69% were found to have AMA of the specific M2 subtype. It was postulated that an abnormal immunological response to rough mutant bacteria in susceptible individuals may predispose to PBC.

Other auto-antibodies

There are several auto-antibodies directed at non-mitochondrial antigens in PBC. Immunofluorescence detects increased levels above background for several non-specific antigens, but in particular reactivity to nuclear antigens stands out (Mackay & Gershwin, 1989; Wesierska-Gadek et al., 1989; Goldenstein et al., 1989; Powell, Scroeter & Dickson, 1987). The strongest reaction is directed to the centromeric antigen, with the same specificity as seen in scleroderma, either with or without the other components of the CREST syndrome. Of patients with PBC 12% have anti-centromere antibodies and a proportion have clinically evident scleroderma. A cDNA for centromeric antigen has been cloned and sequenced. No homologies with cDNAs for M2 antigens are evident (Earnshaw et al., 1987). In addition, 40–50% of PBC sera react by immunofluorescence with other nuclear antigens with speckled patterns, but the nuclear antigens involved are not determined.

Identification of the AMA antigen

In 1987 cloning studies screening a rat liver complementary DNA (cDNA) library with sera from patients with PBC identified a cDNA fragment reactive with the 70 kD M2 auto-antigen in PBC (Gershwin et al., 1987). This led to the identification of the three major M2 antigens as the E2 components (dihydrolipoamide acetyltransferases) of the three mitochondrial oxo-acid dehydrogenase multienzyme complexes; pyruvate dehydrogenase complex (PDC), 2-oxo-glutarate dehydrogenase complex (OGDC) and the branched chain 2-oxo-acid dehydrogenase complex (BCOADC) (Van de Water et al., 1988b; Coppel et al., 1988; Yeaman et al., 1988; Surh et al., 1989). A fourth antigen was then identified, which is designated component X. Although earlier studies suggested auto-antibodies to 2-OADs were largely restricted to IgM and IgG_3 subclasses (Riggione, Stokes & Thompson, 1983), more recent studies suggest a much broader distribution between immunoglobulin classes (Zhang et al., 1992). These antibodies have a potent inhibitory action in vitro on the catalytic function of the enzyme with which they react (Van de Water et al., 1988a).

The role of E2 in primary biliary cirrhosis

PBC is associated with relatively organ specific damage, yet E2 is present in all cells and the role of the anti-E2 antibody remains unexplained. A study identifying AMA on the surface of rat hepatocytes by immunofluorescence

with PBC serum (Ghadiminejad & Baum, 1987) was criticised on methodological grounds (Gerken et al., 1988). A recent study of frozen sections of
liver tissue and portal lymph nodes (Joplin et al., 1991) demonstrated a
distinctive distribution of E2 antigen in PBC subjects compared with healthy
or other liver disease controls. Proliferating bile ductules stained with very
high intensity in PBC (Joplin et al., 1991). The same group also demonstrated a membranous pattern of staining using anti-E2 antibody on cultured
human biliary epithelial cells (BECs) from livers with PBC and no staining
on BECs from healthy control livers processed in an identical manner
(Joplin et al., 1992).

Immunisation of BALB/c mice, rats, rhesus monkeys and rabbits with E2,
stimulated production of AMA in all species (Krams et al., 1989). These
were reactive with the functional site of dihydrolipoamide acetyltransferase.
However, no liver abnormalities developed.

In separate experiments, severe combined immunodeficient (SCID) mice
were injected intraperitoneally with peripheral blood lymphocytes from
patients with PBC (Krams, Dorshkind & Gershwin, 1989), with resultant
humoral changes in all cases, consisting of antibodies to PCD-E2. Histological examination of the livers of these mice revealed changes including portal
tract inflammation and damage to the bile duct morphology. Similar
changes were seen, however, in those mice inoculated with peripheral blood
lymphocytes from control patients without PBC.

Cellular immunity

The major components of the bile duct and periductal infiltrate consist of
$CD4^+$ and $CD8^+$ T lymphocytes. The most prevalent cell type is the $CD8^+$.
Some authors have suggested that the distribution of cells alters with the
stage of disease (Hoffmann et al., 1989), with an increased tendency to
$CD4^+$ in more advanced disease. This is not accepted by all (Hashimoto et
al., 1989), since no alteration in T cell sub-sets was observed between early
and late stage disease.

Ultrastructural studies have shown cytotoxic T cells ($Leu2a^+15$) intimately connected to biliary epithelium in PBC (Yamada et al., 1986). These
cells were often seen within epithelia, breaching the basement membrane.

In vitro studies have demonstrated deficient spontaneous cell-mediated
cytotoxicity (NK cell activity) of peripheral blood lymphocytes (PBLs) to
^{51}chromium labelled Chang K562 target cells, in patients with PBC compared with normal control PBLs, but normal antibody-dependent cytotoxicity (K cell activity) (James & James, 1985). Natural killer activity of
normal lymphocytes was not inhibited by serum or lymphocytes from
patients with PBC. The proportion of NK cells within the PBL population in

PBC patients was normal as assessed by staining reactions with monoclonal antibodies to Leu7 and Leu11.

A more recent study, however, has shown normal NK activity in PBC patients (Muller & Zielinski, 1987), whereas spontaneous NK activity of peripheral blood mononuclear cells (PBMCs) has been shown to be depressed in patients with cirrhosis of other causes (Hirofuji et al., 1987). Cloning studies of T lymphocytes infiltrating liver tissue in PBC, show selection of CD8$^+$ cytotoxic cells in all (Meuer et al., 1988) or some patients (Hoffmann et al., 1989). Such cloning studies provide a spectrum of clones similar to those found within the liver tissue of origin (Saidman et al., 1990). NK and K cell activity is diminished or absent in these clones, although lectin-dependent cell-mediated cytotoxicity (LDCC) is preserved or elevated in CD8$^+$ cells, indicating normal or heightened cytotoxicity of these cells. These studies indicate that not only are CD8$^+$ cytotoxic T lymphocytes an important component of cells infiltrating liver tissue in PBC, but these cells retain their cytotoxicity to cellular targets in vitro. In contrast, not only are NK cells a minor constituent of infiltrating cells in PBC, but their in vitro functional activity is diminished.

Cell adhesion is an important step in many leucocyte-mediated actions and is subserved by specific cell surface molecules. Intercellular adhesion molecule-1 (ICAM-1) binds to members of the LFA-1/MAC-1 family of molecules on leucocytes. Increased expression of ICAM-1 has been demonstrated in the serum of patients with PBC and by immunohistochemical means on the intrahepatic bile ducts of such individuals (Adams et al., 1991; Volpes, Van den Oord & Desmet, 1990), it is not, however, specific to PBC.

Epithelial HLA expression

In normal liver tissue, HLA class I antigens are seen on the surface of bile duct epithelium and sinusoidal cells but not on hepatocytes. In PBC, expression of HLA class I antigens is increased on bile ducts (Ballardini et al., 1984; Van den Oord, Sciot & Desmet, 1986), and focal expression is seen on hepatocytes, mainly in periportal areas, especially those associated with piecemeal necrosis.

Bile duct epithelium of normal liver does not express HLA class II antigens, however, HLA DR was expressed on septal and interlobular bile duct epithelium in 8 of 10 PBC biopsies studied (Ballardini et al., 1984). It was postulated that aberrant expression of HLA DR antigens on bile duct epithelium, may result in presentation of self antigen to sensitised T lymphocytes and promote autorecognition, possibly in response to environmental triggers. Aberrant expression of HLA class II on biliary epithelium, however is not specific to PBC. It also occurs in biliary obstruction, allograft rejection, autoimmune chronic active hepatitis and cirrhosis of viral aetiology.

The factors controlling expression of HLA products on biliary epithelium in PBC remain unclear. *In vitro* studies of vascular endothelial cells, fibroblasts and cell lines have shown elevated mRNA levels and increased surface expression of HLA molecules following treatment with pro-inflammatory cytokines, such as tumour necrosis factor alpha, but again, such occurrences are not unique to primary biliary cirrhosis.

Specific medical therapy and disease modifying drugs

Many therapeutic trials have been performed in primary biliary cirrhosis. So far, convincing evidence of therapeutic benefit is sparse. No drug has been shown to produce the ultimate goal of consistently achieving symptomatic, biochemical and histological remission.

Historically there have been recurrent difficulties in performing clinical trials in PBC, that have detracted from published results. These primarily result from the difficulty in obtaining adequate numbers for trials particularly for those in smaller units. For tertiary or quaternary referral centres there is a risk of introducing bias, since their patient population in likely to have more advanced disease and some of these patients may be entered onto a transplant programme, before drug therapy is fully evaluated.

Corticosteroids

Therapy with corticosteroids has been associated with benefit upon symptoms, serum liver enzymes, serum procollagen III peptide, serum IgG and liver histology in a 1 year double-blind pilot study comparing prednisolone (30 mg/day induction, 10 mg/day maintenance) with placebo (Mitchison *et al.*, 1989). The greatest benefit was seen amongst non-cirrhotic patients, including beneficial effect upon serum biochemistry, immunological markers and histological progression. Unfortunately, bone loss as measured by femoral photon absorption and trabecular biopsy was seen to progress at approximately twice the rate in the treated group, compared with those taking placebo, although this adverse effect was less clear at the three-year review stage (Mitchison *et al.*, 1992).

Most clinicians believe that corticosteroids should not be given alone as specific treatment for PBC, since acceleration of osteoporosis outweighs potential benefit of the drug therapy. Results of further trials are awaited. It will be of particular interest to see if adverse effects on bone density can be mitigated by other concurrent medication, such as diphosphonates.

Azathioprine

Prospective controlled trials of azathioprine in PBC have failed to demonstrate major improvement in serum liver function tests, serial liver biopsies or survival (Christensen *et al.*, 1985; Crowe *et al.*, 1980; Heathcote, Ross & Sherlock, 1976). In a prospective, double-blind placebo controlled trial (Christensen *et al.*, 1985), an improvement in survival was seen following adjustment for differences in severity of disease between treatment and placebo groups. One-third of patients, however, were lost to follow-up or withdrawn from therapy because of side effects.

Azathioprine has not become an established treatment for PBC.

D-Penicillamine

A series of trials of D-penicillamine therapy in PBC have been reported. D-penicillamine has three potential modes of action. It has the potential to act via chelation of copper, an immunomodulatory action or anti-fibrogenic effects (Epstein *et al.*, 1979, 1981). Statistically significant improvement have been reported in serum transaminases, serum immunoglobulin levels and hepatic copper. Improvement in the degree of portal tract inflammation was observed, but not in fibrosis. Claims that treatment with D-penicillamine improved survival (Epstein *et al.*, 1979, 1981) were withdrawn following later studies (Epstein *et al.*, 1984) and a formal review of statistical methods and earlier trial design (Cook & Pocock, 1987). Several controlled trials of D-penicillamine have failed to show benefit in symptoms related to PBC, liver biochemistry, histological progression or survival, in doses ranging from 250–1000 mg/day (Epstein *et al.*, 1984; Matloff *et al.*, 1982; James, 1985; Dickson *et al.*, 1985; Neuberger *et al.*, 1985; Bodenheimer *et al.*, 1985).

Troublesome side-effects are frequent and include dyspepsia, nausea, vomiting, loss of taste, skin reactions and proteinuria. A broad spectrum of haematological side-effects may present including thrombocytopenia, neutropenia, agranulocytosis and aplastic anaemia. Autoimmune disorders may develop, including myasthenia gravis, polymyositis, systemic lupus erythematosus and a Goodpasture-like syndrome (Gollan *et al.*, 1976; Matloff & Kaplan, 1980). Side-effects necessitating withdrawal were seen in 46% (Bodenheimer *et al.*, 1985), 22% (Dickson *et al.*, 1985), and 36% (Neuberger *et al.*, 1985) of patients taking the active agent.

Cyclosporin

Cyclosporin has a marked effect on suppressor inducer T lymphocytes in PBC (Routhier *et al.*, 1980). Improvements in liver enzymes have also been reported, but nephrotoxic side-effects limit its use (Routhier *et al.*, 1980; Wiesner *et al.*, 1987; Minuk *et al.*, 1987). A placebo-controlled trial of low dose cyclosporin (4 mg/kg/day) in patients with pre-cirrhotic disease showed improvement in symptoms, biochemical tests, AMA titre and retardation in progression of histological features (Wiesner *et al.*, 1990). However, nephrotic side-effects were seen in 63% and elevated blood pressure in 47% of patients. A more recent report of European experience in a large multi-centre, placebo controlled trial of cyclosporin (Lombard *et al.*, 1993) suggests benefit with respect to liver-related mortality and biochemical indices of disease progression. There was, however, no statistical benefit in survival overall and nephrotoxicity was a major adverse effect. Long-term risks of malignant lymphoproliferative disease is another potential cause of concern.

Chlorambucil

A randomised, placebo controlled study of chlorambucil (0.5–4 mg/day) therapy in 24 patients with PBC provided serological evidence of improvement in biochemical markers of disease. Liver biopsy showed a reduction of inflammation after 2 years, but not in fibrosis nor histological stage of disease.

The study was discontinued after 2 years because of bone marrow toxicity (Hoofnagle *et al.*, 1986).

Colchicine

Early studies showed improvements in biochemical tests, but not in liver histology or hepatic copper content (Bodenheimer, Schaffner & Pezzulo, 1988; Kaplan *et al.*, 1986). Three prospective double blind studies have shown improvements in serum liver enzymes (Bodenheimer, Schaffner & Pezzulo, 1988; Kaplan *et al.*, 1986; Warnes *et al.*, 1987), and one trial showed improved liver-related mortality (Kaplan *et al.*, 1986). No improvement in histological progression or symptomatology was seen in any of the three prospective trials. The Kaplan study (Neuberger *et al.*, 1985) failed to include two non-hepatic deaths in their survival analysis, which would have resulted in no survival benefit in those receiving active treatment.

The safety profile of the drug is favourable. Treatment is well tolerated, except for the occasional patient with mild diarrhoea. There is a remote risk of serious bone marrow suppression, but in general the drug is well suited to longterm trials in PBC.

Methotrexate and other anti-fibrotics

One study, of a small series of patients, showed temporary improvement in symptoms and serum biochemical tests, which reverted following discontinuation of therapy (Kaplan, 1989). Concerns over its toxicity profile, due to bone marrow suppression and potential hepatotoxicity, were raised.

A trial of the anti-fibrotic agent malotilate, showed no benefit.

Ursodeoxycholic acid

The initial rationale for therapy with ursodeoxycholic acid (UDCA), was in view of its favourable influence upon the bile acid pool and resultant choleresis. Replacement of the relatively cytotoxic bile acid chenodeoxycholic acid, with the relatively cytoprotective ursodeoxycholic acid, might therefore be beneficial.

Early uncontrolled trials confirmed these hypotheses. Serum liver enzymes improved in PBC patients treated with UDCA (Poupon et al., 1987; Kaplan, 1987). Biochemical improvement was most marked at one year, but deteriorated thereafter. More recent uncontrolled (Matsuzaki et al., 1990; Osuga et al., 1989) and controlled (Leuschner et al., 1989; Poupon et al., 1990) studies have confirmed improvement of liver enzymes, but evidence of sustained symptomatic benefit is lacking.

Histological improvement was found in open uncontrolled studies with long-term use of UDCA (Matsuzaki et al., 1990; Osuga et al., 1989; Poupon et al., 1989), but results of controlled double-blind studies have either been unconvincing (Leuschner et al., 1989), or negative at one year (Myszor et al., 1990) or 2 years (Hadziyannis, Hadziyannis & Makris, 1989). The results of long-term studies are awaited.

Therapy with UDCA may confer benefit via means other than choleresis, since it also has immunomodulatory properties. Firstly, it down-regulates aberrant class I (Poupon et al., 1991) and class II (Chapman, Dooley & Fleming, 1993) HLA expression in cholestatic liver disease. Yoshikawa et al. (1992) investigated the effects of UDCA on immunoglobulin and cytokine production. They reported in vitro studies, in which UDCA inhibited IL-2, IL-4 and gamma interferon production, in addition to suppressing production of IgM, IgG and IgA. It was postulated that the beneficial influence of UDCA therapy in PBC, may be partly mediated by immunosuppression.

Liver transplantation for PBC

Orthotopic liver transplantation has become an established treatment. The major acceptance of this treatment, followed the 1983 National Consensus

Meeting at the National Institute of Health, since they declared liver transplantation to be no longer considered experimental, but an appropriate therapeutic procedure for a variety of chronic endstage liver diseases (NIH Consensus Meeting, 1983).

Transplantation for PBC in carefully selected patients is associated with substantially better survival than with conservative management (Adler et al., 1988; Gordon et al., 1986; Neuberger et al., 1986). In one series of 161 patients followed up for a median of 25 months post liver transplantation, survival was 76% and 74% at one and two years respectively (Markus et al., 1989). This compared with 45% and 31% survival at one and two years without transplantation, as predicted by the Mayo model.

Initially, there is a slight excess in mortality associated with liver transplantation, as a result of early deaths. Causes of death following liver transplantation include intra-operative mortality, primary non-function of the allograft, massive haemorrhagic necrosis, hepatic artery thrombosis, infection and chronic rejection. The majority of deaths occur within the first 3 months of transplant. Benefit is most marked therefore, for those transplanted with poor prognostic indicators, who are assessed several years after the procedure.

Survival following transplantation for PBC has improved considerably in recent years. This has occurred for a wide variety of reasons, including surgical and anaesthetic technique, immunosuppressive agents, antibiotics and general experience. Many centres report 1 year survival for patients transplanted for PBC, in excess of 85%. The commonest indication for transplantation in PBC is end-stage disease, often suggested by a serum bilirubin in excess of 150 μmol/l. Occasionally, the disease process is relatively non-cholestatic, in which case hypoalbuminaemia, intractable ascites or chronic encephalopathy, may indicate the need for liver transplantation, despite a comparatively low serum bilirubin. In other patients, intractable variceal bleeding may be an indication, although other techniques may be preferred. Intractable pruritus and symptoms of poor quality of life are more subjective indications.

Patient selection is decided upon the balance of risks and benefits. Selection of those, with a very low operative risk, will result in patients with a reasonable life expectancy being subjected to the threat of premature death, as a result of the transplant. In such cases, however, quality of life may be extremely poor. Alternatively, undue delay may result in the disease entering its terminal stages and transplantation being considered when it is less likely to be successful.

Recurrent primary biliary cirrhosis post-liver transplant

Recurrence of PBC following liver transplantation was first reported by Neuberger et al. (1982). This has not been confirmed by all studies (Starzl et *al.*, 1982; Demetris *et al.*, 1988; Esquivel *et al.*, 1988; Fennell, Shikes & Vierling, 1983) and remains the subject of debate. In a prospective study of 153 patients receiving 175 liver grafts, there was immunological evidence consistent with ongoing primary biliary cirrhosis, in all patients transplanted for this indication (Buist *et al.*, 1989). Histological changes consistent with PBC, however, were seen in liver allografts from both the PBC and the non-PBC groups, with no significant differences.

Interpretation of post transplant biopsies is often complex. One problem is that histological evidence of recurrent PBC may be patchy and therefore missed in a single needle biopsy. Alternatively, biliary features which typify PBC may be mimicked by other processes following liver transplantation, such as chronic rejection in its biliary form, biliary obstruction, ascending cholangitis, hepatitis C and possible drug reactions. Some studies have examined liver biopsies from patients transplanted for conditions other than PBC, yet found them to have histological features consistent with PBC in the allograft (Portmann & Wright, 1987).

Immunological abnormalities usually persist following liver transplantation for PBC. The mitochondrial antibody is usually present in the serum, although the level of IgM often falls. A recent report suggested that histological features of recurrent PBC, were more likely to develop in those receiving FK506 as immunosuppressive therapy (Wong *et al.*, 1993).

Many transplant programmes are able to provide data on much larger series of patients, with longer periods of follow-up. The evidence in favour of recurrent disease occurring in a proportion of allografts appears extremely strong (Hubscher *et al.*, 1993). Perhaps it would be more surprising if liver transplantation did cure the disease?

Conclusion

Primary biliary cirrhosis remains a disease of unknown aetiology. Disease progression from an asymptomatic stage cannot be predicted accurately in any individual case and there is no known pharmacological cure. Despite numerous immunological associations and characterisation of highly specific autoantigens, the stimulus underlying such failure of immune tolerance is unknown.

PBC is considered by many to be an immune-mediated disease, but there are a number of discrepancies, including failure of convincing benefit in response to immunosuppressive therapy and a lack of characteristic HLA association.

Is primary biliary cirrhosis an auto-immune disease? Possibly.

References

Adams, D. H., Hübscher, S. G., Shaw, J. *et al*. (1991). Increased expression of intercellular adhesion molecule 1 on bile ducts in primary biliary cirrhosis and primary sclerosing cholangitis. *Hepatology*, **14**, 426–31.

Adler, M., Gavaler, J. S., Duquesnoy, R. *et al*. (1988). Relationship between the diagnosis, preoperative evaluation and prognosis after orthotopic liver transplantation. *Annals of Surgery*, **208**, 196–202.

Ahrens, E. H., Payne, M. A., Kunkel, H. G., Eisenmenger, W. J. & Blondheim, S. H. (1950). Primary biliary cirrhosis. *Medicine (Baltimore)*, **29**, 299–364.

Alarcón-Segovia, D., Díaz-Jouanen, E. & Fishbein, E. (1973). Features of Sjörgren syndrome in primary biliary cirrhosis. *Annals in Internal Medicine*, **79**, 31–6.

Anthony, P. P. & Scheuer, P. J. (eds.) (1987). *Pathology of the Liver*. 2nd edn. pp. 424–53. Edinburgh: Churchill Livingstone.

Balasubramaniam, K., Grambsch, P. M., Wiesner, R. H., Lindor, K. D. & Dickson, E. R. (1990). Diminished survival in asymptomatic primary biliary cirrhosis. A prospective study. *Gastroenterology*, **98**, 1567–71.

Ballardini, G., Mirakian, R., Bianchi, F. B., Pisi, E., Doniach, D. & Bottazzo, G. F. (1984). Aberrant expression of HLA-DR antigens on bile duct epithelium in primary biliary cirrhosis: relevance to pathogenesis. *Lancet*, **ii**, 1109–13.

Berg, P. A., Doniach, D. & Roitt, I. M. (1967). Mitochondrial antibodies in primary biliary cirrhosis. I: Localisation of the antigen to mitochondrial membranes. *Journal of Experimental Immunology*, **126**, 277–90.

Berg, P. A., Wiedmann, K. H., Sayers, T. J., Klöppel, G. & Linder, H. (1980). Serological classification of chronic cholestatic liver disease by the use of two different types of antimitochondrial antibodies. *Lancet*, **ii**, 1329–32.

Berg, P. A., Klein, R., Lindenborn-Fotinos, J. & Klöppel, G. (1982). ATPase associated antigen (M2): marker antigen for serological diagnosis of primary biliary cirrhosis. *Lancet*, **ii**, 1423–6.

Berg, P. A., Klein, R. & Lindenborn-Fotinos, J. (1985). ELISA techniques for the detection of antimitochondrial antibodies (Letter). *Hepatology*, **6**, 1244–5.

Beswick, D. R., Klatskin, G. & Boyer, J. L. (1985). Asymptomatic primary biliary cirrhosis long-term follow-up and natural history. *Gastroenterology*, **89**, 267–71.

Bodenheimer, H. C. Jr, Schaffner, F., Sternlieb, I., Klion, H. M., Vernace, S. & Pezzullo, J. A. (1985). A prospective clinical trial of D-penicillamine in the treatment of primary biliary cirrhosis. *Hepatology*, **5**, 1139–42.

Bodenheimer, H., Schaffner, F. & Pezzulo, J. (1980). Evaluation of colchicine therapy in primary biliary cirrhosis. *Gastroenterology*, **95**, 124–9.

Buist, L. J., Hübscher, S. G., Vickers, C., Michell, I., Neuberger, J. & McMaster, P. (1987). Does liver transplantation cure primary biliary cirrhosis? *Transplantation Proceedings*, **21**, 2402.

Burroughs, A. K., Rosenstein, I. J., Epstein, O., Hamilton-Miller, J. M. T., Brumfitt, W. & Sherlock, S. (1984). Bacteriuria and primary biliary cirrhosis. *Gut*, **25**, 133–7.

Butler, P., Valle, F., Hamilton-Miller, J. M. T., Brumfitt, W., Baum, H. & Burroughs, A. K. (1993). M2 mitochondrial antibodies and urinary rough mutant bacteria in patients with primary biliary cirrhosis and in patients with recurrent bacteriuria. *Journal of Hepatology*, **17**, 408–14.

Chapman, R. W., Dooley, J. S. & Fleming, K. A. (1993). Aberrant HLA-DR antigen expression by bile duct epithelium in primary sclerosing cholangitisis down-regulated by ursodeoxycholic acid (Abstract). *Gastroenterology*, A943.

Christensen, E., Crowe, J., Doniach, D. *et al.* (1980). Clinical pattern and course of disease in primary biliary cirrhosis based on an analysis of 236 patients. *Gastroenterology*, **78**, 236–46.

Christensen, E., Neuberger, J., Crowe, J. *et al.* (1985). Beneficial effect of azathioprine and prediction of prognosis in primary biliary cirrhosis: final results of an international trial. *Gastroenterology*, **89**, 1084–91.

Clarke, A. K., Galbraith, R. M., Hamilton, E. B. D. & Williams, R. (1978). Rheumatic disorders in primary biliary cirrhosis. *Annals of Rheumatic Diseases*, **37**, 42–7.

Cook, D. G. & Pocock, S. J. (1987). Consultancy in a medical school, illustrated by a clinical trial for treatment of primary biliary cirrhosis. In *The Statistical Consultant in Action*. ed. D. J. Hand & B. S. Everitt. pp. 58–71. Cambridge University Press.

Coppel, R. L., McNeilage, I. J., Smith, C. D. *et al.* (1988). Primary structure of the human M2 mitochondrial autoantigen in primary biliary cirrhosis: dihydrolipoamide acetyltransferase. *Proceedings of the National Academy of Sciences, USA*, **85**, 7317–21.

Crowe, J. P., Christensen, E., Butler, J. *et al.* (1980). Primary biliary cirrhosis: the prevalence of hypothyroidism and its relationship to thyroid autoantibodies and sicca syndrome. *Gastroenterology*, **78**, 1437–41.

Crowe, J. P., Molloy, M. G., Wells, I. *et al.* (1980). Increased Cl_q binding and arthritis in primary biliary cirrhosis. *Gut*, **21**, 418–22.

Crowe, J., Christensen, E., Smith, M. *et al.* (1980). Azathioprine in primary biliary cirrhosis: a preliminary report of an international trial. *Gastroenterology*, **78**, 1005–10.

Culp, K. S., Fleming, C. R., Duffy, J., Baldus, W. P. & Dickson, E. R. (1982). Autoimmune associations in primary biliary cirrhosis. *Mayo Clinical Proceedings*, **57**, 365–70.

Demetris, A. J., Markus, B. H., Esquivel, C. *et al.* (1988). Pathologic analysis of liver transplantation for primary biliary cirrhosis. *Hepatology*, **8**, 939–47.

Dickson, E. R., Fleming, T. R., Wiesner, R. H. *et al.* (1985). Trial of penicillamine in advanced primary biliary cirrhosis. *New England Journal of Medicine*, **312**, 1011–15.

Dickson, E. R., Grambsch, P. M., Fleming, T. R., Fisher, L. D. & Langworthy, A. (1989). Prognosis in primary biliary cirrhosis: model for decision making. *Hepatology*, **10**, 1–7.

Earnshaw, W. C., Machlin, P. S., Bordwell, B. J., Rothfield, N. F. & Cleveland, D. N. (1987). Analysis of anticentromere autoantibodies using cloned autoantigen CENP-B. *Proceedings of the National Academy of Sciences, USA*, **84**, 4979–83.

Elta, G. H., Sepersky, R. A., Goldberg, M. J. *et al.* (1983). Increased incidence of hypothyroidism in primary biliary cirrhosis. *Digest Disease Science*, **28**, 971–5.

Epstein, O., De Villiers, D., Jain, S., Potter, B. J., Thomas, H. C. & Sherlock, S. (1979). Reduction of immune complexes and immunoglobulins induced by D-penicillamine in primary biliary cirrhosis. *New England Journal of Medicine*, **300**, 274–8.

Epstein, O., Jain, S., Lee, R. G., Cook, D. G., Boss, A. M. & Scheuer, P. J. (1981). D-penicillamine treatment improves survival in primary biliary cirrhosis. *Lancet*, **i**, 1275–7.

Epstein, O., Cook, D. G., Jain, S., McIntyre, N. & Sherlock, S. (1984). D-penicillamine and clinical trials in primary biliary cirrhosis (Abstract). *Hepatology*, **4**, 1032.

Eriksson, S. & Lindgren, S. (1984). The prevalence and clinical spectrum of primary biliary cirrhosis in a defined population. *Scandinavian Journal of Gastroenterology*, **19**, 971–6.

Esquivel, C. O., Van Thiel, D. H., Demetris, A. J. *et al.* (1988). Transplantation for primary biliary cirrhosis. *Gastroenterology*, **94**, 1207–16.

Fennell, R. H., Shikes, R. H. & Vierling, J. M. (1983). Relationship of pre-transplant hepatobiliary disease to bile duct damage occurring in the liver allograft. *Hepatology*, **3**, 84–9.

Fox, R. A., Scheuer, P. J. & Sherlock, S. (1973). Asymptomatic primary biliary cirrhosis. *Gut*, **14**, 444–7.

Gerken, G., Manns, M., Ramadori, G., & Meyer zum Büschenfelde, K.-H. To the editor. (1988). *Hepatology*, **8**, 705–6.

Gershwin, M. E., Mackay, I. R., Sturgess, A. & Coppell, R. L. (1987). Identification and specificity of a cDNA encoding the 70 kD mitochondrial antigen recognized in primary biliary cirrhosis. *Journal of Immunology*, **138**, 3525–31.

Ghadiminejad, I. & Baum, H. (1987). Evidence for the cell-surface localization of antibody cross-reacting with the 'Mitochondrial antibodies' of primary biliary cirrhosis. *Hepatology*, **7**, 743–9.

Giovaninni, A., Ballardini, G., Amatetti, S., Bonazzoli, P. & Bianchi, F. B. (1985). Patterns of lachrymal dysfunction in primary biliary cirrhosis. *British Journal of Ophthalmology*, **69**, 832–5.

Goldenstein, C., Rabson, A. R., Kaplan, M. M. & Canoso, J. J. (1989). Arthralgias as a presenting manifestation of primary biliary cirrhosis. *Journal of Rheumatology*, **16**, 681–4.

Gollan, J. L., Hussein, S., Hoffbrand, A. V. & Sherlock, S. (1976). Red cell aplasia following prolonged D-penicillamine therapy. *Journal of Clinical Pathology*, **29**, 135–9.

Gordon, R. D., Shaw, B. W. Jr, Iwatsuki, S., Esquivel, C. O. & Starzl, T. E. (1986). Indications for liver transplantation in the cyclosporine era. *Surgical Clinics of America*, **66**, 541–56.

Gores, G. J., Moore, S. B., Fisher, L. D., Powell, F. C. & Dickson, E. R. (1987). Primary biliary cirrhosis: association with class II major histocompatibility complex antigens. *Hepatology*, **7**, 889–92.

Goudie, B. M., Burt, A. D., Boyle, P. *et al.* (1985). Breast cancer in women with primary biliary cirrhosis. *British Medical Journal*, **291**, 1597–8.

Goudie, B. M., MacFarlane, G., Boyle, P. *et al.* (1987). Epidemiology of antimitochondrial antibody seropositivity and primary biliary cirrhosis in the West of Scotland (Abstract). *Gut*, **28**, A1346.

Grambsch, P. M., Dickson, E. R., Kaplan, M., LeSage, G., Fleming, T. R. & Langworthy, A. L. (1989). Extramural cross-validation of the Mayo primary biliary cirrhosis survival model establishes its generalizability. *Hepatology*, **10**, 846–50.

Hadziyannis, S. J., Hadziyannis, E. S. & Makris, A. (1987). A randomised controlled trial of ursodeoxycholic acid (UDCA) in primary biliary cirrhosis (PBC) (Abstract). *Hepatology*, **10**, 580.

Hamlyn, A. M., Adams, D. & Sherlock, S. (1980). Primary or secondary sicca complex? Investigation in primary biliary cirrhosis by histocompatibility. *British Medical Journal*, **281**, 425–6.

Hamlyn, A. N., Macklon, A. F. & James, O. (1985). Primary biliary cirrhosis: geographical clustering and symptomatic onset seasonality. *Gut*, **24**, 940–5.

Hanik, L. & Eriksson, S. (1977). Presymptomatic primary biliary cirrhosis. *Acta Medica Scandinavica*, **202**, 277–81.

Hashimoto, E., Lindor, K. D., Ludwig, J. *et al.* (1989). Characterization of hepatic inflammatory-cell surface antigens in primary biliary cirrhosis (PBC), primary sclerosing cholangitis (PSC) and chronic active hepatitis (CAH). (Abstract). *Hepatology*, **12**, 108.

Heathcote, J., Ross, A. & Sherlock, S. (1976). A prospective controlled trial of azathioprine in primary biliary cirrhosis. *Gastroenterology*, **70**, 656–60.

Hirofuji, H., Kakumu, S., Fuji, A., Ohtani, A., Murase, K. & Tahara, H. (1987). Natural killer and activated killer activities in chronic liver disease and hepatocellular carcinoma: evidence for a decreased lymphokine-induced activity in effector cells. *Clinical and Experimental Immunology*, **68**, 348–56.

Hoffmann, R. M., Pape, G. E., Spengler, U. *et al.* (1989). Clonal analysis of liver-derived T cells of patients with primary biliary cirrhosis. *Clinical and Experimental Immunology*, **76**, 210–5.

Hoofnagle, J. H., David, G. L., Schafer, D. F. *et al.* (1986). Randomized trial of chlorambucil for primary biliary cirrhosis. *Gastroenterology*, **91**, 1327–34.

Hübscher, S. G. & Harrison, R. F. (1989). Portal lymphadenopathy associated with lipofuscin in chronic cholestatic liver disease. *Journal of Clinical Pathology*, **42**, 1160–5.

Hübscher, S. G., Elias, E., Buckels, J. A. C., Mayer, A. D., McMaster, P. & Neuberger, J. M. (1993). Primary biliary cirrhosis: Histological evidence of disease recurrence after liver transplantation. *Journal of Hepatology*, (in press),

James, O. F. W. (1985). D-penicillamine for primary biliary cirrhosis. *Gut*, **26**, 109–13.

James, S. P. & James, E. A. (1985). Abnormal natural killer cytotoxicity in primary biliary cirrhosis: evidence for a functional deficiency of cytolytic effector cells. *Gastroenterology*, **89**, 165–71.

James, O., Macklon, A. F. & Watson, A. J. (1981). Primary biliary cirrhosis – a revised clinical spectrum. *Lancet*, **i**, 1278–81.

Joplin, R., Lindsay, J. G., Hübscher, S. G. *et al.* (1991). Distribution of dihydrolipoamide acetyltransferase (E2) in liver and portal lymph nodes of patients with primary biliary cirrhosis: an immunohistochemical study. *Hepatology*, **14**, 442–7.

Joplin, R., Lindsay, J. G., Johnson, G. D., Strain, A. & Neuberger, J. (1992). Membrane dihydrolipoamide acetyltransferase (E2) on human biliary epithelial cells in primary biliary cirrhosis. *Lancet*, **339**, 93–4.

Kapelman, B. & Schaffner, F. (1981). The natural history of primary biliary cirrhosis. *Seminars in Liver Diseases*, **1**, 273–81.

Kaplan, M. M. (1987). Primary biliary cirrhosis. *New England Journal of Medicine*, **316**, 521–8.

Kaplan, M. M. (1989). Medical treatment of primary biliary cirrhosis. *Seminars in Liver Diseases*, **29**, 138–43.

Kaplan, M. M., Alling, D. W., Wolfe, H. J. *et al.* (1986). A prospective trial of colchicine for primary biliary cirrhosis. *New England Journal of Medicine*, **315**, 1448–54.

Klöppel, G., Kirchhof, M. & Berg, P. A. (1982). Natural course of PBC. I. A morphological, clinical and serological analysis of 103 cases. *Lancet*, **2**, 141–51.

Krams, S. M., Dorshkind, K. & Gershwin, M. E. (1989). Generation of biliary lesions after transfer of human lymphocytes into severe combined immunodeficient (SCID) mice. *Journal of Experimental Medicine*, **170**, 1919–30.

Krams, S. M., Surh, C. D., Coppel, R. L., Ansari, A., Ruebner, B. & Gershwin, M. E. (1989). Immunization of experimental animals with dihydrolipoamide acetyltransferase, as a purified recombinant polypeptide, generates mitochondrial antibodies but not primary biliary cirrhosis. *Hepatology*, **9**, 411–16.

Lee, R. G., Epstein, O., Jauregui, H., Sherlock, S. & Scheuer, P. J. (1981). Granulomas in primary biliary cirrhosis: a prognostic feature. *Gastroenterology*, **81**, 983–6.

Leuschner, U., Fischer, H., Kurtz, W. *et al.* (1989). Ursodeoxycholic acid in primary biliary cirrhosis: Results of a controlled double-blind trial. *Gastroenterology*, **97**, 1268–74.

Lindgren, S., Laurell, A. B. & Eriksson, S. (1984). Complement components and activation in primary biliary cirrhosis. *Hepatology*, **4**, 9–14.

Logan, R. F. A., Ferguson, A., Finlayson, N. D. C. & Weir, D. G. (1978). Primary biliary cirrhosis and coeliac disease: an association? *Lancet*, **i**, 230–3.

Lombard, M., Portmann, B., Neuberger, J. *et al.* (1993). Cyclosporin A treatment in primary biliary cirrhosis: results of a long-term placebo controlled trial. *Gastroenterology*, **104**, 519–26.

Long, R. G., Scheuer, P. J. & Sherlock, S. (1977). Presentation and course of asymptomatic primary biliary cirrhosis. *Gastroenterology*, **72**, 1204–7.

Mackay, I. R. & Gershwin, M. E. (1989). Primary biliary cirrhosis: Current knowledge, perspectives, and future directions. *Seminars in Liver Diseases*, **9**, 149–57.

MacSween, R. N. M. (1986). Primary biliary cirrhosis. In *Liver Pathology*. ed. R. L. Peters & J. R. Craig, pp. 177–91. New York: Churchill Livingstone.

Manns, M. P., Bremm, A., Schneider, P. M. *et al.* (1991). DRw8 and complement C4 deficiency as risk factors in primary biliary cirrhosis. *Gastroenterology*, **101**, 1367–73.

Markus, B. H., Dickson, E. R., Grambsch, P. M. *et al.* (1989). Efficiency of transplantation in patients with primary biliary cirrhosis. *New England Journal of Medicine*, **320**, 1709–13.

Matloff, D. S. & Kaplan, M. M. (1980). D-penicillamine-induced Goodpasture's-like syndrome in primary biliary cirrhosis – successful treatment with plasmaphoresis and immunosuppressives. *Gastroenterology*, **78**, 1046–9.

Matloff, D. S., Alpert, E., Resnick, R. H. & Kaplan, M. M. (1982). A prospective trial of D-penicillamine in primary biliary cirrhosis. *New England Journal of Medicine*, **306**, 319–26.

Matsuzaki, Y., Tanaka, N., Osuga, T. *et al.* (1990). Improvement of biliary enzyme levels and itching as a result of long-term administration of ursodeoxycholic acid in primary biliary cirrhosis. *American Journal of Gastroenterology*, **85**, 15–23.

Melia, W. M., Johnson, P. J., Neuberger, J., Zaman, S., Portmann, B. C. & Williams, R. (1984). Hepatocellular carcinoma in primary biliary cirrhosis: detection by alpha-feto protein. *Gastroenterology*, **87**, 660–3.

Meuer, S. C., Moebius, U., Manns, M. M. *et al.* (1988). Clonal analysis of human T lymphocytes infiltrating the liver in chronic active hepatitis B and primary biliary cirrhosis. *European Journal of Immunology*, **18**, 1447–52.

Minuk, G., Bohme, C., Burgess, E. *et al.* (1987). A prospective, double-blind, randomized, controlled trial of cyclosporine A in primary biliary cirrhosis. (Abstract) *Hepatology*, **7**, 1119.

Mitchison, H. C., Bassendine, M. F., Hendrick, A. *et al.* (1986). Positive antimitochondrial antibody but normal alkaline phosphate: is this primary biliary cirrhosis? *Hepatology*, **6**, 1279–84.

Mitchison, H. C., Bassendine, M. F., Malcolm, A. J., Watson, A. J., Record, C. O. & James, O. F. W. (1989). A pilot, double-blind, controlled 1-year trial of prednisolone treatment in primary cirrhosis: hepatic improvement but greater bone loss. *Hepatology*, **10**, 420–9.

Mitchison, H. C., Lucey, M. R., Kelly, P. J., Neuberger, J. M., Williams, R. & James, O. F. W. (1990). Symptom development and prognosis in primary biliary cirrhosis: a study in two centres. *Gastroenterology*, **99**, 778–84.

Mitchison, H. C., Palmer, J. M., Bassendine, M. F., Watson, A. J., Record, C. O. & James, O. F. W. (1992). A controlled trial of prednisolone treatment in primary biliary cirrhosis: three year results. *Journal of Hepatology*, **15**, 336–44.

Miyamori, H., Kato, Y., Koboyashi, K. & Hattoi, N. (1983). HLA antigens in primary biliary cirrhosis and autoimmune chronic active hepatitis. *Digestion*, **26**, 211–17.

Myszor, M., Turner, I., Mitchison, H., Bennett, M., Burt, A. D. & James, O. F. W. (1990). No symptomatic or histological benefit from ursodeoxycholic acid treatment in PBC after 1 year controlled pilot study. (Abstract). *Hepatology*, **12**, 415.

Muller, C. & Zielinski, C. C. (1987). Spontaneous and interferon-induced activity of natural killer cells in patients with liver cirrhosis and chronic active hepatitis. *Acta Medica Australia*, **14**, 115–18.

Nakanuma, Y., Terada, T., Doishita, K. & Miwa, A. (1990). Hepatocellular carcinoma in primary biliary cirrhosis: an autopsy study. *Hepatology*, **11**, 1010–16.

National Institutes of Health Consensus Development Conference Statement: Liver transplantation – June 20–23. (1983). *Hepatology*, **4**, 107S–10S.

Neuberger, J., Portmann, B., MacDougall, B. R. D., Calne, R. Y & Williams, R. (1982). Recurrence of primary biliary cirrhosis after liver transplantation. *New England Journal of Medicine*, **306**, 1–4.

Neuberger, J., Christensen, E., Portmann, B. *et al.* (1985). Double blind controlled trial of D-penicillamine in patients with primary biliary cirrhosis. *Gut*, **26**, 114–19.

Neuberger, J., Altman, D. G., Christensen, E., Tygstrup, N. & Williams, R. (1986). Use of a prognostic index in evaluation of liver transplantation for primary biliary cirrhosis. *Transplantation*, **41**, 713–16.

Nyberg, A., Lööf, L. & Hällgren, R. (1985). Serum β_2-microglobulin levels in primary biliary cirrhosis. *Hepatology*, **5**, 282–5.

Osuga, T., Tanaka, N., Matsuzaki, Y. & Aikawa, T. (1989). Effect of ursodeoxycholic acid in chronic hepatitis and primary biliary cirrhosis. *Digest Disease Science*, **34**, 49S–51S.

Parés, A., Rimola, A., Bruguera, M., Mas, E. & Rodes, J. (1980). Renal tubular acidosis in primary biliary cirrhosis. *Gastroenterology*, **78**, 681–6.

Portmann, B. & MacSween, R. N. M. (1987). Diseases of the intrahepatic bile ducts. In *Pathology of the Liver* ed. R. N. M. MacSween, P. P. Anthony & P. J. Scheuer, 2nd edn. pp. 424–53. Edinburgh: Churchill-Livingstone.

Portmann, B. & Wight, D. G. D. (1987). Pathology of liver transplantation. In *Liver Transplantation,* 2nd edn. ed. R. Calne, pp. 437–70. Orlando, Fl: Grune & Stratton.

Portmann, B., Popper, H., Neuberger, J. & Williams, R. (1985). Sequential and diagnostic features in primary biliary cirrhosis, based on serial histologic study in 209 patients. *Gastroenterology*, **88**, 1777–90.

Potter, B. J., Elias, E., Thomas, H. C. & Sherlock, S. (1980). Complement metabolism in chronic liver disease: catabolism of C1q in chronic active liver disease and primary biliary cirrhosis. *Gastroenterology*, **78**, 1034–40.

Poupon, R., Chrétien, Y., Poupon, R. E., Ballet, F., Calmus, Y. & Darnis, F. (1987). Is ursodeoxycholic acid an effective treatment for primary biliary cirrhosis? *Lancet*, **i**, 834–6.

Poupon, R., Balkau, B., Legendre, C., Lévy, V. G. Chrétien, Y. & Poupon, R. E. (1989). Ursodeoxycholic acid improves histologic features and progression of primary biliary cirrhosis (Abstract). *Hepatology*, **10**, 637.

Poupon, R. E., Eschwége, E., Poupon, R. and the UDCA-PBC Study Group. (1990). Ursodeoxycholic acid for treatment of primary biliary cirrhosis; interim analysis of a double-blind multicentre randomized trial. *Journal of Hepatology*, **11**, 16–21.

Poupon, R. E., Balkau, B., Eschwege, E., Poupon, R. and the UDCA-PBC Study Group. (1991). A multicenter, controlled trial of ursodiol for the treatment of primary biliary cirrhosis. *New England Journal of Medicine*, **324**, 1548–54.

Powell, F. C., Scroeter, A. L. & Dickson, E. R. (1987). Primary biliary cirrhosis and the CREST syndrome: a report of 22 cases. *Quarterly Journal of Medicine*, **237**, 75–82.

Riggione, O., Stokes, R. P. & Thompson, R. A. (1983). Predominance of IgG_3 subclass in primary biliary cirrhosis. *British Medical Journal*, **286**, 1015–16.

Roll, J., Boyer, J. L., Barry, D. & Klatskin, G. (1983). The prognostic importance of clinical and histological features in asymptomatic and symptomatic primary biliary cirrhosis. *New England Journal of Medicine*, **308**, 1–7.

Routhier, G., Epstein, O., Janossy, G., Thomas, H. C. & Sherlock, S. (1980). The effects of cyclosporin A on suppressor and inducer T-lymphocytes in primary biliary cirrhosis. *Lancet*, **ii**, 1223–6.

Rudzki, C., Ishak, K. G. & Zimmerman, J. F. (1975). Chronic intrahepatic cholestasis of sarcoidosis. *American Journal of Medicine*, **59**, 373–8.

Saidman, S. L., Demetris, A. J., Zeevi, A. & Duquesnoy, R. J. (1990). Propagation and characterization of lymphocytes infiltrating livers of patients with primary biliary cirrhosis and autoimmune hepatitis. *Human Immunology*, **28**, 237–44.

Sandilands, G. P., Galbraith, I., Reid, F. M., Mills, P. R. & MacSween, R. M. N. (1980). Immune complex inhibition of lymphocytes Fc receptors in primary biliary cirrhosis: a possible immunomodulatory mechanism. *Lancet*, **ii**, 9–13.

Scheuer, P. (1968). Primary biliary cirrhosis. In *Liver Biopsy Interpretation.* 1st edn. pp. 22–29. London: Ballière, Tindall & Cassell.

Shapiro, J. M., Smith, H. & Schaffner, F. (1979). Serum bilirubin: a prognostic factor in primary biliary cirrhosis. *Gut*, **20**, 137–40.

Sherlock, S. (1984). Cirrhosis of the liver. In *Oxford Textbook of Medicine,* 1st edn., ed. D. J. Weatherall, J. G. G. Ledingham, & D. A. Warrell. Vol. **12**, 182–92. Oxford: Oxford University Press.

Sherlock, S. & Scheuer, P. J. (1973). The presentation and diagnosis of 100 patients with primary biliary cirrhosis. *New England Journal of Medicine,* **289**, 674–8.

Starzl, T. E., Iwatsuki, S., Van Thiel, D. H. *et al.* (1982). Evolution of liver transplantation. *Hepatology,* **2**, 614–36.

Surh, C. D., Danner, D. J., Ahmed, A. *et al.* (1989). Reactivity of primary biliary cirrhosis sera with a human fetal liver cDNA clone of branched-chain α-keto acid dehydrogenase dihydrolipoamide acetyltransferase, the 52 kD mitochondrial autoantigen. *Hepatology,* **9**, 63–8.

Tornay, A. S. (1980). Primary biliary cirrhosis. Natural history. *American Journal of Gastroenterology,* **281**, 772–5.

Triger, D. R. (1980). Primary biliary cirrhosis: an epidemiological study. *British Medical Journal,* **281**, 772–5.

Underhill, J., Donaldson, P., Bray, G., Doherty, D., Portmann, B. & Williams, R. (1992). Susceptibility to primary biliary cirrhosis is associated with the HLA-DR8-DQB1*0402 haplotype. *Hepatology,* **16**, 1404–8.

Van den Oord, J. J., Sciot, R. & Desmet, V. J. (1986). Expression of MHC products by normal and abnormal bile duct epithelium. *Journal of Hepatology,* **3**, 310–17.

Van de Water, J., Fregeau, D., Davis, P. *et al.* (1988*a*). Autoantibodies of primary biliary cirrhosis recognize dihydrolipoamide acetyltransferase and inhibit enzyme function. *Journal of Immunology,* **141**, 2321–4.

Van de Water, J., Gershwin, M. E., Leung, P., Ansari, A. & Coppel, R. L. (1988*b*). The autoepitope of the 74-kD mitochondrial autoantigen of primary biliary cirrhosis corresponds to the functional site of dihydrolipoamide acetyltransferase. *Journal of Experimental Medicine,* **167**, 1791–9.

Volpes, R., Van den Oord, J. J. & Desmet, V. J. (1990). Immunohistochemical study of adhesion molecules in liver inflammation. *Hepatology,* **12**, 59–65.

Walker, J. G., Doniach, D., Riott, I. M. & Sherlock, S. (1965). Serological tests in the diagnosis of primary biliary cirrhosis. *Lancet,* **i**, 827–31.

Warnes, T. W., Smith, A., Lee, F. I., Haboubi, N. Y., Johnson, P. J. & Hunt, L. (1987). A controlled trial of colchicine in primary biliary cirrhosis. *Journal of Hepatology,* **5**, 1–7.

Wesierska-Gadek, J., Penner, E., Hitchman, E. & Sauermann, G. (1989). Antibodies to nuclear lamin proteins in liver disease. *Immunology Investigations,* **18**, 365–72.

Wiesner, R. H., Dickson, E. R., Lindor, K. D. *et al.* (1987). A controlled clinical trial evaluating cyclosporine in the treatment of primary biliary cirrhosis: a preliminary report (Abstract). *Hepatology,* **7**, 1025.

Wiesner, R. H., Dickson, E. R., Lindor, K. D. *et al.* (1990). A controlled trial of cyclosporine in the treatment of primary biliary cirrhosis. *New England Journal of Medicine,* **322**, 1419–24.

Wolke, A. M., Schaffner, F., Kapelman, B. & Sacks, H. S. (1984). Malignancy in primary biliary cirrhosis: high incidence of breast cancer affecting women. *American Journal of Medicine,* **76**, 1075–8.

Wong, P. Y. N., Portmann, B., O'Grady, J. G. *et al.* (1993). Recurrence of primary biliary cirrhosis after liver transplantation following FK506-based immunosuppression. *Journal of Hepatology,* **17**, 284–7.

Yamada, S., Hyodo, I., Tobe, K. *et al.* (1986). Ultrastructural immunocytochemical analysis of lymphocytes infiltrating bile duct epithelium in primary biliary cirrhosis. *Hepatology,* **6**, 385–91.

Yamada, S., Howe, S. & Scheuer, P. (1987). Three-dimensional reconstruction of biliary pathways in primary biliary cirrhosis: a computer-assisted study. *Journal of Pathology,* **152**, 317–23.

Yeaman, S. J., Danner, D. J., Mutimer, D. J., Fussey, S. P. M., James, O. F. W. & Bassendine, M. F. (1988). Primary biliary cirrhosis: identification of two major M2 mitochondrial autoantigens. *Lancet*, **i**, 1067–70.

Yoshikawa, M., Tsujii, T., Matsumura, K. *et al.* (1992). Immunomodulatory effects of ursodeoxycholic acid on immune responses. *Hepatology*, **16**, 358–64.

Zhang, L., Weetman, A. P., Jayne, D. R. *et al.* (1992). Antimitochondrial antibody IgG subclass distribution and affinity in primary biliary cirrhosis. *Clinical and Experimental Immunology*, **88**, 56–61.

–16–
Immunology and immunopathology of acute viral hepatitis

G. M. DUSHEIKO and A. J. ZUCKERMAN

Introduction

Five major hepatotrophic viruses causing acute or chronic viral hepatitis have been identified. The viruses causing types A to E have been extensively characterised; other viruses, including Epstein-Barr virus and cytomegalovirus may also cause hepatitis. A giant cell hepatitis, and fulminant hepatitis (Fagan *et al.*, 1989; Phillips *et al.*, 1991), for which viruses are being sought, are recognised. Although the molecular virology and serological response in viral hepatitis have been studied in depth, the immune response to hepatitis A to E remains complex. The immunobiology of type B hepatitis has been most widely studied.

Hepatitis A

Hepatitis A virus (HAV) has a similar particle size, capsid structure and genome organisation to other picornoviruses, but is sufficiently different to be classified as a genus within the picornovirus family. The genomes of several strains of HAV have been sequenced and found to be 7470–7478 nucleotides (nt) in length. Type A hepatitis is spread predominantly by the faecal–oral route, but parenteral transmission has been described. Clinical disease with jaundice is uncommon in infants and young children and the infection may pass unnoticed in this group. Severe hepatitis is correspondingly more common in older persons. In countries where there has been improvement in socio-economic conditions and sanitation, such as southern Europe and China, there has been an increase in the mean age of infection.

There is a high level of conservation of cDNA of human HAV strains at the nucleotide level, but PCR based partial sequencing of regions of HAV has revealed unexpected genetic diversity. At least three genotypes have been delineated, but they appear to represent a single serotype (Cohen *et al.*, 1987). Experimental evidence suggests that there is a single antigenic site within the capsid proteins, comprising several distinct neutralisation epitopes (Stapleton *et al.*, 1993). HAV mutants capable of escape from murine monoclonal antibodies have been isolated from infected cell cultures in the presence of murine monoclonal antibodies (Ping & Lemon, 1992).

The absence of chronic infection indicates the effectiveness of the host immune response to HAV. Serological markers of hepatitis A have been identified. IgM antibody to HAV is detectable in acute hepatitis A. Host antibody responses to recombinantly expressed viral structural and non-structural proteins have been detected in convalescent humans (Summers & Ehrenfeld, 1992; Robertson *et al.*, 1992). Serum neutralising antibodies protect against HAV infection and infection with one strain of HAV provides a high level of protection against genetically divergent strains (Siegl & Lemon 1990). There does not appear to be a major component of intestinal (secretory) immunity in HAV infection and it has proven difficult to detect neutralising antibody in faecal extracts of naturally infected humans (Stapleton *et al.*, 1991). Although anti-HAV has been detected in saliva, HAV neutralising activity is not appreciable. It is of interest that naturally occurring IgG, and IgM anti-IFN-alpha 2a, have been found in up to 50% of patients with acute type A (and B and C) hepatitis (Ikeda *et al.*, 1991).

The pathogenesis of the acute hepatocyte injury in type A hepatitis is unclear. However, only subtle cytopathic change is observed in cell cultures. Experimental evidence suggests that HLA-restricted virus-specific T cells play a significant role in HAV-related hepatocellular injury (Vallbracht & Fleischer, 1992). T cell clones have been described from patients with acute hepatitis A and analysed for their phenotype. During the acute phase of the disease, CD8+ clones predominate over CD4+ clones; these CD8+ clones have cytotoxic activity and show specific cytotoxicity against autologous fibroblasts infected with HAV (Fleischer & Vallbracht, 1991). Human T lymphocytes infiltrating the livers of patients with acute HAV infection have been isolated and expanded *in vitro*. A high proportion of these clones are HLA-restricted and are cytotoxic to HAV-infected skin fibroblasts. Thus, these data support the hypothesis that the liver cell injury, in acute HAV infection, is mediated by HAV-specific CD8+ T lymphocytes and is not entirely due to an intrinsic cytopathic effect of the virus. The molecular targets of these cells are, however, unknown.

Gamma interferon production (IFN) by lymphocytes occurs, but it remains controversial whether interferon alpha or beta are produced (Siegl & Lemon, 1990; Kurane *et al.*, 1985). Natural killer cells can be demonstrated in PBML collected from non-immune donors.

It is uncertain whether cellular immunity protects against re-infection. Recurrent hepatitis has been observed in patients and experimentally inoculated Saimiri monkeys with acute disease. This may be associated with viral shedding in stools (Prevot et al., 1992). The relapses are generally benign, with eventual complete resolution. Rheumatoid factor is present in serum in patients with a relapsing course. Immune manifestations such as purpura, arthritis and nephritis may occur, but these respond to cortico-steroid treatment (Marwick, 1992).

In genetically susceptible individuals, it is possible that hepatitis A may trigger an auto-immune chronic hepatitis. Vento et al. (1991), have identi-fied subjects who possessed a defect in suppressor–inducer T lymphocytes, controlling immune responses to the asialoglycoprotein receptor. These subjects developed a persistent response to the asialoglycoprotein receptor, and auto-immune hepatitis after subclinical hepatitis A.

Vaccination

In many developed countries, the prevalence of antibodies to hepatitis A has fallen; only 5–10% of university students are immune and in many parts of the world, there is a large susceptible population. The diminishing incidence of hepatitis A, is now matched by an increasing incidence of clinically apparent disease and prevention of hepatitis A is justified for public health reasons.

Prophylaxis of HAV infection has until now been achieved by passive means, using human immunoglobulin administration. Pooled human plasma (NHIG) contains neutralising antibodies. (NHIG = normal human immune globulin.) Although passively transferred antibody results in low titres of such neutralising antibody it does not result in a positive test when serum collected after NHIG is tested in a commercial, competitive, anti-HAV assay (Lemon, 1985). Passive immunisation is by a single intramuscu-lar dose of NHIG of 0.02 to 0.06 ml/kg, which gives protection for a few weeks, to a few months, depending on the dose. Post-exposure prophylaxis with NHIG is also effective, if given within two weeks of exposure and will reduce the severity of the disease.

Clearly active immunisation would have obvious advantages. Crude HAV antigen has been prepared from homogenised liver of infected marmosets, and this formalin-inactivated material has been demonstrated to protect immunised monkeys from challenge. Several isolates of HAV, from cell cultures, have been used for the production of formalin-inactivated vaccines. These include, HAV strains CR 326, HM 175, GBM and KRM003.

Safety and immunogenicity studies and partial efficacy trials, with formaldehyde-inactivated, Al(OH)$_3$ adsorbed vaccines (Havrix, Smith Kline Beecham, or Vaqta, Merck Research Laboratories), have been undertaken in human trials (Siegl & Lemon, 1990; Ellerbeck et al., 1992). Both anti-HAV (Abbott RIA) and neutralising antibodies, develop in vaccinated individuals. The currently licensed vaccines appear to be well tolerated and immunogenic at doses of 720–1440 arbitrary 'ELISA' units (SKB) or 125–150 U respectively (Ellerbeck et al., 1992; Flehmig, Heinricy & Pfisterer, 1989). Protection against HAV infection has been demonstrated in chimpanzee studies. Active immunisation actually induces higher levels of both, total and neutralising antibodies, than does ISG.

Three doses of vaccine administered intramuscularly into the deltoid muscle are given at 0, 1, and 6 months, which hopefully will provide long-term protection. Adverse reactions are infrequent and consist primarily of pain or tenderness at the injection site. Hypersensitivity reactions or changes in serum ALT, have not been observed.

Several live, attenuated and recombinant vaccines are also under study. The observation that the cell-mediated responses to HAV infection may be responsible for the liver damage accompanying type A hepatitis, has considerable implications for the development of attenuated vaccines (Lemon, 1985). Synthetic peptides have not proven successful immunogens.

Currently, the immune status of individuals exposed to hepatitis A, is determined by assays which measure antibodies against capsid proteins of HAV, that could result from infection or vaccination. Antibody titres may differ, if different test methods for measurement are used (Barnaba et al., 1992).

Protocols for administering HAV vaccine have not been finalised and policies will differ in different regions. In developed countries, the vaccine should be given to travellers to countries where HAV infection is endemic, armed forces personnel, diplomats, staff of children's day-care centres and of institutions for intellectually handicapped individuals, male homosexuals, intravenous drug abusers, haemophiliacs and sewage workers. If immediate protection is required, travellers will require passive immunisation with immunoglobulin, as well as vaccine to confer protection, or possibly a single dose of 1440 ELISA units. The cost–benefit ratio of HAV vaccination is probably optimal when vaccine is given to frequent travellers to endemic areas. Where practical, testing for antibodies to hepatitis A prior to immunisation may be indicated in those aged 50 years or over, those born in areas of high endemicity and those with a history of jaundice.

Hepatitis B

Acute hepatitis B (HBV) is defined as acute inflammation and hepatocellular necrosis, in association with a transient HBV infection. The diagnosis generally rests upon the finding of hepatitis B surface antigen (HBsAg) and IgM antibody to hepatitis B core antigen (anti-HBc), in the serum of patients with clinical and serum biochemical evidence of acute hepatitis.

HBV exists as a 42 nm particle in serum, containing an outer envelope component of HBsAg and an inner nucleocapsid component of hepatitis B core antigen (HBcAg). The genome of HBV has been cloned and four open reading frames, delineating the four gene products of HBV, have been identified (Galibert *et al.*, 1979); all of which appear to represent functional genes. The three envelope regions of the genome encode HBsAg, pre-S1 and pre-S2 polypeptides. Pre-S polypeptides may play a role in attachment of HBV to hepatocyte receptors. The C region encodes HBcAg and the HBeAg, P gene encodes the viral polymerase and the X gene encodes a small protein with transactivating activity (HBxAg) (Siddiqui, Jameel & Mapoles, 1986). The polymerase, encoded by the viral P gene, has both DNA-dependent and RNA-dependent polymerase activity.

The C region of the HBV includes two start codons. The N-terminus of the pre-core protein encodes a signal peptide that directs the protein to the endoplasmic reticulum, where the signal peptide is removed and, after further modification, is secreted as HBeAg. In contrast, the polypeptide synthesised from the core region is directed to the nucleus and, after post-translational modification, assembles into core particles (Ou, Lamb & Rutter, 1986). HBcAg can be detected in liver, usually in the nuclei of hepatocytes. HBeAg is detectable as a soluble 17 kD protein in serum.

Although serious hepatitis may occur as a result of acute hepatitis B, the optimal outcome of acute hepatitis B is eradication of infected hepatocytes, curtailment of viral replication, and rapid hepatic regeneration. While acute and chronic infection are undoubtedly due to viral infection, the nature and pattern of infection suggest that immunologic factors are important. There is little correlation between the severity of illness and the amount or level of viral replication or viral antigen production. Peak HBV replication occurs well before peak cellular injury in acute hepatitis, suggesting that the disease represents immune lysis of infected hepatocytes.

Varying levels of HBV replication may be found during chronic infection. There is a spectrum of disease in patients, ranging from minimal hepatitis to rapidly progressive liver injury and cirrhosis. Patients with the highest level of virus in liver and serum, typically, have the mildest disease. Large amounts of HBsAg and HBcAg can be found in liver biopsies, with minimal evidence of cellular necrosis. These findings suggest that HBV is not cytopathic and that failure of clearance of virus is due to a failure of an adequate immune response. The subsequent expression of the disease involves a complex interplay between viral and host factors.

If cell injury in hepatitis is immunologically mediated, it remains unclear what specific immune reaction is responsible for cell lysis, or what failure of the immune response leads to viral persistence. Furthermore, it is probably an oversimplification to say that host factors alone determine the outcome of HBV infection, or that the virus is totally non-cytopathic. For example, in transplanted, immunosuppressed patients, high levels of HBsAg may be associated with a syndrome of fibrosing cholestatic hepatitis (Lau *et al.*, 1992).

Acute hepatitis B

Intense hepatocyte lysis occurs in acute hepatitis B, apparently as a result of a polyclonal, multispecific, immune response. The observed increase in serum ALT levels is the discernable manifestation of this phenomenon. Serum bilirubin concentrations increase in proportion to the severity of the hepatic damage. The immune response in acute hepatitis B is targeted to envelope, nucleocapsid and non-structural polypeptides of HBV (Mishra *et al.*, 1992; Mondelli *et al.*, 1982). S, Pre-S, antigens, HBcAg and HBeAg, have all been detected along the cell membrane (Saito *et al.*, 1992; Chu & Liaw, 1992). Envelope encoded antigens are recognised by cytotoxic T cells, in a transgenic mouse model (Moriyama *et al.*, 1990). HBV envelope-specific B cells, may internalise and process virions and present HBcAg epitopes to HBcAg-specific T cells. These cells, may in turn, provide help to envelope specific B cells for the production of anti-envelope antibodies (Milich *et al.*, 1985*a*). Peptide-stimulated T lymphocytes, show a response to conformation-dependent pre-S epitopes (Ferrari *et al.*, 1992). During this phase, IgM anti-HBc in serum correlates with active hepatitis in patients. Antibodies to pre-S components appear early in the disease and correlate with the disappearance of serological markers of HBV replication, suggesting a role in immunological clearance of HBV (Alberti *et al.*, 1990; Milich *et al.*, 1985*a*; Cupps *et al.*, 1990). Both anti-preS1, preS2 and anti-HBs have neutralising activity. Antibodies to the RNAse-H domain of the HBV P protein, are found in the sera of both chimpanzees and humans early in infection, shortly after the IgM anti-HBc response. They persist in chronic carriers with ongoing viral replication, but decline and disappear at the time of virus clearance from the sera (Weimer *et al.*, 1990).

Immune complexes may be responsible for some of the manifestations of the acute disease. A mild decrease in serum C3 and C4 concentrations occurs in acute hepatitis B and may reflect antigen–antibody complex formation. The composition and specificity of these are unresolved, but they may contain complexes of HBsAg and anti-HBs, or other antigens of HBV, complexed with antibody. Auto-antibodies, including abnormalities in rheumatoid factor and anti-nuclear and anti-smooth muscle antibodies, are also detectable in acute hepatitis. In fulminant hepatitis, extremely rapid clearance of HBeAg and HBsAg may occur.

The cell-mediated, immune response in acute hepatitis B, has been less easily studied. Attempts to develop immunoassay techniques to measure immunological function, directed at specific viral or hepatocyte antigens, are difficult to perform, but recently have met with more success. The weight of available evidence suggests that the T cell response to HBV epitopes accounts for cellular injury and viral clearance in acute hepatitis B. In addition, experimental evidence suggests that elimination of virus-infected hepatocytes is dependent on the recognition of viral determinants, in association with HLA proteins on the infected hepatocytes, by cytotoxic T cells.

HLA protein display is modulated by interferon proteins, which may also regulate the cytotoxic T cell and NK lytic processes. However, most investigators have not found detectable levels of alpha interferon in the serum of patients with acute hepatitis, and HBV is not an efficient, interferon inducer. HLA markers have not been associated conclusively with the chronicity of HBV interferon. There is evidence of depressed cellular immune function and decreases in helper-inducer T lymphocytes (CD4+) in peripheral blood and an increase in the number of CD8+ or suppressor T lymphocytes. These defects improve as the acute disease resolves. Natural killer cell activity is increased. An impaired production of interleukin-1 by patients with acute hepatitis B has been observed (Muller, Knoflach & Zielinski, 1993).

Mechanisms of chronicity and immunological injury: Acute hepatitis B

Immunological defects are responsible for the failure to eradicate HBV and the subsequent hepatocyte injury in persistent infection, is a result of immune-mediated damage (Peters *et al.*, 1991). The precise impairments of humoral and cellular immunity that determine the development and outcome of hepatitis B have not been categorised. Chronic disease is unusual in patients with acute, icteric, hepatitis B and the majority of cases of chronic hepatitis will not have been preceded by an epidose of icteric hepatitis, suggesting that clearance of HBV requires a hepatitis illness. This, in turn, demands an appropriate cellular immune response limb, the action of neutralising antibodies and an interplay between the immune and interferon system.

The majority of experiments which have analysed the proliferative response to envelope, core and HBeAg, indicate a strong polyclonal and multispecific proliferative immune response in patients with acute hepatitis B, but a lower T cell responsiveness to HBeAg and HBcAg in patients with chronic hepatitis B (Ferrari *et al.*, 1990; Jung *et al.*, 1991). A number of immunodominant recognition sites have been characterised, by measuring cytotoxic lymphocyte (CTL) proliferation to synthetic peptides spanning the core, envelope and non-structural regions. The specific epitopes recognised by B as well as T cells are currently being mapped. In recent years, several experimental systems have been devised to evaluate immune responsiveness to selected epitopes. CTL can be expanded *in vitro* by stimulation with HBV-derived synthetic peptides and then selected by restimulation with a panel of HLA-matched, stable transfectants, that express the corresponding HBV protein. In these experiments, it has proven possible to amplify the frequency of precursor cells, to detect a CTL response in the peripheral blood from patients with acute hepatitis B. The experimental evidence supports cytotoxicity to both exogenous and endogenously synthesised nucleocapsid antigens (Penna *et al.*, 1992*a*).

Several investigators have reported peptide regions from the core region of HBV that are recognised by a majority of patients with acute hepatitis B. These regions include peptide 50–69, 1–20 and 117–131, in reactions which are HLA class II restricted (Penna *et al.*, 1992*b*). Other investigators have noted PBML responses to P120–131 (Ishikawa *et al.*, 1992). The response to amino acid 11–27 of the core protein, which is shared by secretory HBeAg, is CD8+ mediated and is specific for an endogenously synthesised HBV nucleocapsid antigen (Bertoletti *et al.*, 1991). Residues 11–27 of HBcAg, contain a cytotoxic T cell epitope, that is recognised by T cells from virtually all HLA-A2 positive patients with acute hepatitis B. The optimal stimulatory sequence is a 10 mer (18–27), containing the predicted peptide binding motif for HLA-A2. There are recent reports of a CTL epitope located between HBcAg residues 141 and 151, a region that completely overlaps a critical domain in the viral nucleocapsid protein that is essential for its nuclear localisation and genome packaging functions. The CTL response to this epitope is restricted by the HLA-A31 and HLA-Aw68 alleles (Missale *et al.*, 1993). The polyclonal nature of this response argues against the emergence of CTL escape mutants as a significant problem during acute HBV infection, especially at this locus, where mutations might be incompatible with viral replication.

Although patients with acute disease mount a T cell response to several motifs, patients with chronic hepatitis B fail to mount a T cell response to the same epitopes (Bertoletti *et al.*, 1993). The identification of an HLA-A2 restricted epitope located within the amino terminal of the HBcAg (which is shared with HBeAg) and recognised by patients with self-limited acute hepatitis B, but less efficiently in patients with chronic hepatitis, supports an association between the HBV-specific CTL response and viral clearance (Penna *et al.*, 1991). This finding may have implications for the design of immunotherapeutic strategies to terminate HBV infection in chronically infected patients (Missale *et al.*, 1993).

The absence of a similar polyclonal response in chronically infected patients may be due to a defect in processing of peptides and presentation at cell-membranes, rather than a T cell defect, but the evidence favours the latter, at least in neonates.

This propensity to cause chronic infection is a property of hepadna viral infections, particularly in those mammalian or avian hosts affected early in life. An inverse relationship exists between the age of infection and the probability of chronic disease. In neonates, specific suppression of the cell-mediated immune response may favour infection, perhaps because of transplacental exposure to maternal HBeAg, inducing tolerance (within the thymus) to epitopes that are usually the target of the cytotoxic T cell response at a time when the immune system is ontogenically 'immature'. It has been suggested that a peptide fragment of HBeAg, or intact HBeAg, crosses the placenta and induces T cell tolerance to HBeAg and HBcAg in the newborn (Milich *et al.*, 1990). HBeAg and HBcAg appear cross reactive at the T cell level, but not at the B cell level, different peptides leading to anti-HBc and anti-HBe responses. HBcAg is significantly more immunogenic when compared to particulate or non-particulate forms of HBeAg. This disparity may be explained by the fact that HBcAg can function as a T cell independent antigen, whereas HBeAg is a T cell-dependent antigen (Milich, 1988; Milich *et al.*, 1988). Maternal anti-HBc, which is transported across the placenta, may modulate the lysis of infected hepatocytes by T cells. T cells, but not B cells are tolerised by HBeAg in neonatal mice and T cell tolerance elicited by HBeAg also extends to HBcAg specific T cells (Milich *et al.*, 1989). The combination of T cell tolerance to the nucleocapsid antigens in the presence of a B cell response to HBcAg (anti-HBc), may mimic the outcome in newborns of chronic carrier mothers with HBsAg and HBeAg in serum.

Despite the profound immunological tolerance present in neonates, it appears that this may be overcome later in life. This altered T cell tolerance may coincide with the appearance of raised ALT levels (Hsu *et al.*, 1992).

These theories do not, however, explain the mechanism of chronic infection in children who acquire the disease by horizontal transmission (Thomas *et al.*, 1988). Chronic infection is also more common in immunosuppressed individuals, particulary renal dialysis, kidney transplant patients and children with Down's syndrome, leprosy or leukaemia and homosexuals with HIV infection. A heterogenous group of immunoregulatory defects may exist in these groups. A B-lymphocyte defect may explain impaired synthesis of anti-HBs after induction by non-specific mitogens; *in vitro* synthesis of anti-HBc and immunoglobulin remain normal in chronic carriers (Dusheiko *et al.*, 1983). The high concentrations of HBsAg in the serum may lead to a state of tolerance. Antibody to HBcAg (anti-HBc) may blunt the expression of nucleocapsid antigens on the surface of hepatocytes (Mondelli *et al.*, 1982). Alternatively, selective killing of antigen-specific B cells, delivering HBsAg envelope proteins to class I restricted cytotoxic T cells, may suppress the antibody response. The immune response may also be blunted by HBV infection in bone marrow, lymphocytes or macrophages (Pontisso *et al.*, 1984; Barnaba *et al.*, 1992).

During chronic HBV infection, there is some evidence of failure of interferon production and activation of the infected liver cells, so that viral protein synthesis is not decreased and there is poor enhancement of HLA protein display. Such a mechanism might result in failure of presentation of HLA antigens on the cell surface and hence poor presentation of viral peptides to the immune system. Peripheral blood leucocyte production of alpha interferon has been found to be suboptimal in chronic carriers, although there is considerable overlap in individual carriers. There is decreased production of interferon by PBML from children with chronic hepatitis B (Tolentino *et al.*, 1992). (Gamma interferon production remains normal). Experimental HBV transfection, and integration, may affect the ability of the cell to respond to interferon (Twu *et al.*, 1988).

This virus-specific mechanism of resistance may reflect nucleotide homology between HBV DNA and sequences regulating the interferon-induced antiviral system, or involve transcription or translation products of HBV (Twu *et al.*, 1988). Arguing against a defect in interferon synthesis or production, however, is the fact that β-2-microglobulin expression on hepatocyte membranes, reflecting the display of HLA antigen, has indeed been observed in patients with acute hepatitis, chronic active hepatitis and cirrhosis and in patients treated with interferon. The degree of interferon deficiency does not correlate with the severity of the illness, however. Moreover, other investigators have not found support for the hypothesis that there is an inherent deficiency in the interferon system in acute or chronic hepatitis B; serial $2'5'$- oligoadenylate synthetase (2–5 AS) levels, have not identified those patients who progressed from acute to chronic hepatitis: and patients with chronic hepatitis B infection, regardless of liver histology, have been found to have normal basal lymphocyte 2–5 AS levels (Heathcote *et al.*, 1989). Also, recombinant gamma IFN, administered to patients with chronic hepatitis B, causes an increase in $\beta 2$ microglobulin and 2–5 AS (Quiroga *et al.*, 1988).

Chronic hepatitis B

A detailed discussion of the immunopathology of chronic hepatitis B is beyond the scope of this article (Desmet, 1991). A number of defects have been characterized in patients with chronic hepatitis B, which has a complex natural history. The weight of evidence from these studies suggests that in chronic infection, the hepatic injury may be the result of an immune response of the host to one or more antigenic components of HBV

(Pignatelli *et al.*, 1986). However, HBV may produce cell lysis by a direct cytopathic action.

HBcAg can be demonstrated in both the nucleus and the membrane of the hepatocyte in chronically infected persons. Membranous or cytoplasmic, rather than nuclear expression of HBcAg, may correlate with disease activity. Recently, membrane bound HBeAg has been detected and the relative presentation of HBeAg versus HBcAg may modulate immune injury. Investigators seem to agree that suppressor cytotoxic (CD8+) T lymphocytes predominate in portal and lobular inflammatory infiltrates in the liver, in patients with acute and chronic hepatitis B. CD4+ cells predominate in areas of single cell necrosis and focal inflammation in the hepatic parenchyma. Irrespective of histologic classifications, HBeAg positive patients contain predominantly CD8+ cells, whereas in anti-HBe positive patients, CD4+ helper T cells and B cells are more common in the portal areas. This pattern of mononuclear cell infiltrates in the liver in patients with chronic HBV infection suggests that T cell-mediated cytotoxicity to HBV-infected hepatocytes is diminished in accordance with the decrease of active HBV replication. This decrease is shown by seroconversion from HBeAg to anti-HBe (Yamada *et al.*, 1985).

In patients with a high level of HBV replication, nuclear HBcAg has been detected with relatively faint HLA expression. In contrast, in patients with limited virus replication (anti-HBe positive), nuclear HBcAg has been found to be absent and membrane expression of HLA A, B and C antigens, to be intense. The finding of increased HLA class I and II antigen expression in association with cytoplasmic HBcAg, and active chronic hepatitis B, adds credence to the possibility that nucleocapsid antigens of HBV, may be the focus of immunologically mediated injury (Pignatelli *et al.*, 1986).

Recently, the correlation between liver reaction patterns and molecules mediating binding between cells and adhesion molecules involved in the recruitment of lymphocytes, has been studied. ICAM-1 and LFA-1, which are not normally found in liver cells, can be upregulated in acute hepatitis and in some patients with chronic active hepatitis. In acute hepatitis, intercellular adhesion molecule 1 (ICAM-1) and human leucocyte antigen DR are strongly expressed throughout liver parenchyma (Volpes, van den Oord & Desmet, 1990). These molecules may facilitate the accumulation of lymphocytes into inflammatory regions. The reactions, which are enhanced by gamma interferon, may be an important facet of a coordinated immune and inflammatory response.

Hepatitis B virus variants

The natural history of chronic hepatitis is variable, but many patients show a gradual or rapid transition from predominantly 'replicative' to predominantly 'non-replicative' infection. HBV DNA has been found to be integrated into chromosomal DNA of hepatocytes. Integrated sequences have been detected in acute HBV infection, but detectable integration may increase with the duration of infection (Shafritz *et al.*, 1981). Integration may disrupt the transcription and packaging of nucleocapsid proteins, but allow continued transcription of envelope proteins (Brechot *et al.*, 1981). In general, predominantly episomal HBV DNA is detectable in carriers with high levels of viral replication, and integrated HBV DNA genomes are detectable in those with less active viral replication. In most patients, there is a requirement for active viral replication in the pathogenesis of liver injury and improvement in histology follows interferon-induced or spontaneous seroconversion to anti-HBe. Conversely, cells which do not express nucleocapsid antigens, may be protected from the host immune response.

T cell cytotoxity, with an increase in T cell response during exacerbations of chronic hepatitis and increase in precursor T cell frequencies during these exacerbations, has been noted (Tsai *et al.*, 1992). A cluster of changes in the core region codons 84–101, has been found in patients with chronic active hepatitis, which may mean that these mutations evolved under immune selection pressure (Ehata *et al.*, 1992).

The nucleocapsid antigens (HBcAg and HBeAg) are expressed on the cell membrane and are important targets of the immune response and cytolytic T cells in acute hepatitis B. These antigens are products of a single gene region on the virion genome (Stahl *et al.*, 1982). The C gene has two initiation codons and therefore two gene regions (pre-core and core) and two potential molecular forms (HBcAg and HBeAg). Initiation of translation at the first site (nucleotide 1814), produces a 321 amino acid (aa) polypeptide (p25), which has a signal peptide directing it to the endoplasmic reticulum. There the signal piece is removed by signal peptidase, to cleave the N terminal 19 aa residues, as well as the C terminal 34 residues, the resultant polypeptide of 159 amino acids, is secreted as HBeAg (p15–18), a soluble protein that is the product of 10 residues coded by the pre-core region and 149 residues coded by the C gene (Ou, Laub & Rutter, 1986). Translation from second initiation codon (nucleotide 1901), results in unprocessed polypeptides (p23, 183 amino acids), which are assembled into core particles within the liver (P21). HBcAg, is a 27 nm particulate nucleocapsid protein. HBcAg is not detected in serum, but is an intracellular virion-associated nucleocapsid antigen, that is the product of the C gene alone. HBeAg therefore, has substantial amino acid homology to HBcAg, and the proteins are cross-reactive at the T cell level.

Spontaneous mutations in the genome are not uncommon and may explain the variation in disease expression in some patients (Brunetto *et al.*, 1991a; Bonino *et al.*, 1991). An immune response to HBeAg may explain the decline in virus titre through viral elimination (Schlicht, von Brunn &

Theilmann, 1991). Genetic mutants of HBV have recently been described in serum of anti-HBe and HBV DNA positive patients, who have HBcAg in hepatocytes and histological evidence of chronic active hepatitis, but who lack HBeAg in serum (Hadziyannis *et al.*, 1983). Polymerase chain reaction amplification and subsequent sequencing of DNA from such virions in serum, has revealed one or more nucleotide substitutions in the pre-core region of the HBV genome. A point mutation from guanine (G) to adenine (A) at nucleotide 83 (1896), creating an in-frame TAG stop codon converting codon 28 for tryptophan (TGG) to a stop codon (TAG) has been the most common finding, with or without additional point mutations in succeeding codons (Carman *et al.*, 1989; Brunetto *et al.*, 1991*b*; Akahane *et al.*, 1990; Okamoto *et al.*, 1990). This substitution prevents the production and secretion of HBeAg. It is not clear whether these represent *de novo* infections with a mutant type virus, or, perhaps more likely, whether these mutations have arisen during infection, as a result of immune selection pressure. It has been hypothesised that hepatocytes infected with wild type HBV produce HBeAg molecules, which would be exposed on the hepatocyte surface in the process of secretion. However, hepatocytes infected with pre-core defective mutants would not be able to produce HBeAg. Immune selection may thus assist pre-C defective mutants, with an HBeAg-negative phenotype to exceed HBeAg-positive phenotypes.

The mechanism of active hepatitis in these patients is not clear; these variants may be cytotoxic, or the immunopathogenicity of the host response may be affected. It has been proposed that cytotoxic T-cells primed with anti-HBc/anti-HBe, might selectively attack hepatocytes harbouring defective mutants, because of the lack of blocking HBeAg. Pre-C region defects are also found in patients with fulminant hepatitis; these variants may have altered virulence.

Coursaget and co-workers (Coursaget *et al.*, 1987; Coursaget *et al.*, 1990), reported unusual serological patterns in Senegalese children, whose sera showed transient reactivity for HBsAg, but lacked anti-HBc, anti-HBe and anti-HBs on follow up. Pre-S2 reactivity was sometimes detected and virus particles similar to HBV were detected. It was suggested that this is a new HBV-related virus, HBV-2. However, it is possible that these individuals have an aberrant immune response and do not produce anti-HBc. Most investigators report that the absence of anti-HBc in carriers is due to an immune defect, rather than viral mutations, which affect the expression of HBcAg (Lee *et al.*, 1992). Delayed seroconversion to anti-HBc has been reported in HBsAg-positive neonates, born to HBsAg-positive mothers (Ni *et al.*, 1993).

Superinfection

When there is delta virus superinfection in a carrier of chronic HBV, there is an acceleration of the rate of progression of the liver disease (Rizzetto, 1983; Rizzetto *et al.*, 1983). Superinfection by hepatitis A virus, HIV and possibly hepatitis C, may also affect HBV replication.

Drug treatment

Hepatic failure may develop in patients with chronic hepatitis B, after stopping cytotoxic therapy. Drugs which modify the immune response, such as interferon, levamisole and corticosteroids, may in fact affect hepatitis B expression. A treatment response during alpha interferon, is characterised by a transient increase in the serum aminotransferases (Dusheiko *et al.*, 1985). This is the discernable manifestation of an immune response targeted to hepatocytes expressing nucleocapsid epitopes. During high dose prednisolone therapy, there is a decrease in immunoglobulin synthesis by peripheral blood mononuclear cells and in lymphocyte proliferation to all mitogens. Following the withdrawal of prednisolone therapy in chronic HBV carriers, lymphocyte function rapidly returns to baseline levels and is associated with, in some carriers, a subsequent rebound increase in serum aminotransferase activities. This has been shown to be accompanied by a striking increase in suppressor T lymphocyte activity, without significant changes in either helper T cell or B cell function. The close correlation between changes in helper and suppressor T lymphocyte function and serum aminotransferase activities during and after immunosuppressive therapy, suggests that immunoregulatory T lymphocytes may play an important role in the pathogenesis of chronic type B hepatitis.

Vaccination against hepatitis B

Hepatitis B virus infection can be prevented by administration of recombinant DNA vaccines. The first generation of hepatitis B vaccines were derived from HBsAg particles in human plasma. These vaccines have been superseded in developed countries by recombinant HBV vaccines, but are still in use in some countries such as Korea and China and some African countries. Two recombinant vaccines are available (Engerix B, Smith Kline Beecham and Heptavax B, Merck Sharpe and Dohme). Both are produced in yeast cells and are derived from the S gene region of HBV. Both vaccines are highly immunogenic and induce anti-HBs in approximately 90% of individuals.

The recombinant HBV vaccines are well tolerated and few serious side effects have been reported. The most common side effects are local reactions at the injection site.

The human antibody response to HBsAg is HLA-complex related. Individuals homozygous for HLA-B8, SC01 DR31 lack an immune response gene to HBsAg; this is inherited in a dominant fashion (Kruskall *et al.*, 1992; Alper *et al.*, 1989). Non-responders to hepatitis B vaccine, have an increased frequency of HLA D7 and lack HLA D1, or possibly a higher frequency of an HLA-linked immune suppressor gene for HBsAg, in linkage disequilibrium with HLA-Bw54-DR4-Drw53 haplotype.

In vivo antibody production to HBsAg in the mouse, is regulated by at least two immune response genes, mapping to different loci. The HBsAg specific T cell proliferative response of congenic mouse strains parallels the *in vivo* anti-HBs production and may also be genetically restricted. The pre-S2 region is significantly more immunogenic than the S region at the T cell level. Pre-S2 region specific T cell activation is regulated by immune response genes and correlates with genetic restriction of *in vivo* antibody production to the pre-S2 region. Immunisation of an S-region-nonresponder, pre-S2-region T-cell-responder strain with HBV envelope particles containing both the pre-S2 and S region can circumvent non-responsiveness to the S region through pre-S2-specific T-cell helper function (Milich *et al.*, 1985*a*; Milich *et al.*, 1985*b*; Milich *et al.*, 1985*c*).

Vaccination with hepatitis B surface antigen (HBsAg), has shown that antibody directed against the common 'a' determinant of this antigen is protective against infection with hepatitis B virus (HBV). The antigenic epitopes of the 'a' determinant have been analysed by competitive inhibition assays and by binding studies to synthetic peptides (Waters *et al.*, 1992). Several investigators have reported the detection of antibody escape mutants in children vaccinated against hepatitis B. These mutations are associated with an apparent alteration in antigenicity of a component of HBsAg and induce escape from conventional vaccine which results in antibody to wild type HBsAg, or from passive antibody from immunoglobulin. The common type of antibody escape mutant is a gly–arg mutation at the 145 colon of the S gene (Fujii *et al.*, 1992), or a missense mutation at the 126 codon of the S gene (Okamoto *et al.*, 1992).

HIV positive patients have an impaired response to HBV vaccine, indicative of diminishing immunological function (Bruguera *et al.*, 1992).

Antibody concentrations fall progressively with the passage of time. The need for booster doses of vaccine in the population, will be determined by long-term follow-up of immunised cohorts (Delage, Remy-Prince & Montplaisir, 1993). Comprehensive strategies for the elimination of hepatitis B vaccination, will involve vaccination of all newborn children, or school children at the age of 12 years.

Hepatitis C

In 1989, the molecular cloning of an RNA virus responsible for most cases of post-transfusion non-A, non-B hepatitis was reported. This virus has been given the nomenclature of hepatitis C virus (HCV). Infection with hepatitis C is most clearly seen after transfusion of whole-blood products, but in many countries the disease has been acquired by community acquired transmission. Expressed proteins of this virus protein are now used as antigens in enzyme-linked immunoassays to detect diagnostic antibodies in serum. In some regions, for example Southern Europe, Africa, or Japan, the prevalence of hepatitis C is relatively high.

HCV may cause acute disease, which is frequently asymptomatic and unnoticed. The acute disease may resolve in 25–50% of cases, but it is well known that hepatitis C has a disturbing propensity to lead to chronic hepatitis C. The natural history of the chronic disease is variable. The persistent infection may lead progressively to chronic active hepatitis, cirrhosis, portal hypertension and hepatocellular carcinoma. Typically, patients have an indolent disease and the onset of cirrhosis is slow, over 10–20 years in most. However, rapidly progressive disease, leading to cirrhosis has been noted.

HCV is an enveloped RNA virus. The complete nucleotide sequence of the HCV genome has been determined in a number of isolates and shown to be a positive strand RNA, of approximately 9400 nucleotides. This consists of one long open reading frame encoding a polyprotein of 3010–3033 amino acids, which is cleaved into functionally distinct polypeptides, during or after translation. The virus has similar organisation to pestiviruses and flaviviruses of the family Flaviviridae, but is sufficiently distinct to be classified within its own genus. The nucleocapsid and envelope proteins are encoded at the 5′ end of the genome, while the non-structural elements are downstream of this region. The total or partial nucleotide sequences, obtained from a number of isolates, indicate that hepatitis C can be divided into at least six major types, with component subtypes, based upon nucleotide homology. There are hypervariable regions, especially in the E1 and E2 domains. These regions, especially those of the envelope glycoproteins, may be important antigenic sites and their variability may be critical to persistence of infection and immunopathogenesis. Considerable microheterogeneity has been found in the sequence of genomic regions in clones obtained from patients and chimpanzees, who have been studied longitudinally.

To date, it has not been possible to detect viral antigens routinely. Thus, the detection of antibodies to HCV has become important as an indication of past or present infection. The first generation ELISA assay, based on antibody capture, detected antibodies to c100-3 a 363 amino acid fusion polypeptide, representing part of the NS4 region of the HCV genome.

The second generation of antibody assays incorporate extra HCV-derived recombinant proteins, which improve the sensitivity of the assay. C22-3 represents the majority of 22-kD nucleocapsid protein. Antibodies to C22 are an earlier finding and occur more frequently than those to c100-3 during the course of HCV infection. This is probably due to conservation of amino acid sequence in this region, together with greater immunogenicity of the core peptide. These antibodies are probably not neutralising, in that they are found throughout chronic infection. The third generation of antibody assays also incorporate epitopes derived from the NS5 region.

A transient IgM anti-HCV response has been observed in acute hepatitis C (Chen *et al.*, 1992). IgM responses to c1003 and C22-3 have also been detected in acute and chronic disease. Their significance in distinguishing acute from chronic disease is not yet established. In alpha-interferon treated patients, anti-HCV IgM positivity was significantly lower in good responders, than in non-responders or transient responders (Kikuchi *et al.*, 1992; Quiroga *et al.*, 1992; Brillanti *et al.*, 1992). Antibody profiles may be related to epidemiological or clinical features of chronic infection or to viral replication (Chemello *et al.*, 1993).

Antibodies to E1 and E2 can be detected in patients with chronic infection. The detection is dependent upon sequence heterogeneity found in these regions. These antibodies may be neutralising, but this is not yet established (Yokosuka *et al.*, 1992). The N-terminal E2 region may encode protective epitopes that are subject to immune selection. Antibody-epitope binding studies have shown isolate-specific linear epitopes located in the E2 hypervariable region, suggesting that the hypervariable domain is a target for the human immune response (Weiner *et al.*, 1992). Variability in the E2 hypervariable domain may result from immune selection, whereby particular variants may predominate during different episodes of disease. Antibodies against particular motifs present in pre-existing clones, have been detected in patients and chimpanzees who have been studied longitudinally.

It is clear that HCV is a systemic disease, which may be associated with disorders with an immunological basis. In particular, mixed essential cryoglobulinaemia (Dammacco & Sansonno, 1992), and membraneous glomerulonephritis, may be associated with HCV infection.

Frequent episodes of hepatitis are observed, which may be due to reinfection or reactivation. In chimpanzees, re-inoculation with the same strain of virus resulted in re-appearance of viraemia, which suggests that immunity to HCV is not readily elicited (Farci *et al.*, 1992). These episodes of hepatitis may be due to the emergence of mutants of HCV not neutralised by circulating antibody. However, this hypothesis has to be proven by careful assessment of nucleotide sequence change in patients with hepatitis C and corresponding antibody reactivity to viral epitopes.

There is an overlap between hepatitis C infection and autoimmune hepatitis. The humoral response to a host cellular, gene-derived epitope GOR (anti-GOR), has been reported to be associated with chronic hepatitis C virus (HCV) infection (Mishiro *et al.*, 1990; Mehta *et al.*, 1992). Anti-Gor has been found in a high proportion of anti-LKM1 antibody-positive patients with anti-HCV, but not in anti-LKM-positive patients negative for anti-HCV (type IIb vs IIa autoimmune chronic hepatitis (Michel *et al.*, 1992). Immune cross-reaction of P450IID6 epitopes and hepatitis C proteins, may explain the occurrence of anti-LKM antibodies in patients (Manns *et al.*, 1991).

There does not seem to be a correlation between the clinical features, response to interferon or histological features (Lau *et al.*, 1993). Although false positive anti-HCV tests were encountered in first generation immunoassays in patients with auto-immune hepatitis (McFarlane *et al.*, 1990), recent studies have suggested that true antibodies to hepatitis C are presently found in approximately 50% of patients with auto-immune hepatitis type 2 (LKM antibody positive) (Lunel *et al.*, 1992).

Geographical differences may exist in this spectrum of overlap disease. The pattern is less common in patients studied in the US, and the proportion of patients with type II auto-immune hepatitis and anti-HCV varies in UK, versus Italian patients (Czaja, Manns & Homburger, 1992; Lenzi *et al.*, 1990; Lenzi *et al.*, 1991).

An auto-immune diathesis may be aggravated in patients with a high level of auto-antibodies after treatment with interferon; a thyroid disease accompanied by anti-thyroid antibodies may also occur with treatment.

Tissue damage in hepatitis C infection

The pathogenic mechanisms that result in hepatitis are unknown. Lymphocytes are typically observed within the hepatic parenchyma, but the functional characteristics of these cells have not been fully defined. However, in the liver, CD8+ cell subsets predominate over CD4+ subsets in patients with chronic hepatitis C (Onji *et al.*, 1992). The mechanism of hepatitis in acute hepatitis C has not been well studied. T cell clones, reactive with non-A, non-B infected hepatocytes, from patients with chronic hepatitis, have been identified (Imawari *et al.*, 1989). Liver-infiltrating lymphocytes, from subjects with chronic HCV hepatitis, have been cloned at limiting dilution and tested for HCV-specific, cytolytic activity, using autologous target cells infected with vaccinia viruses expressing recombinant HCV Ag or sensitised with synthetic HCV peptides. HCV-specific, HLA class I-restricted CTL, were identified that recognised epitopes in variable regions of either the envelope or non-structural proteins. Thus, HCV-specific CTL can be demonstrated at the site of tissue damage in persons with chronic HCV hepatitis, which may have a pathogenic role (Koziel et al., 1992). Minutello and colleagues have established that NS4 non-structural protein stimulated CD4 T cells obtained from liver biopsies, suggesting that proteins from this region are highly immunogenic (Minutello et al., 1993).

A CD4+ proliferative T-lymphocyte response to recombinant viral antigens has been found in infected individuals with different clinical courses. Several viral proteins are immunogenic for T cells, although NS4 has been the most immunogenic. There may be a correlation between the presence of CD4+ T cell responses to HCV core and a benign course of infection, in viraemic carriers with minimal hepatitis (Botarelli et al., 1993).

Beta 2-microglobulin epitopes are evident on hepatocytes from patients with chronic active hepatitis C. Interferon therapy could down-regulate this expression through its effect in reducing the histological activity, resulting from the lysis of virus-infected hepatocytes by cytotoxic T cells (Garcia-Buey et al., 1993).

Vaccination

The worldwide prevalence of hepatitis C and the current morbidity from the disease, point to the importance of a vaccine to prevent the spread of the disease. However, the genotype diversity of the virus indicates that vaccine development is likely to be difficult and will require multivalent vaccines. The envelope proteins are potential components of an HCV vaccine. Initial experiments with recombinantly produced proteins were discouraging. Recently, Ralston et al., 1993 reported the effect of purified E1 and E2 glycoproteins extracted from the endoplasmic reticulum of infected HeLa cells. Anti-E1 and E2 antibodies developed in the vaccinated animals; five of seven chimpanzees inoculated with these proteins, were protected after a small (and homologous) infectious challenge dose.

Hepatitis D

Hepatitis D (delta) is caused by a defective virus or virusoid, the hepatitis D virus (HDV). The propagation of HDV depends upon the presence of helper hepadnavirus (Rizzetto et al., 1986). Four particles can be detected in the serum of HDV infected persons: the Dane particle, two non-infectious HBsAg-positive particles and the delta particle in serum (Rizzetto, 1989). The delta particle uses HBsAg to make its own coat and the HDV virus is therefore classifiable as a satellite virus or virusoid. The delta antigen is found both within virions and in the nucleus of infected cells. The protein binds HDV RNAs. There appear to be two major forms of the delta antigen, 195 and 214 amino acids in length (Chao, Hsieh & Taylor, 1990; Chao *et al.*, 1991). The functional motifs essential for RNA binding, and replication, including putative leucine zippers are being studied (Chang *et al.*, 1992; Chang *et al.*, 1993; Taylor, 1991).

The genome of the HDV is a single stranded RNA molecule about 1700 nucleotides in length. It has a closed circular conformation and can fold on itself by base pairing, which is similar to that of plant satellite RNAs. A second, complementary molecule of the genome (the anti-genome), is present in liver of infected animals, but is not efficiently packaged into viruses. The coding region for the delta antigen is on the antigenome. A self-cleavage reaction has been demonstrated, which is proposed to involve a rolling circle method of genome replication (Wu *et al.*, 1992; Smith, Gottlieb & Dinter-Gottlieb, 1992). It has been possible to infect primary monolayer cells from woodchuck and chimpanzees and to transfect cultured cells with cDNA clones of the entire HDV genome (Sureau *et al.*, 1991).

Transmission of HDV infection is by parenteral or inapparent parenteral routes, as for HBV.

IgA antibodies may correlate with hepatic injury in patients with chronic hepatitis D (McFarlane *et al.*, 1991). Monomeric IgM, anti-HD (7S), predominates in patients with chronic hepatitis D.

It has long been held that HDV is pathogenic and that the liver injury in hepatitis D is related to HDV itself. Fulminant hepatitis may occur in acute HDV and HBV infection and outbreaks of severe hepatitis have been reported in Indians of the Amazon basin and areas of Central Africa. Degenerative changes were observed in these patients, characterised by fine steatotic vacuolisation of hepatocytes, in keeping with a cytotoxic inflammatory lesion. Antigenic diversity has been observed in the HDV genome, associated with an outbreak of fulminant hepatitis in Bangui. A single, 28 kD protein was detected, instead of the 24 and 27 kD proteins seen in wild-type, hepatitis D infection.

Severe hepatitis D infection may involve disruption of cellular metabolic processes, as a result of sequence homology between two conserved regions of HDV RNA and human 7SL RNA (cytoplasmic RNA associated with the signal recognition particle) (Negro *et al.*, 1989; Negro & Rizzetto, 1993). However, it is apparent that there is a spectrum of disease. Carriers of HDV and experimentally infected chimpanzees, may have relatively minor hepatitis (Rizzetto *et al.*, 1986; Hadziyannis *et al.*, 1987).

The postulate that HDV is cytopathic has recently been challenged with the observation that HDV re-occurs in liver transplanted patients soon after grafting, but without signs of HBV recurrence or evidence of liver damage. In these persons, HDV may establish latent infection, that is not dependent upon HBV for replication and which is only associated with recrudescent liver injury, after the acquisition of HBV (Ottobrelli *et al.*, 1991; Mason & Taylor, 1991). It is possible the agent cannot be propagated without a surface envelope, which HDV is unable to produce.

It is known that hepatitis D may result in interference of HDV, but the intrahepatic molecular or immunological mechanism has not been established.

Increased viral replication has been noted in HDV and HIV infection but not necessarily with evidence of more severe hepatitis (Buti *et al.*, 1991).

Host-related factors may contribute to the tissue injury in patients with chronic disease. Autoantibodies have been detected in 50% of patients with chronic hepatitis D. These include anti-thymocyte, liver and kidney microsomes (LKM3). The concomitant influence of hepatitis C infection upon hepatitis D is being closely studied.

Vaccination

Hepatitis D can be prevented by vaccination against hepatitis B. There have been attempts to produce recombinant HDV vaccines (Karayiannis *et al.*, 1990; Karayiannis *et al.*, 1993).

Hepatitis E

An enterically transmitted form of hepatitis was first recognised following epidemics of hepatitis in India, unrelated to HAV or HBV. Epidemics of infection with the hepatitis E virus (HEV), have also been observed in South East and Central Asia, in Eastern, Northern and Western Africa and in Central America. In these epidemics, attack rates have been higher in males than females and for adults rather than children. Evidence of secondary intrafamilial spread is uncommon (Naik *et al.*, 1992). The disease is also a common cause of acute sporadic hepatitis in these countries (el-Zimaity *et al.*, 1993). Sporadic cases have been observed in developed countries, among migrant labourers and travellers returning from such areas. In contrast to prior epidemics of enterically transmitted non-A, non-B hepatitis, HEV has been found to be a common cause of acute hepatitis in a paediatric population in Egypt (Hyams *et al.*, 1992). Seroprevalence studies in Hong Kong, suggest that hepatitis E accounts for a third of non-A, non-B, non-C hepatitis and that coinfection of hepatitis A and E can occur (Lok *et al.*, 1992).

The hepatitis E virus has been molecularly cloned and sequenced and has a single-stranded, positive-sense RNA genome of approximately 7200 nucleotides, followed by a poly(A) tail. There are three open reading frames. The non-structural gene, approximately 5 kb, is located at the 5' end, while the structural gene, approximately 2 kb, is located at the 3' end of the genome. There is relative sequence homogeneity in the 3′ end of Asian strains of HEV (Aye *et al.*, 1992*a*; Aye *et al.*, 1992*b*).

The diagnosis could until recently only be made with a history of exposure, in an appropriate epidemiologic setting, and the exclusion of other causes of viral hepatitis. Recently, research-based serological tests were developed to test for antibody to hepatitis E virus (anti-HEV) (Krawczynski, 1993). The first of these, was a fluorescent antibody completion assay against native HEV Ag, in liver sections. Recombinant HEV proteins derived from the Burmese or Mexican isolates have been used in enzyme-linked and immunoblotting assays. The fusion protein C2 expressed from a 1700 bp cDNA fragment of the ORF2, can be used to capture IgG and IgM, anti-HEV in patients. More comprehensive assays are in development.

Western blot assays are able to detect IgM, anti-HEV. The diagnosis can be confirmed by the polymerase chain reaction on faecal material, from acutely infected patients. Bile, from experimentally infected monkeys, is also positive by PCR (Jameel *et al.*, 1992). Stool specimens contain HEV, when tested by immune electron microscopy (IEM) and reveal 27–32 nm virus-like particles.

Macaca monkeys develop changes in acute viral hepatitis associated with a rise in liver enzymes, the presence of HEV specific viral particles in the stool and histological changes in the liver, from 21 to 45 days after HEV inoculation. In general, the disease in humans is self-limited, with no evidence of chronic infection. Liver biopsies obtained during the acute illness in humans show portal inflammation and cytoplasmic cholestasis. HEVAg has been identified in the cytoplasm of hepatocytes of experimentally infected primates, with immunofluorescent antibody prepared from convalescent phase serum.

Ultrastructural changes in the livers of experimental monkeys include infiltration of lymphocytes and polymorphonucleocytes around the necrotic area, swelling of mitochondria, dilation of smooth endoplasmic reticulum (ER) and presence of 27–34 nm virus particles during the acute phase of the disease (Gupta, Iyenger & Tandon, 1993). It is not known whether these changes reflect cytopathic liver injury or immune-mediated damage.

High fatality rates in infected pregnant women are characteristic of the disease. This uniquely deleterious effect, resulting in fulminant hepatic failure, has not been explained. Fulminant hepatitis has been reported in the UK, but appears to be a relatively infrequent cause elsewhere.

Immunity to HEV

Household contact has been reported to result in transmission in 29% of cases. Immunoglobulin, from an Indian source, did not prevent transmission (Khuroo & Dar, 1992). Antibody development supports the assumption that humans become immunised once they contact hepatitis E. However, perhaps because of low infectivity or waning immunity, adult populations in endemic areas are susceptible to hepatitis E, with high attack rates in epidemics.

Vaccines for hepatitis E are in development.

References

Akahane, Y., Yamanaka, T., Suzuki, H. *et al.* (1990). Chronic active hepatitis and hepatitis B virus DNA and antibody against e antigen in the serum. Disturbed synthesis and secretion of e antigen from hepatocytes due to a point mutation in the precore region. *Gastroenterology*, **99**, 1113–19.

Alberti, A., Cavalletto, D., Chemello, L. *et al.* (1990). Fine specificity of human antibody response to the PreS1 domain of hepatitis B virus. *Hepatology*, **12**, 199–203.

Alper, C. A., Kruskall, M. S., Marcus-Bagley, D. *et al.* (1989). Genetic prediction of nonresponse to hepatitis B vaccine. *New England Journal of Medicine*, **321**, 708–12.

Aye, T. T., Uchida, T., Ma, X. *et al.* (1992a). Sequence comparison of the capsid region of hepatitis E viruses isolated from Myanmar and China. *Microbiology and Immunology*, **36**, 615–21.

Aye, T. T., Uchida, T., Ma, X. Z. *et al.* (1992b). Complete nucleotide sequence of a hepatitis E virus isolated from the Xinjiang epidemic (1986–1988) of China. *Nucleic Acids Research*, **20**, 3512.

Barnaba, V., Franco, A., Paroli, M., Benvenuto, R., Santilio, I. & Balsano, F. (1992). T cell recognition of hepatitis B envelope proteins [Review]. *Archives of Virology – Supplementum*, **4**, 19–22.

Bertoletti, A., Ferrari, C., Fiaccadori, F. *et al.* (1991). HLA class I-restricted human cytotoxic T cells recognize endogenously synthesized hepatitis B virus nucleocapsid antigen. *Proceedings of the National Academy of Sciences, USA*, **88**, 10445–9.

Bertoletti, A., Chisari, F. V., Penna, A. *et al.* (1993). Definition of a minimal optimal cytotoxic T-cell epitope within the hepatitis B virus nucleocapsid protein. *Journal of Virology*, **67**, 2376–80.

Bonino, F., Brunetto, M. R., Rizzetto, M. & Will, H. (1991). Hepatitis B virus unable to secrete e antigen [editorial]. *Gastroenterology*, **100**, 1138–41.

Botarelli, P., Brunetto, M. R., Minutello, M. A. *et al.* (1993). T-lymphocyte response to hepatitis C virus in different clinical courses of infection. *Gastroenterology*, **104**, 580–7.

Brechot, C., Hadchouel, M., Scotto, J. *et al.* (1981). Detection of hepatitis B virus DNA in liver and serum: a direct appraisal of the chronic carrier state. *Lancet*, **ii**, 765–8.

Brillanti, S., Masci, C., Ricci, P., Miglioli, M. & Barbara, L. (1992). Significance of IgM antibody to hepatitis C virus in patients with chronic hepatitis C. *Hepatology*, **15**, 998–1001.

Bruguera, M., Cremades, M., Salinas, R., Costa, J., Grau, M. & Sans, J. (1992). Impaired response to recombinant hepatitis B vaccine in HIV-infected persons. *Journal of Clinical Gastroenterology*, **14**, 27–30.

Brunetto, M. R., Giarin, M., Oliveri, J. *et al.* (1991b). 'e' Antigen defective hepatitis B virus and course of chronic infection. *Journal of Hepatology*, **13**, Suppl. 4, S82–6.

Brunetto, M. R., Giarin, M. M., Oliveri, F. *et al.* (1991a). Wild-type and e antigen-minus hepatitis B viruses and course of chronic hepatitis. *Proceedings of the National Academy of Sciences, USA*, **88**, 4186–90.

Buti, M., Esteban, R., Espanol, M. T. *et al.* (1991). Influence of human immunodeficiency virus infection on cell-mediated immunity in chronic D hepatitis. *Journal of Infectious Diseases*, **163**, 1351–3.

Carman, W. F., Jacyna, M. R., Hadziyannis, S. *et al.* (1989). Mutation preventing formation of hepatitis B e antigen in patients with chronic hepatitis B infection. *Lancet*, **ii**, 588–91.

Chang, M.-F., Chang, S. C., Chang, C.-I., Wu, K. & Kang, H.-Y. (1992). Nuclear localization signals, but not putative leucine zipper motifs, are essential for nuclear transport of hepatitis delta antigen *Journal of Virology*, **66**, 6019–27.

Chang, M.-F., Sun, C.-Y., Chen, C. J. & Chang, S. C. (1993). Functional motifs of delta antigen essential for RNA binding and replication of hepatitis delta virus. *Journal of Virology*, **67**, 2529–36.

Chao, M., Hsieh, S.-Y. & Taylor, J. (1990). Role of two forms of hepatitis delta virus antigen: Evidence for a mechanism of self-limiting genome replication. *Journal of Virology*, **64**, 5066–9.

Chao, M., Hsieh, S.-Y., Luo, G. & Taylor, J. (1991). The antigen of human hepatitis delta virus: The significance of the two major electrophoretic forms. *Progress in Clinical Biology Research*, **364**, 275–81.

Chemello, L., Cavalletto, D., Pontisso, P. *et al.* (1993). Patterns of antibodies to hepatitis C virus in patients with chronic non-A, non-B hepatitis and their relationship to viral replication and liver disease. *Hepatology*, **17**, 179–82.

Chen, P. J., Wang, J. T., Hwang, L. H. *et al.* (1992). Transient immunoglobulin M antibody response to hepatitis C capsid antigen in posttransfusion hepatitis C: putative serological marker for acute viral infection. *Proceedings of the National Academy of Sciences, USA*, **89**, 5971–5.

Chu, C. M. & Liaw, Y. F. (1992). Intrahepatic expression of pre-S1 and pre-S2 antigens in chronic hepatitis B virus infection in relation to hepatitis B virus replication and hepatitis delta virus superinfection. *Gut*, **33**, 1544–8.

Cohen, J. I., Rosenblum, B., Ticehurst, J. R., Daemer, R. J., Feinstone, S. M. & Purcell, R. H. (1987). Complete nucleotide sequence of an attenuated hepatitis A virus: comparison with wild-type virus. *Proceedings of the National Academy of Sciences, USA*, **84**, 2497–501.

Coursaget, P., Yvonnet, B., Bourdil, C. *et al.* (1987). HBsAg positive reactivity in man not due to hepatitis B virus. *Lancet*, **ii**, 1354–8.

Coursaget, P., Yvonnet, B., Bourdil, C. *et al.* (1990). Hepatitis B surface antigen reactivity in man due to a new variant of hepatitis B virus. *Vaccine*, **8** Suppl, S15–17.

Cupps, T. R., Hoofnagle, J. H., Ellis, R. W., Miller, W. J., Gerin, J. L. & Volkman, D. J. (1990). In vitro immune response to hepatitis B surface antigens S and preS2 during acute infection by hepatitis B virus in humans. *Journal of Infectious Diseases*, **161**, 412–19.

Czaja, A. J., Manns, M. P. & Homburger, H. A. (1992). Frequency and significance of antibodies to liver/kidney microsome type I in adults with chronic active hepatitis. *Gastroenterology*, **103**, 1290–5.

Dammacco, F. & Sansonno, D. (1992). Antibodies to hepatitis C virus in essential mixed cryoglobulinaemia. *Clinical and Experimental Immunology*, **87**, 352–6.

Delage, G., Remy-Prince, S. & Montplaisir, S. (1993). Combined active-passive immunization against the hepatitis B virus: five-year follow-up of children born to hepatitis B surface antigen-positive mothers. *Pediatric Infectious Disease Journal*, **12**, 126–30.

Desmet, V. J. (1991). Immunopathology of chronic viral hepatitis [Review]. *Hepato-Gastroenterology*, **38**, 14–21.

Dusheiko, G., Dibisceglie, A., Bowyer, S. *et al.* (1985). Recombinant leukocyte interferon treatment of chronic hepatitis B. *Hepatology*, **5**, 556–60.

Dusheiko, G. M., Hoofnagle, J. H., Cooksley, W. G., James, S. P. & Jones, E. A. (1983). Synthesis of antibodies to hepatitis B virus by cultured lymphocytes from chronic hepatitis B surface antigen carriers. *Journal of Clinical Investigations*, **71**, 1104–13.

Ehata, T., Omata, M., Yokosuka, O., Hosoda, K. & Ohto, M. (1992). Variations in codons 84-101 in the core nucleotide sequence correlate with hepatocellular injury in chronic hepatitis B virus infection. *Journal of Clinical Investigation*, **89**, 332–8.

el-Zimaity, D. M., Hyams, K. C., Imam, I. Z. *et al*. (1993). Acute sporadic hepatitis E in an Egyptian pediatric population. *American Journal of Tropical Medicine and Hygiene*, **48**, 372–6.

Ellerbeck, E. F., Lewis, J. A., Nalin, D. *et al*. (1992). Safety profile and immunogenicity of an inactivated vaccine derived from an attenuated strain of hepatitis A. *Vaccine*, **10**, 668–72.

Fagan, E. A., Ellis, D. W., Tovey, G. M., Portmann, B., Williams, R. & Zuckerman, A. J. (1989). Virus-like particles in liver in sporadic non-A, non-B fulminant hepatitis. *Journal of Medical Virology*, **27**, 76–80.

Farci, P., Alter, H. J., Govindarajan, S. *et al*. (1992). Lack of protective immunity against reinfection with hepatitis C virus. *Science*, **258**, 135–40.

Ferrari, C., Penna, A., Bertoletti, A. *et al*. (1990). Cellular immune response to hepatitis B virus-encoded antigens in acute and chronic hepatitis B virus infection. *Journal of Immunology*, **145**, 3442–9.

Ferrari, C., Cavalli, A., Penna, A. *et al*. (1992). Fine specificity of the human T-cell response to the hepatitis B virus preS1 antigen. *Gastroenterology*, **103**, 255–63.

Flehmig, B., Heinricy, U. & Pfisterer, M. (1989). Immunogenicity of a killed hepatitis A vaccine in seronegative volunteers. *Lancet*, **i**, 1039–41.

Fleischer, B. & Vallbracht, A. (1991). Demonstration of virus-specific cytotoxic T lymphocytes in liver tissue in hepatitis A – a model for immunopathological reactions. *Behring Institute Mitteilungen*, **89**, 226–30.

Fujii, H., Moriyama, K., Sakamoto, N. *et al*. (1992). Gly 145 to Arg substitution in HBs antigen of immune escape mutant of hepatitis B virus. *Biochemical and Biophysical Research Communications*, **184**, 1152–7.

Galibert, F., Mandart, E., Fitoussi, F., Tiollais, P. & Charnay, P. (1979). Nucleotide sequence of the hepatitis B virus genome (subtype ayw) cloned in *E. coli*. *Nature*, **281**, 646–50.

Garcia-Buey, L., Lopez-Botet, M., Garcia-Sanchez, A. *et al*. (1993). Variability in the expression of a beta 2-microglobulin epitope on hepatocytes in chronic type C hepatitis on treatment with interferon. *Hepatology*, **17**, 372–82.

Gupta, H., Iyenger, B. & Tandon, B. N. (1993). Localization of a new enteric non-A, non-B [HEV] virus in target organ liver. *Gastroenterologia Japonica*, **28**, 46–50.

Hadziyannis, S. J., Lieberman, H. M., Karvountzis, G. G. & Shafritz, D. A. (1983). Analysis of liver disease, nuclear HBcAg, viral replication and hepatitis B virus DNA in liver and serum of HBeAg versus anti-HBe positive carriers of hepatitis B virus. *Hepatology*, **3**, 656–62.

Hadziyannis, S. J., Hatzakis, A., Papaioannou, C., Anastassakos, C. & Vassiliadis, E. (1987). Endemic hepatitis delta virus infection in a Greek community. *Progress in Clinical and Biological Research*, **234**, 181–202.

Heathcote, J., Kim, Y. I., Yim, C. K., LeBrocq, J. & Read, S. E. (1989). Interferon-associated lymphocyte 2'5'-oligoadenylate synthetase in acute and chronic viral hepatitis. *Hepatology*, **9**, 105–9.

Hsu, H. Y., Chang, M. H., Hsieh, K. H. *et al*. (1992). Cellular immune response to HGcAG in mother-to-infant transmission of hepatitis B virus. *Hepatology*, **15**, 770–6.

Hyams, K. C., McCarthy, M. C., Kaur, M. *et al*. (1992). Acute sporadic hepatitis E in children living in Cairo, Egypt. *Journal of Medical Virology*, **37**, 274–7.

Ikeda, Y., Toda, G., Hashimoto, N., Umeda, N., Miyake, K. & Yamanaka, M. (1991). Naturally occurring anti-interferon-alpha 2a antibodies in patients with acute viral hepatitis. *Clinical and Experimental Immunology*, **85**, 80–4.

Imawari, M., Nomura, M., Kaieda, T. *et al.* (1989). Establishment of a human T-cell clone cytotoxic for both autologous and allogenic hepatocytes from chronic hepatitis patients with type non-A, non-B virus. *Proceedings of the National Academy of Sciences, USA*, **86**, 2883–7.

Ishikawa, T., Kakumu, S., Yoshioka, K., Wakita, T., Takayanagi, M. & Olido, E. (1992). Immune response of peripheral blood mononuclear cells to antigenic determinants within hepatitis B core antigen in HB virus-infected man. *Liver*, **12**, 100–5.

Jameel, S., Durgapal, H., Habibullah, C. M., Khuroo, M. S. & Panda, S. K. (1992). Enteric non-A, non-B hepatitis: epidemics, animal transmission, and hepatitis E virus detection by the polymerase chain reaction. *Journal of Medical Virology*, **37**, 263–70.

Jung, M. C., Spengler, U., Schraut, W. *et al.* (1991). Hepatitis B virus antigen-specific T-cell activation in patients with acute and chronic hepatitis B. *Journal of Hepatology*, **13**, 310–17.

Karayiannis, P., Saldanha, J., Monjardino, J. *et al.* (1990). Immunization of woodchucks with recombinant hepatitis delta antigen does not protect against hepatitis delta virus infection. *Hepatology*, **12**, 1125–8.

Karayiannis, P., Saldanha, J., Monjardino, J., Jackson, A., Luther, S. & Thomas, H. C. (1993). Immunisation of woodchucks with hepatitis delta antigen expressed by recombinant vaccinia and baculoviruses, controls HDV superinfection. *Progress in Clinical and Biological Research*, **382**, 193–9.

Khuroo, M. S. & Dar, M. Y. (1992). Hepatitis E: evidence for person-to-person transmission and inability of low dose immune serum globulin from an Indian source to prevent it. *Indian Journal of Gastroenterology*, **11**, 113–16.

Kikuchi, T., Onji, M., Michitaka, K. & Ohta, Y. (1992). Anti-hepatitis C virus immunoglobulin M antibody in patients with chronic hepatitis type C. *Hepato-Gastroenterology*, **39**, 525–8.

Koziel, M. J., Dudley, D., Wong, J. T., Dienstag, J., Houghton, M. & Ralston, R. (1992). Intrahepatic cytotoxic T lymphocytes specific for hepatitis C virus in persons with chronic hepatitis. *Journal of Immunology*, **149**, 3339–44 [published erratum appears in *Journal of Immunology* 1993 **150**, 2563].

Krawczynski, K. (1993). Hepatitis E. *Hepatology*, **17**, 932–41.

Kruskall, M. S., Alper, C. A., Awdeh, Z., Yunis, E. J. & Marcus-Bagley, D. (1992). The immune response to hepatitis B vaccine in humans: inheritance patterns in families. *Journal of Experimental Medicine*, **175**, 495–502.

Kurane, I., Binn, L. N., Bancroft, W. H. & Ennis, F. A. (1985). Human lymphocyte responses to hepatitis A virus-infected cells: interferon production and lysis of infected cells. *Journal of Immunology*, **135**, 2140–4.

Lau, J. Y., Bain, V. G., Davies, S. E., O'Grady, J. G., Alberti, A. & Alexander, G. J. (1992). High-level expression of hepatitis B viral antigens in fibrosing cholestatic hepatitis. *Gastroenterology*, **102**, 956–62.

Lau, J. Y., Davis, G. L., Orito, E., Qian, K. P. & Mizokami, M. (1993). Significance of antibody to the host cellular gene derived epitope GOR in chronic hepatitis C virus infection. *Journal of Hepatology*, **17**, 253–7.

Lee, J. H., Paglieroni, T. G., Holland, P. V. & Zeldis, J. B. (1992). Chronic hepatitis B virus infection in an anti-HBc-nonreactive blood donor: variant virus or defective immune response? *Hepatology*, **16**, 24–30.

Lemon, S. M. (1985). Type A viral hepatitis. New development in an old disease. [Review]. *New England Journal of Medicine*, **313**, 1059–67.

Lenzi, M., Ballardini, G., Fusconi, M., Cassani, F., Selleri, L., Volta, U. & Bianchi, F. B. (1990). Type 2 autoimmune hepatitis and hepatitis C virus infection. *Lancet*, **335**, 258–9.

Lenzi, M., Johnson, P. J., McFarlane, I. G. *et al.* (1991). Antibodies to hepatitis C virus in autoimmune liver disease: evidence for geographical heterogeneity. *Lancet*, **338**, 277–80.

Lok, A. S., Kwan, W. K., Moeckli, R. *et al.* (1992). Seroepidemiological survey of hepatitis E in Hong Kong by recombinant-based enzyme immunoassays. *Lancet*, **340**, 1205–8.

Lunel, F., Abuaf, N., Frangeul, L. *et al.* (1992). Liver/kidney microsome antibody type 1 and hepatitis C virus infection. *Hepatology*, **16**, 630–6.

Manns, M. P., Griffin, K. J., Sullivan, K. F. & Johnson, E. F. (1991). LKM-1 autoantibodies recognize a short linear sequence in P450IID6, a cytochrome P-450 monooxygenase. *Journal of Clinical Investigation*, **88**, 1370–8.

Marwick, C. (1992). Hepatitis A vaccines considered for licensing [news]. *Journal of the American Medical Association*, **267**, 2007–8.

Mason, W. S. & Taylor, J. M. (1991). Liver transplantation: A model for the transmission of hepatitis delta virus. *Gastroenterology*, **101**, 1741–3.

McFarlane, I. G., Smith, H. M., Johnson, P. J., Bray, G. P., Vergani, D. & Williams, R. (1990). Hepatitis C virus antibodies in chronic active hepatitis: pathogenetic factor or false-positive result? *Lancet*, **335**, 754–7.

McFarlane, I. G., Chaggar, K., Davis, S. E., Smith, H. M., Alexander, G. J. & Williams, R. (1991). IgA class antibodies to hepatitis delta virus antigen in acute and chronic hepatitis delta virus infections. *Hepatology*, **14**, 980–4.

Mehta, S. U., Mishiro, S., Sekiguchi, K. *et al.* (1992). Immune response to GOR, a marker for non-A, non-B hepatitis and its correlation with hepatitis C virus infection. *Journal of Clinical Immunology*, **12**, 178–84.

Michel, G., Ritter, A., Gerken, G., Meyer zum Buschenfelde, K. H. & Decker, R. (1992). Anti-GOR and hepatitis C virus in autoimmune liver disease. *Lancet*, **339**, 267–9.

Milich, D. R., Thornton, G. B., Neurath, A. R., Kent, S. B., Michel, M.L., Tiollais, P. & Chisari, F. V. (1985*a*). Enhanced immunogenicity of the pre-S region of hepatitis B surface antigen. *Science*, **228**, 1195–9.

Milich, D. R. (1988). T and B cell recognition of hepatitis B viral antigens. *Immunology Today*, **9**, 380–6.

Milich, D. R., McLachlan, A., Stahl, S., Wingfield, P., Thornton, G., Hughes, J. L. & Jones, J. E. (1988). Comparative immunogenicity of hepatitis B virus core and e antigens. *Journal of Immunology*, **141**, 3617–24.

Milich, D. R., Jones, J. E. McLachlan, A., Houghten, R., Thornton, G. B. & Hughes, J. L. (1989). Distinction between immunogenicity and tolerogenicity among HBcAg T cell determinants. Influence of peptide-MHC interaction. *Journal of Immunology*, **143**, 3148–56.

Milich, D. R., Jones, J. E., Hughes, J. L., Price, J., Raney, A. K. & McLachlan, A. (1990). Is a function of the secreted hepatitis B e antigen to induce immunologic tolerance *in utero*. *Proceedings of the National Academy of Sciences, USA*, **87**, 6599–603.

Milich, D. R., McNamara, M. K., McLachlan, A., Thornton, G. B. & Chisari, F. V. (1985*b*). Distinct H-2-linked regulation of T-cell responses to the pre-S and S regions of the same hepatitis B surface antigen polypeptide allows circumvention of nonresponsiveness to the S region. *Proceedings of the National Academy of Sciences, USA*, **82**, 8168–72.

Milich, D. R., Peterson, D. L., Leroux-Roels, G. G., Lerner, R. A. & Chisari, F. V. (1985*c*). Genetic regulation of the immune response to hepatitis B surface antigen (HBsAg). VI. T cell fine specificity. *Journal of Immunology*, **134**, 4203–11.

Minutello, M. A., Pileri, P., Unutmaz, D. *et al.* (1993). Compartmentalization of T lymphocytes to the site of disease: Intrahepatic CD4$^+$ T cells specific for the protein NS4 of hepatitis C virus in patients with chronic hepatitis C. *Journal of Experimental Medicine*, **178**, 17–25.

Mishiro, S., Hoshi, Y., Takeda, K. *et al.* (1990). Non-A, non-B hepatitis specific antibodies directed at host-derived epitope: implication for an autoimmune process. *Lancet*, **336**, 1400–3. [published erratum appears in *Lancet* 1990; **337**, 252].

Mishra, A., Durgapal, H., Manivel, V., Acharya, S. K., Rao, K. V. & Panda, S. K. (1992). Immune response to hepatitis B virus surface antigen peptides during HBV infection. *Clinical and Experimental Immunology*, **90**, 194–8.

Missale, G., Redeker, A., Person, J., Fowler, P., Guilhot, S., Schlicht, H. J. and Chisari, F. V. (1993). HLA-A31- and HLA-Aw68-restricted cytotoxic T cell responses to a single hepatitis B virus nucleocapsid epitope during acute viral hepatitis. *Journal of Experimental Medicine*, 177, 751–62.

Mondelli, M., Vergni, G. M., Alberti, A. *et al.* (1982). Specificity of T lymphocyte cytotoxicity to autologous hepatocytes in chronic hepatitis B virus infection: evidence that T cells are directed against HBV core antigen expressed on hepatocytes. *Journal of Immunology*, 129, 2773–8.

Moriyama, T., Guilhot, S., Klopchin, K. *et al.* (1990). Immunobiology and pathogenesis of hepatocellular injury in hepatitis B virus transgenic mice. *Science*, 248, 361–4.

Muller, C., Knoflach, P. & Zielinski, C. C. (1993). Reduced production of immunoreactive interleukin-1 by peripheral blood monocytes of patients with acute and chronic viral hepatitis. *Digestive Diseases and Sciences*, 38, 477–81.

Naik, S. R., Aggarwal, R., Salunke, P. N. & Mehrotra, N. N. (1992). A large waterborne viral hepatitis E epidemic in Kanpur, India. *Bulletin of the World Health Organization*, 70, 597–604.

Negro, F., Gerin, J. L., Purcell, R. H. & Miller, R. H. (1989). Basis of hepatitis delta virus disease? *Nature*, 341, 111.

Negro, F. & Rizzetto, M. (1993). Pathobiology of hepatitis delta virus. *Journal of Hepatology*, 17 Suppl. 3, S149–53.

Ni, Y. H., Hsu, H. Y., Chang, M. H., Chen, D. S. & Les, C. Y. (1993). Absence or delayed appearance of hepatitis B core antibody in chronic hepatitis B surface antigen carrier children. *Journal of Hepatology*, 17, 150–4.

Okamoto, H., Yotsumoto, S., Akahane, Y. *et al.* (1990). Hepatitis B viruses with precore region defects prevail in persistently infected hosts along with seroconversion to the antibody against e antigen. *Journal of Virology*, 64, 1298–303.

Okamoto, H., Yano, K., Nozaki, Y. *et al.* (1992). Mutations within the S gene of hepatitis B virus transmitted from mothers to babies immunized with hepatitis B immune globulin and vaccine. *Pediatric Research*, 32, 264–8.

Onji, M., Kikuchi, T., Kumon, I. *et al.* (1992). Intrahepatic lymphocyte subpopulations and HLA class I antigen expression by hepatocytes in chronic hepatitis C. *Hepato-Gastroenterology*, 39, 340–3.

Ottobrelli, A., Marzano, A., Smedile, A. *et al.* (1991). Patterns of hepatitis delta virus reinfection and disease in liver transplantation. *Gastroenterology*, 101, 1649–55.

Ou, J., Lamb, O. & Rutter, W. (1986). Hepatitis B virus gene function: the precore region targets the core antigen to cellular membranes and causes the secretion of the e antigen. *Proceedings of the National Academy of Sciences, USA*, 83, 1578–82.

Penna, A., Fowler, P., Bertoletti A. *et al.* (1992*a*). Hepatitis B virus (HBV)-specific cytotoxic T-cell (CTL) response in humans: characterization of HLA class II-restricted CTLs that recognize endogenously synthesized HBV envelope antigens. *Journal of Virology*, 66, 1193–8.

Penna, A., Chisari, F. V., Bertoletti, A. *et al.* (1991). Cytotoxic T lymphocytes recognize an HLA-A2-restricted epitope within the hepatitis B virus nucleocapsid antigen. *Journal of Experimental Medicine*, 174, 1565–70.

Penna, A., Bertoletti, A., Cavalli, A. *et al.* (1992*b*). Fine specificity of the human T cell response to hepatitis B virus core antigen. *Archives of Virology – Supplementum*, 4, 23–8.

Peters, M., Vierling, J., Gershwin, M. E., Milich, D., Chisari, F. V. & Hoofnagle, J. H. (1991). Immunology and the liver. *Hepatology*, 13, 977–94.

Phillips, M. J., Blendis, L. M., Poucell, S. *et al.* (1991). Syncytial giant-cell hepatitis – sporadic hepatitis with distinctive pathological features, a severe clinical course, and paramyxoviral features. *New England Journal of Medicine*, 324, 455–60.

Pignatelli, M., Water, J., Lever, A. M. L. et al. (1986). HLA class I antigens on hepatocyte membrane: Increased expression during interferon therapy of chronic hepatitis B. *Hepatology*, **6**, 349–53.

Ping, L.-H. & Lemon, S. M. (1992). Antigenic structure of human hepatitis A virus defined by analysis of escape mutants selected against murine monoclonal antibodies. *Journal of Virology*, **66**, 2208–16.

Pontisso, P., Poon, M. C., Tiollais, P. & Brechot, C. (1984). Detection of hepatitis B virus DNA in mononuclear blood cells. *British Medical Journal of Clinical Research*, **288**, 1563–6.

Prevot, S., Marechal, J., Pillot, J. & Prevot, J. (1992). Relapsing hepatitis A in Saimiri monkeys experimentally reinfected with a wild type of hepatitis A virus (HAV). *Archives of Virology – Supplementum*, **4**, 5–10.

Quiroga, J. A., Mora, I., Porres, J. C. & Carreno, V. (1988). Elevation of 2′,5′-oligoadenylate synthetase activity and HLA-I associated beta 2-microglobulin in response to recombinant interferon-gamma administration in chronic HBeAg-positive hepatitis. *Journal of Interferon Research*, **8**, 755–63.

Quiroga, J. A., Bosch, O., Gonzalez, R., Marriott, E., Castillo, I. & Bartolome, J. (1992). Immunoglobulin M antibody to hepatitis C virus during interferon therapy for chronic hepatitis C. *Gastroenterology*, **103**, 1285–9.

Ralston, R., Thudium, K., Berger, K., Quo, C., Gervase, B., Hall, J., Selby, M. et al. (1993). Characterization of hepatitis C virus envelope glycoprotein complexes expressed by recombinant vaccinia viruses. *Journal of Virology*, **67**, 6753–61.

Rizzetto, M. (1983). The delta agent. *Hepatology*, **3**, 729–37.

Rizzetto, M. (1989). Hepatitis delta virus (HDV) infection and disease. *Ric Clin Lab*, **19**, 11–26.

Rizzetto, M., Verme, G., Recchia, S. et al. (1983). Chronic hepatitis in carriers of hepatitis B surface antigen, with intrahepatic expression of the delta antigen. An active and progressive disease unresponsive to immunosuppressive treatment. *Annals of Internal Medicine*, **98**, 437–41.

Rizzetto, M., Verme, G., Gerin, J. L. & Purcell, R. H. (1986). Hepatitis delta virus disease. *Progress in Liver Disease*, **8**, 417–31.

Robertson, B. H., Jia, X. Y., Tian, H., Margolis, H. S., Summers, D.F. & Ehrenfeld, E. (1992). Serological approaches to distinguish immune response to hepatitis A vaccine and natural infection. *Vaccine*, **10** Suppl. 1, S106–9.

Saito, T., Kamimura, T., Ishibashi, M., Shinzawa, H. & Takahashi, T. (1992). Electron microscopic study of hepatitis B virus-associated antigens on the infected liver cell membrane in relation to analysis of immune target antigens in chronic hepatitis B. *Gastroenterologia Japonica*, **27**, 734–44.

Schlicht, H. J., von Brunn, A. & Theilmann, L. (1991). Antibodies in anti-HBe-positive patient sera bind to an HBe protein expressed on the cell surface of human hepatoma cells: implications for virus clearance. *Hepatology*, **13**, 57–61.

Shafritz, D. A., Shouval, D., Sherman, H. I., Hadziyannis, S. J. & Kew, M. C. (1981). Integration of hepatitis B virus DNA into the genome of liver cells in chronic liver disease and hepatocellular carcinoma. Studies on percutaneous liver biopsies and post-mortem tissue specimens. *New England Journal of Medicine*, **305**, 1067–73.

Siddiqui, A., Jameel, S. & Mapoles, J. (1986). Transcriptional control elements of hepatitis B surface antigen gene. *Proceedings of the National Academy of Sciences, USA*, **83**, 566–70.

Siegl, G. & Lemon, S. M. (1990). Recent advances in hepatitis A vaccine development. [Review]. *Virus Research*, **17**, 75–92.

Smith, J. B., Gottlieb, P. A. & Dinter-Gottlieb, G. (1992). A sequence element necessary for self-cleavage of the antigenomic hepatitis delta RNA in 20 M formamide. *Biochemistry*, **31**, 9629–35.

Stahl, S., MacKay, P., Magazin, M., Bruce, S. A. & Murray, K. (1982). Hepatitis B virus core antigen: synthesis in *Escherichia coli* and application in diagnosis. *Proceedings of the National Academy of Sciences, USA*, **79**, 1606–10.

Stapleton, J. T., Lange, D. K., LeDuc, J. W., Binn, L. N., Jansen, R. W. & Lemon, S. M. (1991). The role of secretory immunity in hepatitis A virus infection. *Journal of Infectious Diseases*, **163**, 7–11.

Stapleton, J. T., Raina, V., Winokur, P. L. *et al.* (1993). Antigenic and immunogenic properties of recombinant hepatitis A virus 14S and 70S subviral particles. *Journal of Virology*, **67**, 1080–5.

Summers, D. F. & Ehrenfeld, E. (1992). Host antibody response to viral structural and nonstructural proteins after hepatitis A virus infection. *Journal of Infectious Diseases*, **165**, 273–80.

Sureau, C., Jacob, J. R., Eichberg, J. W. & Lanford, R. E. (1991). Tissue culture system for infection with human hepatitis delta virus. *Journal of Virology*, **65**, 3443–50.

Taylor, J. (1991). Hepatitis delta virus. *Journal of Hepatology*, **13** Suppl. 4, S114–15.

Thomas, H. C., Jacyna, M., Waters, J. & Main, J. (1988). Virus–host interaction in chronic hepatitis B virus infection. *Seminars in Liver Disease*, **8**, 342–9.

Tolentino, P., Dianzani, F., Zucca, M. & Giacchino, R. (1992). Decreased interferon response by lymphocytes from children with chronic hepatitis. *Journal of Interferon Research*, Spec. No. 3–6.

Tsai, S. L., Chen, P. J., Lai, M. Y. *et al.* (1992). Acute exacerbations of chronic type B hepatitis are accompanied by increased T cell responses to hepatitis B core and e antigens. Implications for hepatitis B e antigen seroconversion. *Journal of Clinical Investigation*, **89**, 87–96.

Twu, J. S., Lee, C. H., Lin, P. M. & Schloemer,, R. H. (1988). Hepatitis B virus suppresses expression of human beta-interferon. *Proceedings of the National Academy of Sciences, USA*, **85**, 252–6.

Vallbracht, A. & Fleischer, B. (1992). Immune pathogenesis of hepatitis A. *Archives of Virology – Supplementum*, **4**, 3–4.

Vento, S., Garofano, T., Di Perri, G., Dolci, L., Concia, E. & Bassetti, D. (1991). Identification of hepatitis A virus as a trigger for autoimmune chronic hepatitis type 1 in susceptible individuals. *Lancet*, **337**, 1183–7.

Volpes, R., van den Oord, J. J. & Desmet, V. J. (1990). Hepatic expression of intercellular adhesion molecule-1 (ICAM-1) in viral hepatitis B. *Hepatology*, **12**, 148–54.

Waters, J. A., Brown, S. E., Steward, M. W., Howard, C. R. & Thomas, H. C. (1992). Analysis of the antigene epitopes of hepatitis B surface antigen involved in the induction of a protective antibody response. *Virus Research*, **22**, 1–12.

Weimer, T., Schodel, F., Jung, M. C. *et al.* (1990). Antibodies to the RNase H domain of hepatitis B virus P protein are associated with ongoing viral replication. *Journal of Virology*, **64**, 5665–8.

Weiner, A. J., Geysen, H. M., Christopherson, C. *et al.* (1992). Evidence for immune selection of hepatitis C virus (HCV) putative envelope glycoprotein variants: potential role in chronic HCV injections. *Proceedings of the National Academy of Sciences, USA*, **89**, 3468–72.

Wu, H.-N., Wang, Y.-J., Hung, C.-F., Lee, H.-J. & Lai, M. M. C. (1992). Sequence and structure of the catalytic RNA of hepatitis delta virus genomic RNA. *Journal of Molecular Biology*, **223**, 233–45.

Yamada, G., Hyodo, I., Nishihara, T. & Nagashima, H. (1985). Intrahepatic lymphocyte subpopulation defined by monoclonal antibodies in anti-HBe positive type B chronic active hepatitis. *Gastroenterology, Japan*, **20**, 441–6.

Yokosuka, O., Ito, Y., Imazeki, F., Ohto, M. & Omata, M. (1992). Detection of antibody to hepatitis C E2/NS1 protein in patients with type C hepatitis. *Biochemical and Biophysical Research Communications*, **189**, 565–71.

–17–
Immunology of liver transplantation

S. A. SADEK

Introduction

The past three decades have witnessed the evolution of orthotopic liver transplantation from a pioneering procedure with a prohibitive mortality and morbidity to a standardised therapeutic measure for end-stage liver disease. Currently, one year survival for elective cases are often in excess of 80% with an excellent quality of life (Tarter *et al.*, 1988). Equally important, long-term patient and graft survival in non-malignant cases, is excellent (Iwatsuki, Shaw & Starzl, 1985).

Issues in graft selection

ABO groups

The majority of transplant centres regard blood group compatibility as the prime immunological selection criterion. Transplantation of a liver from a donor with an incompatible ABO blood group is feasible, with well-documented reports of this being performed usually in urgent situations (Gordon *et al.*, 1986). However, it soon became clear that results were quite poor, with a substantial number of grafts rapidly failing and requiring urgent retransplantation (Rego *et al.*, 1987; Gugenheim *et al.*, 1990).

On the other hand, transplantation of compatible but not identical livers is common practice, especially for recipients with the less common blood groups. Interestingly, the results of ABO identical grafts were slightly better than the ABO compatible but non-identical organs (White *et al.*, 1987; Gugenheim *et al.*, 1990). An occasional complication with compatible, non-identical grafts, is the occurrence of a form of graft-versus-host disease, where the immunocompetent passenger lymphocytes within the transplanted liver produce antibodies against the recipient erythrocytes. The ensuing haemolysis is usually mild and self-limiting in the majority of cases (Gordon et al., 1986), but occasionally may be severe enough to manifest clinically, with extreme cases requiring massive transfusion and may even lead to patient death. Diagnosis is straight forward, with a positive direct Coombs test and it is possible to characterise the specific anti-erythrocyte antibodies.

Cross matching

It is well established that renal transplantation in the presence of donor-specific cytotoxic antibodies, demonstrated by a positive cross-match, will result in rapid graft loss. The liver behaves in a totally contrary manner. Not only is transplantation possible in presence of a positive cross-match with no adverse outcome, but donor-specific cytotoxic antibodies rapidly disappear after transplantation, permitting renal transplant from the same donor in sensitised patients (Fung et al., 1988; Starzl et al., 1989). The resistance of the liver, to the presence of pre-existing cytotoxic antibodies, will be discussed with the topic of hyperacute rejection.

The role of histocompatibility antigen

The major histocompatibility antigens have a well-documented role in renal transplantation. Beneficial matches improve graft survival or at least reduce the incidence of acute rejection and hence influence long-term graft function (Opelz, 1987). However, early studies of liver transplantation in pigs, implied that the liver may be a privileged organ exhibiting minimal rejection, with some grafts surviving without immunosuppression. This concept, when coupled with the relatively small waiting list pool of liver transplant recipients, prompted transplant surgeons to ignore HLA matching in patient selection. This process generated retrospective data, which up to now has consistently failed to show any clear survival advantage of good HLA matching. Interestingly, several of these studies suggest that there is a clear disadvantage with certain aspects of HLA matching. One such study indicated that Class I matched with a Class II antigen mismatch, increases the incidence of chronic rejection, as manifested by the vanishing bile duct syndrome (Donaldson et al., 1987). The largest series from Pittsburgh involving 500 transplants, suggests that overall graft survival is actually reduced in grafts matched for Class I or Class II antigens. Conversely, they also suggest that graft failure due to rejection is associated with poor matching (Markus et al., 1988). The mechanisms underlying these observations are far from clear.

Rejection

Hyperacute rejection

This form of rejection is well documented in renal transplantation, where it occurs almost immediately following transplantation in patients with pre-formed antibodies, resulting in invariable graft loss (Starzl *et al.*, 1968). This process remains a rather ambiguous phenomenon in hepatic transplantation. In animal models, hyperacute rejection can be reliably demonstrated if the recipient is presensitised against the donor (Gubernatis *et al.*, 1987). In humans, the situation remains mainly limited to a few case reports (Merion & Colletti, 1990; Hanto *et al.*, 1987), where graft loss occurred within hours of implantation and, as discussed before, liver transplantation is regularly performed in sensitised patients, without any substantial adverse effects.

The situation is even more ambiguous when it comes to the so-called accelerated rejection phenomenon, where graft loss occurs within a few days. Hubscher (1989), on behalf of the Birmingham group, described six patients with distinct clinical and pathological criteria, where rapid graft loss occurred within the first three weeks of transplantation. Acute graft failure was accompanied by massive haemorrhagic necrosis of the liver, with minimal evidence of rejection as demonstrated by the paucity of the cellular infiltrates. It is presumed that this is another form of delayed fulminant or hyperacute rejection, possibly attributed to humoral mechanisms (Gubernatis *et al.*, 1989).

Acute rejection

The rejection process is an inflammatory cascade, which is initiated by presentation of the transplant antigens (MHC) to the host immune system, resulting in immune activation and subsequently the recruitment of the effector mechanisms, leading to graft damage (Ascher *et al.*, 1984; Adams & Neuberger, 1990; Adams, 1990). Medawar (1944), first described the immunological phenomenon associated with the rejection of foreign tissues and attributed it to the difference in genetic constitution between donor and recipient. Since then, the major interests, in clinical and immunological study of the allograft, have primarily concentrated on the effector mechanisms mediating the rejection process, which is largely T cell dependent and MHC antigen restricted.

Interestingly, Batchelor, Welch & Burgos (1984), found that MHC antigens alone are relatively weak immunological stimuli. Hence, to provoke an adequate recipient T cell response, a second or co-stimulus is required. The donor accessory cells, such as the dendritic or passenger leucocytes, are not only capable of fulfilling the role of antigen presentation to the recipient cell, but also are capable of producing such a second signal (Steinman *et al.*, 1986).

The exact mechanisms that initiate the cascade, which culminates in acute graft rejection, remain to be fully elucidated. The effector mechanisms, however, are much better documented and understood. Several mechanisms are postulated: the first which has been mentioned above is direct antibody and complement-mediated damage and is primarily implicated in the rare phenomenon of hyperacute rejection.

The T-cell mediated responses play the central role in the acute rejection process. During acute rejection, the inflammatory infiltrate is concentrated around the portal tract and the central vein. There is little or no infiltrate within the hepatic lobule. Thus, the main brunt of the process is directed toward the bile ducts and the endothelial cell, which express MHC antigens.

Normally hepatocytes, at most, weakly express MHC class I antigens, while Kuppffer cells and endothelial cells strongly express both class I and class II antigens (Steinhoff, Wonigeit & Pichlmayer, 1988). During the acute rejection process, there is undoubtedly increased hepatocyte expression of MHC class I antigen (So *et al.*, 1987). However, this phenomenon is also present during episodes of cholangitis and other infections such as CMV hepatitis and thus may be a secondary phenomenon, probably due to local release of cytokines.

The phenotype of inflammatory cells in the portal tracts during the rejection process is well defined. There is primarily a clear predominance of T lymphocytes with minimal B-cell infiltrates (Lautenschlager *et al.*, 1988). There is normally an initial predominance of activated CD4 (helper) cells expressing DR antigen and are hence, implicated in the initiation of the rejection process (Markus *et al.*, 1987). Subsequently, CD8 cell (suppressor and cytotoxic) are seen in the portal tracts, restoring the normal CD4/CD8 ratio.

Immunological indices of rejection

A simple, non-invasive, reproducible and reliable marker of acute rejection still eludes us. However, there are many indirect markers of graft dysfunction, that provide an indication of ongoing rejection and perhaps response to therapy. Lymphocyte activation is associated with expression of specific membrane markers and the secretion of cytokines. It is well recognised that interleukin-2 (IL2), plays a central role in lymphocyte activation. However, attempts at measuring any increase in its serum level during rejection have been disappointing (Tilg *et al.*, 1990). The IL2 receptor is shed in a stable soluble form and although it was clearly shown to be elevated during rejection, this was found to be a non-specific marker, as it was also noted to be elevated during infective processes (Adams *et al.*, 1989*a*, Perkins *et al.*, 1989). Other substances such as gamma interferon, beta-2-microglobulin and neopterin have also been disappointingly non-specific and relatively insensitive.

An alternative approach is to examine the product of target organ damage. In the case of the liver, these are primarily the biliary epithelium and the venous endothelium. Two proteins specific to biliary epithelium, are epithelial membrane antigen and secretory component. Only the latter's level rose in bile during rejection but again this was found to be non-specific (Adams *et al.*, 1987). As mentioned before, there is increased expression of class I MHC antigens on biliary epithelium during rejection. They are expressed on the cell surface in association with beta-2-microglobulin (β2M). Serum and bile levels of soluble Class I antigens and β2M were found to be significantly elevated during rejection (Tilg *et al.*, 1990; Adams *et al.*, 1988; Pollard, Davies & Calne, 1989). Evidence of endothelial damage can be detected by measuring hyaluronic acid, circulating levels of which were found to be elevated 24 hours prior to the onset of rejection (Adams *et al.*, 1989*b*).

Chronic rejection

Although the term 'chronic' implies a slow and prolonged phenomenon, in actual fact chronic rejection is a clear-cut syndrome, which can in some cases manifest within a few weeks from transplantation. The hallmarks of chronic rejection are occlusive arteriopathy and bile duct loss, which appear to be closely related (Oguma *et al.*, 1989). The mechanisms responsible are still not fully elucidated, but it appears to be a combination of arterial ischaemia and immunological damage to the biliary tree. The arteriopathy is of particular relevance, as it appears to be a common phenomenon in various forms of allografts, such as renal and cardiac. In liver transplantation, the distinctive association between arterial occlusive damage and bile duct destruction is not surprising, as the arterial system is the prime source of blood for the biliary tree (Mika, 1966). Parenchymal damage is less extensive and hence the synthetic function of the liver remains largely intact (Wiesner *et al.*, 1991). Histologically, a progressive loss of bile ducts led to what is often termed the 'vanishing bile duct syndrome' (VBDS) (Vierling & Fennel, 1985). Unlike acute rejection, this process is associated with minimal portal infiltrates, which are predominantly lymphocytes, plasma cells and macrophages.

The exact aetiology of VBDS is not known. However, there are some well documented predisposing and associated factors. O'Grady *et al.* (1988) found a strong association between VBDS and the combination of a good HLA-DR match, coupled with cytomegalovirus (CMV) infection. One possible mechanism, is that CMV infection induces cellular expression of class II antigens in the graft. Following transplantation, there is increased expression of Class I antigens (primarily on hepatocytes) and Class II antigens (primarily on bile ducts). Failure of regression of expression towards baseline levels has been associated with chronic rejection (Hubscher, Adams & Elias, 1990). Most of the cellular infiltrates are T cells. Predominance of the cytotoxic CD8 phenotype, has been associated with chronic rejection (McCaugan et al., 1990). There are as yet no conclusive data implicating humoral factors in chronic rejection. However, there is evidence of increased plasma cells in the portal tracts with deposition of IgM immunoglobulins within the arterial wall (Demetrius et al., 1987).

Graft versus host disease

The transplanted liver contains a broad spectrum of potentially immunologically active cells: these include lymphocytes, dendritic cells and Kupffer cells. The continued survival of these cells within the host can potentially result in graft-versus-host disease (GVH). The full clinical syndrome, as seen in bone marrow transplant patients, is quite rare. However, various minor forms can be clinically and immunologically documented. The most common is the haemolytic reaction, seen in some patients with ABO compatible but not identical transplants (*vide supra*). A few case reports exist of the severe form which can potentially respond to increasing immunosuppression (Burdick et al., 1988). In this case, there was clear HLA chimerism within the bone marrow of the host.

Immunosuppression

In spite of substantial advances in the past three decades, the ideal immunosuppressant is yet to be found. The methods, by which the immune system is suppressed, are gradually shifting from the blanket-type general suppression of all leukocytes, to the more specific suppression of T cells and to selection of certain T cell subsets for immunomodulation. Attempts are being made to evaluate drugs that would help induce tolerance.

Drugs

The clinical introduction of cyclosporin (Cya), coincided with a rapid proliferation in the number of liver transplants and substantial improvement in clinical outcome. Cya is the first routinely employed immunosuppressant, that selectively inhibits T lymphocyte proliferation. It acts by suppressing IL2 production at the genome level, hence preventing the immunological cascade that follows antigen presentation and preventing clonal expansion of immunocompetent T cells. FK506 is very similar in action to Cya but is substantially more potent. Both drugs have substantial clinical side effects.

Currently, a plethora of new drugs are being introduced and evaluated in various clinical trials. The most salient feature, they all share, is the paucity of well-conducted clinical trials to evaluate their true potential. A few examples of such drugs include rapamycin which also inhibits T cell activation, RS-61443 a purine synthesis inhibitor and hence, inhibits both T and B cell proliferation, 15-deoxyspergualin and brequinar.

Monoclonal antibodies

The recent explosion in the development of molecular biological techniques has enabled us for the first time to start examining methods of lymphocyte activation and the associated expression of surface markers. This inevitably led to the testing and development of many monoclonal antibodies (mAB), which bind to these surface markers in the hope of inhibition and modulation of lymphocyte responses to alloantigens. One major advance which significantly reduces side-effects, is the humanisation of the mAB by grafting the structural framework of a human antibody to the variable segment or antigen-specific segment of the mAB (Winter & Milstein, 1991).

OKT3 is currently the most widely used monoclonal antibody, which binds to part of the T cell receptor (CD3) complex. The major impact of this, very potent, murine, monoclonal antibody, has been in the reversal of steroid-resistant, acute rejection (Cosimi et al., 1981). Many centres also choose to use it in induction regimens, particularly in North America. Its primary, immediate side-effect, following initial administration, is the cytokine-release syndrome, when the antibody combines with the CD3 receptor on the T cells resulting in their stimulation and release of IL2 and TNF, leading to a flu-like illness, which can be severe. Fatal, acute, pulmonary oedema is well documented. Other anti-CD3, mAB are being developed and may have less side-effects (Waid et al., 1991).

New monoclonal antibodies

The clinical success, of OKT3, was inevitably followed by the development of a substantial number of new monoclonal antibodies. Many are currently undergoing experimental evaluation in vitro and in animal models. Anti-CD4 is more specific in its binding than OKT3, combining with one T cell subset (helper/inducer), which plays a pivotal role in the development of inflammatory responses. Although human data are very limited (Morel *et al.*, 1990) and long-term side-effects are unknown, an exciting experimental finding is the induction of tolerance (Qin *et al.*, 1989). This has particularly been noted when anti-CD4 is given in conjunction with donor antigen prior to transplantation (Pearson *et al.*, 1991).

Anti-CD7, in its chimeric or humanised form, was developed in the UK at the Royal Free Hospital and has undergone clinical trials (Akbar *et al.*, 1990). It is expressed primarily on naive T cells. It was successful in abolishing the CD7 expression on lymphocytes over a substantial period of time, although it had no significant outright effect on the incidence of rejection. Anti-CD25, which binds to part of the interleukin-2 receptor, is currently undergoing clinical trials.

Xenotransplantation

Clinical aspects

Organ shortage is rapidly imposing a major restricting factor on liver transplant programmes. The consistent growth of transplantation, will invariably lead to significant shortages in the next few years. In 1992 in the UK, almost 500 liver transplants were performed, with a potential organ surplus of less than 200 livers. Hence, clinicians are often faced with the difficult prospect of rationing organs. In addition, transplantation of urgent cases is often delayed, occasionally with fatal outcome, until a suitable organ becomes available. Using animals as donors (xenotransplantation), is a theoretically attractive solution, as it offers a potentially inexhaustible source of organs, allowing careful planning and timing of transplantation. This is of particular relevance in patients with fulminant liver failure, requiring urgent transplantation. Certain countries such as Japan, have no cadaveric programmes and xenotransplantation may be the only avenue.

Another potential use of xenografts, is to capitalise on the fact that certain animals are immune to viruses, that may reinfect a human organ transplant. Hepatitis B being a case in point. Xenotransplantation is now a clinical reality. Starzl's team at Pittsburgh, have at the time of writing, transplanted two baboon livers in human subjects (Starzl *et al.*, 1993). The first in an HIV-positive patient, where the patient regained normal liver function, but died of cerebral haemorrhage approximately 3 months later, the second was in a patient with hepatitis B infection, the baboon being immune to Hepatitis B virus.

Although the first patient eventually died, he did so with good graft function and therefore there is every indication, that this may well result in further development of this approach.

Immunological aspects

White (1993), has recently reviewed the immunology of xenotransplantation. In 1970, Calne attempted to classify xenotransplantation into two-broad categories, based on whether or not grafts were hyper-acutely rejected (Calne, 1970). Organs transplanted between unrelated species, e.g. sheep and dog, were rapidly rejected within minutes or hours and were termed discordant grafts, while organs transplanted across closely related species, behaved similarly as allografts and hence were termed concordant.

This classification often fails to reflect reality. Within the so-called concordant group, the full spectrum of rejection can be demonstrated with grafts that survive without immunosuppression, e.g. wolf to dog (Hameer, Saumweber & Kronback, 1989), those requiring standard T-cell immuno-suppression (Kemp *et al.*, 1988; Chen *et al.*, 1992), and some who reject in spite of substantial immunosuppression, e.g. hamster to rat (Thomas *et al.*, 1991). The latter phenomenon is secondary to the presence of anti-species antibodies and can be experimentally overcome by pre-treatment with cyclophosphamide or methotrexate (Hasan *et al.*, 1992). White (1993) has proposed the hypothesis that the spectrum of rejection emanates from the relative involvement of T and B cells in the rejection process. He suggests that where rejection is primarily a T cell-dependent process, those species are relatively easy to immunosuppress, while B-cell dependent ones are more resistant to conventional therapy.

The future of clinical xenotransplantation will ultimately depend on the success of several strategies that are primarily directed at the first stumbling block, namely hyper-acute rejection. The first approach is to deal with the host natural, anti-species antibodies; for example Hasan *et al.* (1992), used methotrexate and cyclophosphamide prior to transplantation. A second approach is to deal with the targets of these antibodies. Currently, work is largely directed towards understanding endothelial activation and the various epitopes for antibody binding (Platt & Bach, 1991). A third approach deals with complement activation, which plays a crucial part in hyperacute rejection. White *et al.* (1992) demonstrate that transferring human regulators of complement activation (RCA) to animal tissue can protect from complement-mediated tissue destruction. Work is under way to develop genetically modified donor species exhibiting human RCAs, in the hope that this will obviate hyperacute rejection (Cary *et al.*, 1993).

References

Adams, D. H., Burnett, D., Stockley, R. A. *et al.* (1987). Markers of biliary epithelial damage in liver allograft rejection. *Transplant Proceedings*, **19**, 3820–1.

Adams, D. H., Burnett, D., Stockley, R. A. *et al.* (1988). Biliary beta-2-microglobulin in liver allograft rejection. *Hepatology*, **8**, 1565–70.

Adams, D. H., Wang, L., Hubscher, S. G. *et al.* (1989*a*). Soluble interleukin-2 receptors in serum and bile of liver transplant recipients. *Lancet*, **i**, 469–72.

Adams, D. H., Wang, L., Hubscher, S. G. *et al.* (1989*b*). Hepatic endothelial cells: targets in liver allograft rejection? *Gastroenterology*, **97**, 433–8.

Adams, D. H. (1990). Mechanisms of human liver allograft rejection. *Clinical Science*, **78**, 343–50.

Adams, D. H. & Neuberger, J. M. (1990). Patterns of liver allograft rejection. *Journal of Hepatology*, **10**, 113–19.

Akbar, A. N., Amlot, P., Ivory, K. *et al.* (1990). Inhibition of alloresponsive naive and memory T cells by CD7 and CD25 antibodies and by Cyclosporin. *Transplantation*, **50**, 823–5.

Ascher, N. L., Hoffman, R. A., Hanto, D. W. *et al.* (1984). Cellular basis of allograft rejection. *Immunology Review*, **77**, 217–32.

Batchelor, J. R., Welch, K. I. & Burgos, H. (1984). Transplantation antigens *per se* are poor immunogens within a species. *Nature*, **273**, 54–6.

Burdick, J. F., Vogelsang, G. B., Smith, W. J. *et al.* (1988). Severe graft versus host disease in a liver transplant recipient. *New England Journal of Medicine*, **318**, 689–91.

Calne, R. Y. (1970). Organ transplantation between disparate species. *Transplant Proceedings*, **2**, 550–4.

Cary, N., Moody, J., Yannoutsos, N. *et al.* (1993). Tissue expression of human decay accelerating factor, a regulator of complement activation expressed in mice: a potential approach to inhibition of hyperacute xenograft rejection. *Transplant Proceedings*, **25**, 400–1.

Chen, Z., Cobold, S., Metcalfe, S. *et al.* (1992). Tolerance in the mouse to MHC mismatched heart allografts and for rat heart xenografts using monoclonal antibodies to CD4 and CD8. *European Journal of Immunology*, **22**, 805–10.

Cosimi, A. B., Burton, R. C., Colvin, R. B. *et al.* (1981). Treatment of acute renal allograft rejection with OKT3 monoclonal antibody. *Transplantation*, **32**, 535–9.

Demetrius, A. J., Markus, B. H., Burnham, J. *et al.* (1987). Antibody deposition in liver allografts with chronic rejection. *Transplant Proceedings*, **19**, 121–5.

Donaldson, P. T., Alexander, G. J. M., O'Grady, L. *et al.* (1987). Evidence for an immune response to HLA class I antigens in the vanishing-bile duct syndrome after liver transplantation. *Lancet*, **i**, 945–8.

Fung, J., Makowaka, L., Tzakis, A. *et al.* (1988). Combined liver and kidney transplantation: Analysis of patients with preformed lymphocytotoxic antibodies. *Transplant Proceedings*, **20**(suppl. 1), 88–91.

Gordon, R., Iwatsuki, S., Esquivel, C. O. *et al.* (1986). Liver transplantation across ABO groups. *Surgery*, **100**, 342–8.

Gubernatis, G., Lauchart, W., Jonker, M. *et al.* (1987). Signs of hyperacute rejection of liver grafts in rhesus monkeys after donor-specific presensitisation. *Transplant Proceedings* **19**, 1082–1083.

Gubernatis, G., Kemnitz, J., Bornscheuer, A. *et al.* (1989). Potential various appearances of hyperacute rejection in human liver transplantation. *Langenbecks Archives Chirurgie*, **374**, 240–4.

Gugenheim, J., Samuel, D., Reynes, M. *et al.* (1990). Liver transplantation across ABO blood group barriers. *Lancet*, **336**, 519–23.

Hanto, D. W., Snover, D. C., Sibley, R. K. *et al.* (1987). Hyperacute rejection of a human orthotopic liver allograft in a presensitised recipient. *Clinical Transplantation*, **1**, 3004–10.

Hameer, C., Saumweber, D. & Kronback, F. (1989). Xenotransplantation in canines. In ed. M. A. Hardy, pp. 115–24. Amsterdam: Elsevier.

Hasan, R., Van Den Bogaerde, J. B., Wallwork, J. *et al.* (1992). Evidence that long-term survival of concordant xenografts is achieved by inhibition of antispecies antibody production. *Transplantation*, **54**, 408–13.

Hubscher, S. G., Adams, D. H., Neuberger, J. M. *et al.* (1989). Massive haemorrhagic necrosis of the liver following transplantation. *Journal of Clinical Pathology*, **42**, 360–70.

Hubscher, S. G., Adams, D. H. & Elias, E. (1990). Changes in the expression of major histocompatibility complex antigens in liver allograft rejection. *Journal of Pathology*, **162**, 165–71.

Iwatsuki, S., Shaw, B. W. Jr, Starzl, T. E. (1985). Five-year survival after liver transplantation. *Transplant Proceedings*, **17**, 259–63.

Kemp, E., Starklin, T. H., Larsen, S. *et al.* (1988). Cyclosporin in concordant renal hare to rabbit xenotransplantation: prolongation and modification of rejection and adverse effects. *Transplant Proceedings*, **17**, 1351–6.

Lautenschlager, I., Hockerstedt, K., Ahonen, J. *et al.* (1988). Fine-needle aspiration biopsy in the monitoring of liver allografts. *Transplantation*, **46**, 47–52.

McCaugan, G. M., Davies, J. S., Waugh, J. A. *et al.* (1990). A quantitative analysis of T lymphocyte populations in human liver allografts undergoing rejection: the use of monoclonal antibodies and double immunolabelling. *Hepatology*, **12**, 1305–13.

Markus, B. H., Fung, J. J., Zeevi, A. *et al.* (1987). Analysis of T lymphocytes infiltrating human hepatic allografts. *Transplant Proceedings*, **19**, 2470–3.

Markus, B. H., Duquesnoy, R. J., Gordon, R. D. *et al.* (1988). Histocompatibility and liver transplant outcome. Does HLA exert a dualistic effect? *Transplantation*, **46**, 372–7.

Medawar, P. B. (1944). The behaviour and fate of skin autografts and skin homografts in rabbits. *Journal of Anatomy*, **78**, 176–99.

Merion, R. M. & Colletti, L. M. (1990). Hyperacute rejection in porcine liver transplantation. *Transplantation*, **49**, 861–8.

Mika, S. K. (1966). The terminal distribution of the hepatic artery with special reference to arterio-portal anastomosis. *Journal of Anatomy*, **100**, 651–63.

Morel, P., Vincent, C., Corgier, G. *et al.* (1990). Anti CD4 monoclonal administration in renal transplanted patients. *Clinical Immunology and Immunopathology*, **56**, 311–20.

O'Grady, J. G., Alexander, G. J. M., Sutherland, S. *et al.* (1988). Cytomegalovirus infection and donor/recipient HLA antigens: interdependent co-factors in pathogenesis of vanishing bile duct syndrome after liver transplantation. *Lancet*, **ii**, 302–5.

Oguma, S., Belle, S., Starzl, T. E. *et al.* (1989). A histometric analysis of chronically rejected liver allografts: Insights into the mechanisms of bile duct loss: direct immunologic and ischaemic. *Hepatology*, **9**, 204–9.

Opelz, G. (1987). Effect of HLA matching on 10 000 cyclosporin-treated cadaver kidney transplants. *Transplant Proceedings*, **19**, 641.

Pearson, T., Madson, J., Morris, P. *et al.* (1991). Effect of anti-CD4 monoclonal antibody dosage when combined with donor antigen for the induction of transplantation tolerance. *Transplant Proceedings*, **23**, 565–6.

Perkins, J. D., Nelson, D. L., Rakela, J. *et al.* (1989). Soluble interleukin-2 receptor level as an indicator of liver allograft rejection. *Transplantation*, **47**, 77–81.

Platt, J. L. & Bach, F. H. (1991). Discordant xenografting challenges and controversies. *Current Opinions in Immunology*, **3**, 735–9.

Pollard, S. G., Davies, H. F. F. S. & Calne, R. Y. (1989). Soluble class I antigen in human bile. *Transplantation*, **48**, 712–14.

Qin, S., Cobbold, S., Benjamin, R. *et al.* (1989). Induction of classical transplantation tolerance in the adult. *Journal of Experimental Medicine*, **169**, 779–94.

Rego, J., Prevost, F., Rumeau, J. L. *et al.* (1987). Hyperacute rejection after ABO-incompatible orthotopic liver transplantation. *Transplant Proceedings*, **19**, 4589–90.

So, S. K. S., Platt, J. L., Ascher, N. L. *et al.* (1987). Increased expression of class I major histocompatibility complex antigens on hepatocytes in rejecting human liver allografts. *Transplantation*, **43**, 79–84.

Starzl, T. E., Lerner, R. A., Dixon, F. S. *et al.* (1968). Schwartzmann reaction after human renal transplantation. *New England Journal of Medicine*, **278**, 642–8.

Starzl, T. E., Tzakis, A., Makowka, L. *et al.* (1989). Combined liver and kidney transplantation: with particular reference to positive cytotoxic cross matches. In *Progress and Prevention of Uraemia* eds. C. Giordano & E. Friedman, Vol. II, pp. 24–29. Philadelphia: Field & Wood.

Starzl, T. E., Fung, J., Tzakis, A. *et al.* (1993). Baboon-to-human liver transplantation. *Lancet*, **341**, 65–71.

Steinhoff, G., Wonigeit, K. & Pichlmayer, R. (1988). Analysis of sequential changes in major histocompatibility complex expression in human liver grafts after transplantation. *Transplantation*, **45**, 394–401.

Steinman, R. M., Inaba, K., Schuler, G. *et al.* (1986). Stimulation of the immune response: contributions of dendritic cells. In *Mechanisms of Host Resistance to Infectious Agents, Tumours, and Allografts.* ed. R. M. Skinman & R. J. North, pp. 71–97. New York: Rockefeller University Press.

Tarter, R. E., Erb, S., Biller, P. *et al.* (1988). The quality of life following liver transplantation: a preliminary report. *Gastroenterology Clinics of North America*, **17**, 207–17.

Thomas, F. T., Marchman, A., Corribi, D. *et al.* (1991). Immunobiology of xenograft response: xenograft rejection in immunodeficient animals. *Transplant Proceedings*, **23**, 208.

Tilg, H., Vogel, W., Aulitsky, W. E. *et al.* (1990). Evaluation of cytokines and cytokine-induced secondary messages in sera of patients after liver transplantation. *Transplantation*, **49**, 1074–82.

Vierling, J. M. & Fennel, R. H. (1985). Histopathology of early and late human hepatic allograft rejection: evidence of progressive destruction of interlobular bile ducts. *Hepatology*, **5**, 1076–82.

Waid, T. H., Lucas, B. A., Thompson, J. S. *et al.* (1991). Treatment of acute rejection with anti-T-cell antigen receptor complex alpha-beta (T10B9.1A-31) or anti CD3 (OKT3) monoclonal antibody. *Transplant Proceedings*, **23**, 1062–5.

White, D. L. G., Gore, S. M. *et al.* (1987). The significance of ABO blood groups in liver transplant patients. *Transplant Proceedings*, **19**, 4571–4.

White, D. J. G., Oglesby, T. J., Liszewski, M. K. *et al.* (1992). Expression of human decay accelerating factor or membrane cofactor protein genes on mouse cells inhibits lysis by human complement. *Transplant International*, **5**, S648–50.

White, D. J. G. (1993). Xenotransplantation. *Clinical and Experimental Perspectives in Sandimmune therapy*, **3**, 29–31.

Wiesner, R. H., Ludwig, J., Van Hoek, B. *et al.* (1991). Current concepts in cell-mediated hepatic allograft rejection leading to ductopenia and liver failure. *Hepatology*, **14**, 721–9.

Winter, G. & Milstein, C. (1991). Man-made antibodies. *Nature*, **349**, 293–9.

Further reading

Immunology of Liver Transplantation (1993), Ed. J. Neuberger and D. Adams. London: Edward Arnold.

–18–
Clinical correlates with hepatic diseases

JAMES NEUBERGER

Introduction

Involvement of immune mechanisms in the pathogenesis of liver diseases is complex and poorly understood. It is often difficult to determine whether abnormalities in the immune system in patients with liver disease are due to a primary pathogenetic mechanism, arise as a consequence of the liver disease, or else whether immunological mechanisms modify the disease process. The advent of molecular biological techniques has allowed for major advances in the understanding of the role of the immune system in the pathogenesis of a variety of liver diseases but mechanisms still remain poorly understood. The earlier approaches which were limited to assessing phenotypic markers of peripheral lymphocyte subsets, have been overtaken by more sophisticated approaches where phenotypic, morphological and functional assessment of lymphocyte target/cell interactions have allowed elucidation of possible pathways of disease. None the less, extrapolation of *in vitro* observations to *in vivo* mechanisms is fraught with problems; availability of appropriate material for study is often limited by obvious clinical and ethical considerations. The *in vitro* reactions of cells from peripheral blood do not necessarily reflect the situation within the liver itself.

Of the various liver diseases in which immune mechanisms have been implicated, acute, cellular allograft rejection is probably the most clear-cut model, and therefore will be discussed in greater detail. In contrast, in primary biliary cirrhosis, patients have many immunological abnormalities and the disease is thought to belong in the 'auto-immune' group of disorders, yet immunosuppressive therapy is largely ineffective.

Liver transplantation

In many respects, liver allograft rejection is merely one manifestation of acute inflammation. This concept is supported by the observation that

Table 18.1. *Sensitivity and specificity of immunological tests for liver allograft rejection*

	Sensitivity	Specificity
Blood		
Bilirubin	+	−
Protein F	++	+
Glutathione-S-transferase	++	+
IL2R	+++	+
B$_2$M	+++	+
sICAM	++	+
TNF	+	++
IL-6	++	+
Neopterin	+	+
Hyaluronic acid	+++	++
Amyloid A	+	+
C-Reactive protein	++	+
Eosinophilia	+++	++
Bile		
IL2R	++	+++
B$_2$M	+++	++
sICAM-1	++	+++
Lymphocyte chemotaxis	+++	+++
Secretory component	+++	++
IL-6	++	++

markers of acute inflammation are present in patients with liver allograft rejection and are similar to those in infection. Those which are more specific focus on the bile and therefore reflect events within the portal tracts (Table 18.1). As described elsewhere, acute cellular rejection occurs in up to 70% of patients and in the majority, a short course of high-dose corticosteroids, effectively resolves the rejection process. A small proportion of patients, about 10–15%, will develop chronic ductopenic rejection, which is usually unresponsive to therapy, and requires regrafting. Hyper-acute or fulminant rejection, defined as graft failure due to preformed cytotoxic antibodies occurring within hours of transplantation, has been described in liver transplantation only rarely, even in the presence of ABO blood group incompatibility and a positive cross-match (Adams & Neuberger, 1990). Hyper-acute rejection is seen more commonly in renal grafting.

The features of acute cellular rejection are based on a characteristic clinical picture of the patient developing pyrexia and jaundice. The diagnosis is confirmed on liver histology which shows the triad of (a) a mixed inflammatory infiltrate of the portal tracts, (b) bile duct damage with infiltration by lymphocytes, neutrophils, eosinophils and polymorphs and (c) hepatic and venous endolialitis. Fine needle aspiration can be used to make this diagnosis. Chronic ductopenic rejection is usually manifest within the first year after transplantation and is characterised by progressive cholestasis and loss of bile ducts and arterial changes, with the presence of foamy macrophages, intimal thickening, sclerosis and peri-venular hepatocyte loss. Although later stages of the disease show a very scanty cell infiltrate, in the early stage, there is an intense lymphocytic portal infiltrate. In contrast to acute cellular rejection, ductopenic rejection rarely responds to immunosuppressive therapy and re-grafting remains the only therapeutic option. Those grafted for ductopenic rejection are at greatest risk of developing the same syndrome in subsequent grafts.

The immune mechanisms of rejection remain poorly understood. Rejection occurs when the host immune system recognises any allogeneic antigen in the graft liver; the most important of these are the histocompatibility determinants, as encoded by the MHC. These antigens act as recognition signals in lymphocyte reactions and are crucial in the development of both cell-mediated and humoral responses. The expression of MHC antigens varies between tissues and is determined not only by the cell type but can be up- or down-regulated in the presence of inflammation. In the liver, HLA class I and HLA class II antigens are strongly expressed on sinusoidal lining cells; on vascular endothelium there is HLA DR expression and weak class I expression. On biliary epithelial cells, class I and occasionally class II antigens are seen. Hepatocytes are usually negative for both class I and class II. During rejection, however, there is increased HLA antigen expression: hepatocytes show a membranous pattern of focal staining for both class I and class II, vascular endothelial cells show intense staining for class I and some class II antigens are indeed P but not DQ and biliary epithelium shows a similar increased pattern of antigen expression (Daar *et al.*, 1984; Steinhoff, 1989). *In vitro*, increased membrane MHC expression in response to a variety of pro-inflammatory cytokines can be demonstrated, and it is possibly this mechanism which is responsible for the increased antigen expression after transplantation. Nonetheless, it must not necessarily be assumed that MHC expression equates with rejection, since MHC expression can be found in cholestasis, where there is no evidence of immune-mediated damage to the graft (Dustin *et al.*, 1986). It has also been suggested that class II MHC expression, in the absence of antigen presentation, may induce tolerance rather than an immune cell damaging response.

Other, non-MHC products, may also be implicated in the pathogenesis of allograft rejection. The role of the minor histocompatibility complex antigens, and the blood group antigens, may all play a role in the generation of the immune response.

In recent years, the importance of adhesion processes in the inflammatory response has been realised. Amongst the different processes involving adhesion of lymphocytes to other endothelial cells or target cells, a number of interactions must occur. For example, the lymphocyte adherence receptor CD2 interacts with the lymphocyte function associated antigen 3 (LFA-3) and LFA-1 interacts with the ligands ICAM-1 and ICAM-2. This ICAM1/LFA-1 pathway is also implicated in the interaction of monocytes and neutrophils with target cells (Pattarroyo & Makgoba, 1989). ICAM-1 is expressed on target cells during allograft rejection and this can be induced *in vitro* by pro-inflammatory cytokines. Corticosteroids themselves are not associated with down-regulation of ICAM-1 expression *in vitro*; their rapid disappearance in treated allograft rejection is likely to represent, therefore, a secondary effect presumably related to reduction of the pro-inflammatory cytokines.

Transplantation antigens are presented to the recipient immune system either by the host antigen presenting cells (APCs) in conjunction with class II, or presented directly by the donor APCs directly to the primed, alloantigen specific host T cells, without the need for antigen processing. It is thought that the latter process is most important for acute allograft rejection, although some have suggested that the former pathway may be involved with ductopenic rejection (Rubenstein, Roska & Lipsky, 1987). Both the dendritic cells from the portal tract and the Kupffer cells which line the sinusoids are effective antigen-presenting cells. After human liver transplantation the donor Kupffer cells are replaced by recipient cells, as shown by phenotypic studies. In patients with severe rejection this process occurs rapidly whereas in those who tolerate grafts this occurs more gradually. The control of this process is not properly understood. It has been suggested that biliary epithelial cells and vascular endothelial cells are also capable of presenting antigens; yet there remains no convincing evidence that this is indeed the case.

The presentation of donor MHC antigens results in the activation of T cells with a subsequent stimulation of the inflammation cascade. Both CD4 and CD8 positive T cells are involved, with generation of cytotoxic T lymphocytes, and a delayed-type-hypersensitivity reaction, with recruitment and stimulation of eosinophils and monocytes. Antibody production is probably also implicated in the pathogenesis of disease. Analysis of the phenotype of infiltrating T lymphocytes shows that T cells are the most common usually of the alpha beta T cell receptor lineage; both CD4 and CD8 lymphocytes are found in the inflammatory infiltrate. One study has suggested that a predominantly CD4 infiltrate is associated with reversible rejection, whereas CD8 infiltration is associated more with severe acute rejection and progression to chronic rejection (McCaughan *et al.*, 1990). These cells are mainly primed cells as they express the CD45 RO antigen; many also express activation markers. Eosinophils and neutrophils are also involved in disease pathogenesis.

The role of humoral antigens has been eluded to briefly above.

In those with fulminant rejection, there is deposition of immunoglobulin with complement components on endothelium in association with MHC expression on the hepatocyte membrane. Whilst this fulminant rejection has been found in certain animal experiments, it remains unclear whether massive haemorrhagic necrosis remains a form of liver rejection. However, in acute rejection, two humoral mechanisms may be involved, since there are increased levels of anti-class I cytotoxic antibodies in those with rejection and IgM in particular, is deposited on arterial walls.

In order to further understand the mechanism of allograft rejection and in order to look for serological markers of allograft rejection to obviate the need for liver histology, attention has focused on serological correlates with rejection. As shown in Table 18.1 there are many peripheral changes which occur in rejection. However, many of these are non-specific for rejection and may be found in other forms of inflammation such as infection or infarction.

In contrast to the relatively well-defined mechanisms of acute allograft rejection, the mechanisms of chronic ductopenic rejection are less well understood. Although in the early stages of the process, there is increased histological activity, with a mixed cellular response around the portal tracts and increased serum levels of immune markers, as the condition progresses, the inflammatory infiltrate decreases and serum markers of inflammation tend to return to basal levels. Concomitant with the reduction in inflammation, the bile ducts become increasingly scarce and intimal hyperplasia of small and middle-sized arteries becomes more apparent and cholestasis increases. Response to immunosuppressive therapy is usually disappointing, although claims have been made for therapeutic efficacy of the newer immunosuppressive agent FK506.

The mechanisms underlying ductopenic rejection are less clear. The targets of the immune responses are uncertain; it has been suggested the bile duct loss and consequent cholestasis occurs secondarily to vascular immune mediated vascular damage. The association between chronic rejection and CMV infection remains controversial, as does the role of HLA matching. Many centres are now reporting a decline in the incidence of ductopenic rejection with time; the reasons for this are unclear and do not appear to be related simply to changes in immunosuppressive regimes.

Immunosuppression

Most immunosuppression regimes are broad-based and relatively non-specific. Although there are no proper trials to suggest the optimal method of immunosuppression, most are based on a combination of corticosteroids, azathioprine and cyclosporin. Some centres use anti-lymphocyte globulin

Table 18.2. *Possible role of antibodies in rejection*

Stage of inflammation	Antibody
Antigen presentation	Anti-CD45
CD4 Lymphocyte activation	Anti-CD4
Activation and recruitment	Anti-CD3 (OKT3) Anti-IL2R Anti-CD7 Anti-CD5
Induction of cells Recruitment Transendothelial migration	Anti-IFN Anti-TNF Anti-LFA-1 Anti-ICAM-1 Anti-B7

or monoclonal antibodies to CD3 (OKT3) in the short term, but their superiority has yet to be confirmed (Neuberger & Adams, 1993).

In general, immunosuppression involves a delicate balance between over-immunosuppression, resulting in sepsis and under-immunosuppression, resulting in rejection. With under-immunosuppression, the graft may be lost whereas with sepsis, the patient may die. Over-immunosuppression renders the patient at risk of developing *de novo* malignancy.

Understanding of the mechanisms of allograft rejection, has allowed a more specific and targeted approach. In particular, the use of monoclonal antibodies, and their availability by commercial production, has resulted in the possibility of more specific intervention. As shown in Table 18.2, monoclonal antibodies can be used both for the prevention of rejection (anti-CD45), or interference with specific areas of the immune response. Clearly, such principles also apply to other aspects of inflammation. As yet, prevention of rejection remains an imprecise science. Whilst acute rejection can usually be well treated, chronic rejection remains resistant to therapy other then transplantation.

Primary biliary cirrhosis

In contrast to liver allograft rejection, primary biliary cirrhosis remains an intriguing disease in which the involvement of the immune system remains uncertain. The recent identification of dihydrolipoamide acetyl transferase, as a major target antigen of the anti-mitochondrial antibodies, has allowed further insight into the pathogenesis of this disease, although the aetiology, the pathophysiology and the treatment remain as uncertain today as they were 15 years ago.

There are many immunological abnormalities, both in patients and their relatives, yet the extent to which these changes are either a cause of the liver disease, a consequence of the liver disease or modifying processes in the liver, remains uncertain. If immune mechanisms are involved in the pathogenesis of the disease, then the response to immunosuppressive therapy has been overall disappointing. Although there remains controversy as to how clinical studies should be evaluated in this disease, the many investigations looking at different immunosuppressive agents in the treatment of PBC, have failed overall to show any major clinically significant effects on survival. Thus, prednisolone, cyclosporin, azathioprine – all potent immunosuppressive agents – have not been associated with great success in modifying the immune response in a way that corticosteroids, for example, have been shown to control auto-immune chronic active hepatitis (Mitchison & Bassendine, 1993). Furthermore, PBC has been reported to recur following liver transplantation, even though patients are maintained on otherwise adequate immunosuppression using either cyclosporin or FK506 (see Chapter 15).

None the less, the association with other auto-immune diseases such as thyroid disease, pernicious anaemia and coeliac disease, all suggests that PBC is part of this auto-immune spectrum. Although certain HLA phenotypes are reported in increased frequency in PBC, especially C4B2 and DRw8, the association overall is weak. Clinically, it is apparent that PBC is a heterogenous disease. The rate of progression varies considerably. Although the disease is nine times more frequent in women than men, the clinical course of disease is similar between the two groups. As yet, no clear-cut immunological feature has been identified, which explains the difference in rate of progression.

A common paradigm for the disease, as with many other presumed immune-mediated disease, is that there is an initial trigger which, in a susceptible individual, results in a breakdown of tolerance and chronic disease. Whether the trigger is infectious, toxic or other has not been established. The reports of PBC developing after drug ingestion, such as the analgesic benoxaprofen or phenothiazines (Stricker, 1992), suggests that there may be a potential for a toxin to trigger the immune response: conversely, it may be that the association is coincidental or that the drug exacerbates a pre-existing but undiagnosed disease. Other agents, including penicillins, are associated with progressive bile-duct damage, which may mimic PBC. The overlap of PBC with sarcoid, also suggests that the two diseases may share a similar aetiological trigger. The initial presentation of PBC in pregnancy or in women using the oral contraceptive, may merely

Table 18.3. *Possible scheme of progression and treatment of PBC (based on MacKay & Gershwin, 1989)*

Lesion	Possible treatment
Immune mediated bile duct damage	Immunosuppression (e.g. prednisolone, azathioprine, cyclosporine)
↓	
Bile duct loss	Methotrexate
↓	
Cholestasis	Ursodeoxycholic acid
↓	
Fibrosis	Colchicine
↓	
Cirrhosis	Methotrexate
↓	
Liver failure	Transplantation

reflect the cholestasis increase with raised circulating oestrogens; thus, pre-existing disease becomes manifest at this time.

The association between PBC and the auto-antigen E2, and the appearance of low titre of anti E-2 in patients with asymptomatic bacteruria (Hopf, Miller & Stermerowicz, 1989; Chapter 15), has raised the hypothesis that a common infective agent, such as *E. coli*, may trigger the disease process. These intriguing observations have yet to be confirmed, but preliminary data are convincing. Furthermore, rough forms of *E. coli* have been associated with primary biliary cirrhosis although not all units (including ours) have been able to confirm this observation (Butler *et al.*, 1993). Until a definitive serotype of *E. coli* can be associated with the disease process, the association must remain, at present speculative.

The pathogenic mechanisms suggest that the trigger stimulates an immune response, resulting in an immune attack upon the bile duct. This leads to cholestasis, which in turn leads to fibrosis, portal hypertension, cirrhosis and ultimately end-stage disease (MacKay & Gershwin, 1989) (Table 18.3). It is likely this hypothesis is over simple. As indicated elsewhere (Chapter 15), immunosuppressive agents have little therapeutic affect in halting or arresting the disease. Furthermore, evidence of immunological abnormalities persist during the course of the disease process. The extent to which these abnormalities occur, as a consequence of ischaemic or toxic damage to middle-sized bile ducts, is not clear. Whether E2 is a marker of the disease or is implicated in the pathogenesis is uncertain. While studies have shown that

E2 is expressed on the membrane of biliary epithelial cells, it is possible that this represents the target of an immune attack. However, the recognition that AMA negative PBC, or autoimmune cholangitis, behaves in a manner similar to AMA positive PBC suggests that either AMA is not clinically detectable in serum, which is unlikely, or that alternative antigens are important in the pathogenesis.

In PBC, in contrast to primary sclerosing cholangitis, the middle-sized bile ducts are the prime target for the damage. Studies have shown there is phenotypic heterogeneity of bile ducts within the biliary tree (Tavoloni *et al.*, 1987). If immune mechanisms are involved in the pathogenesis of the disease, then the immune system must recognise an antigen present on the middle-sized bile duct only, but this remains to be established.

The difficulties in dissecting the various components of the disease is exemplified by the effect of the bile-acid, ursodeoxycholic acid (UDCA). As shown earlier (Chapter 15), there are many studies on the effect of UDCA in PBC. There is general agreement that UDCA is associated with a significant improvement in many of the important prognostic factors in PBC; an effect on survival, in the absence of transplantation, has yet to be shown. In addition to its choleretic effect, UDCA both *in vivo* and *in vitro* is associated with an improvement in the immune abnormalities induced by bile acids as lithocholic acid (Yoshikawa, Tsuji & Matsumura, 1992). It cannot be assumed that any effect of UDCA is mediated by its immune activity, since the agent is reported to be effective in other non-immune cholestatic diseases, such as cystic fibrosis. In patients with primary sclerosing cholangitis, the Oxford group reported no clinical effect, yet they did find a reduction in the class II MHC expression on bile ducts (Lo *et al.*, 1993). Thus, the alterations in immune function, associated with UDCA, may be a consequence of its effects on bile acids, rather than a primary action on the immune system. If so, the extent to which the immune abnormalities are a consequence of the cholestasis remains unclear.

Drug related liver disease

The involvement of immune mechanisms in liver damage, associated with drugs, is suggested by a number of features including the idiosyncratic nature of the response, the association with fever, eosinophilia (both circulating and intra-hepatic) and the association with other auto-immune phenomena such as haemolytic anaemia, pyrexia and arthralgia. Clearly, none of these features is specific nor do they provide clear evidence of an immune mechanism.

Of the various drugs in which immune mechanisms are postulated to result in liver damage, halothane is probably the most well studied. Patients

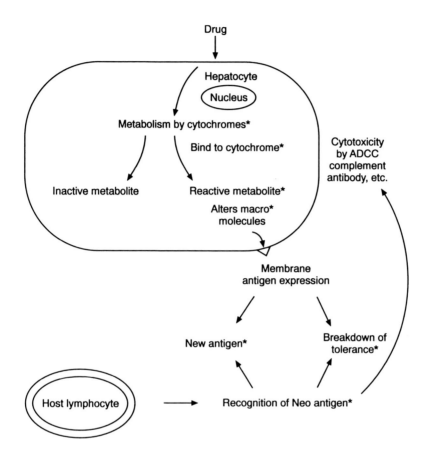

*Areas of possible idiosyncracy.

Fig. 18.1. Scheme of possible mechanisms of immune mediated drug reaction.

with severe hepatic failure, following halothane anaesthesia, have circulating antibodies which react with a trifluroacetylated antigen (TFA) (a product of halothane oxidative metabolism) present on the surface of isolated hepatocytes. Furthermore, leucocytes from such patients can be shown *in vivo* to be sensitised to these TFA-adduct antigens (Pohl, 1990). It is now becoming clear that cytochromes may be present on cell plasma membranes (Loeper *et al.*, 1993) and thus it is possible to construct a scenario whereby a drug is metabolised with the generation of reactive metabolites. Such reactive metabolites bind covalently to cellular macromolecules, possibly including cytochromes. If these are translocated on the cell membrane, then it is possible that susceptible individuals will recognise these antigens present on hepatocytes and the resulting immune response induce liver cell necrosis (Fig. 18.1).

The nature of the susceptibility has yet to be identified: certainly HLA studies have not been rewarding but this does not exclude an immune response. Studies have been small and include a heterogeneous group of patients; stereotyping rather than phenotyping has been employed. In anecdotal reports, corticosteroids have been tried in patients with liver failure associated with halothane but there has been no clinical response. While it is possible that the cellular and humoral responses to halothane-altered antigens occur as a consequence of liver damage, this is less likely in view of the observation that patients who are exposed to halothane and develop liver failure from other unrelated causes, such as ischaemia, fail to demonstrate such immune responses.

Chronic drug ingestion may also lead to a chronic hepatitis. This is well recognised in the cases associated with a now discarded laxative oxyphenisatin, alpha methyl dopa and uricosuric diuretic tienilic acid (Lafay *et al.*, 1976). The latter drug has been associated with the presence of circulating antibodies to the cytochrome P450 responsive for metabolising the drug, resulting in the appearance of the liver/kidney microsomal antibody type-II. Although cellular and humoral responses suggest immune mechanisms are responsible, the treatment is drug withdrawal, whereupon the histological damage regresses.

Alcohol related liver damage

While the evidence for immune mediated drug induced liver damage is relatively clear, the involvement of immune mechanisms in alcoholic liver disease is less well defined. The possible involvement of immune mechanisms in alcoholic liver disease has been suggested by a number of observations, including the great variation in the clinical response to alcohol, the possible association of the HLA B8 phenotype with accelerated progression of cirrhosis, the hypergammaglobulinaemia (especially IgA), abnormalities of T-cell function, increased incidence of auto-antibodies including anti-LSP (liver specific proteins) and anti-nuclear antibodies and functional changes to functional lymphocyte responses. It is difficult to clarify whether these changes occur as a consequence or a cause of liver disease, the effects of ethanol *per se* on the immune system or resulting from associated malnutrition.

Analogous to the halothane altered antigens, studies have shown that patients with alcoholic liver disease have an increased incidence of antibodies reacting with ethanol altered liver cell determinants (Tuma & Klassen, 1992). Subsequent studies demonstrated that these are related to acetaldehyde metabolism and are of IgA sub-class. Further studies have revealed evidence of lymphocyte sensitisation to a 200 kD acetaldehydeadduct, possibly related to procollagen, but other targets, including cytochromes, cytosolic or mitochondrial protein, have been postulated.

Acetaldehyde is central to the generation of liver damage, Barry and coworkers have shown that acetaldehyde adducts may themselves directly lead to complement activation (Barry, McGiven & Hayes, 1981) and so result in cellular damage.

Thus, as yet there are alternative explanations for the variation in susceptibility, including unreliability of the drinking history, differences in patterns of drinking, differences in the volume of distribution, variations in the activity of alcohol metabolising enzymes and the effect of malnutrition on enzyme activity, and differences in enzyme activities (Day & Bassendine, 1992). Demonstration of *in vitro* autologous cytotoxicity, of lymphocytes to hepatocytes, may represent a secondary phenomenon and does not necessarily imply a primary action. Thus, there is conflicting evidence to suggest immune mechanisms in the pathogenesis of alcoholic cirrhosis.

In contrast, alcoholic hepatitis is characterised by a peripheral and hepatic neutrophilia, with evidence of activation of lymphocytes and increased expression of adhesion molecules and their ligands within the liver. The reasons for these changes are not clear; endotoxin, TNF and other proinflammatory cytokines may be involved. Hyaline may act as a trigger, since it can activate lymphocytes and stimulate neutrophils. Again, it is unclear whether these changes occur as a consequence or are causal in the pathogenesis of alcohol hepatitis. Deposition of hyaline is not specific for alcoholic hepatitis. Alcohol withdrawal may be associated with an exacerbation of the syndrome, rather than a reduction. Although corticosteroids have some effect in improving at least short-term survival, they appear to have little effect in switching off the immune response in a way analogous to autoimmune chronic active hepatitis. The histological similarity between alcoholic hepatitis and the non-alcoholic steatohepatitis syndromes, associated with a variety of different agents such as perhexiline, amiodarone, obesity and diabetes mellitus suggests that a toxic rather than immune factor may be involved.

Auto-immune chronic active hepatitis

There is little that can be added to the discussions from previous chapters on auto-immune chronic active hepatitis. This syndrome, which may better be termed autoimmune hepatitis, is associated with a wide spectrum of specific and non-specific autoimmune responses.

Patients with untreated autoimmune hepatitis have high levels of circulating immunoglobulins and autoantibodies; these markers rapidly return to normal with successful treatment and may be the first sign of reactivation, rising before the serum transaminases become abnormal. Most of these antibodies react with organ non-specific, intra-cellular antigens. Of the various liver specific antigens associated with autoimmune hepatitis, LSP (liver specific protein) contains the human asialoglycoprotein receptor (ASGPR); anti-ASGPR appears to be a relatively sensitive marker for the disease (Treichel *et al.*, 1990).

The division of autoimmune hepatitis according to the type of circulating antibody may lead to a further clarification of the events that result in this syndrome. The role of sensitisation to the different antigens (including soluble liver antigen (SLA), liver/kidney microsomal antigen type I or II (LKM), and anti-nuclear antibodies (ANA)), is not yet apparent.

Although the early clinical trials can be criticised in the light of modern clinical practice, there is little clinical doubt that the introduction of corticosteroids and azathioprine is associated with a major clinical response and reduction or correction of the immunological abnormalities. Trials have suggested that use of corticosteroids is associated with a significant improvement in survival, although these studies were performed before the identification of auto-immune chronic active hepatitis.

Viral hepatitis

Perhaps the most intriguing association of auto-immunity is with chronic viral hepatitis. The mechanisms and pathogenesis of chronic hepatitis B viral (HBV) infection is discussed earlier. Although the immune response is clearly central to the pathogenesis of chronic liver disease associated with chronic hepatitis B, mechanisms are now becoming better understood. While it is generally accepted that the hepatitis B virus is not directly cytopathic, the mechanisms which determine the severity of disease and viral persistence remain uncertain. The severity of infection may be determined in part by the immune response and by the virus itself, since mutant virus seem, in some series, to be associated with fulminant disease. Persistence of virus, and hence development of chronic liver disease, may be due to a combination of factors (Peters *et al.*, 1991), including alteration of viral replication, alteration of immune function or avoidance of immune surveillance. The extent to which each of these factors may be responsible for persistence is unclear, but the differing responses in adults and neonates and the increased risk in males have still not been fully explained.

Chronic HBV infection contrasts with that of auto-immune chronic active hepatitis, in that treatment is directed towards eradication of infected cells; the development of a hepatitis is seen as a therapeutic goal, reflecting immune mediated clearance of virally infected hepatocytes. Interferon is effective in only a selected sub-group of patients; therapy is expensive, the mode of administration is unpleasant for the patient and side-effects are common and may be serious. Recent trials assessing anti-viral agents (rather than immune modifiers), may lead to more effective and less toxic therapeutic regimes. The potentially adverse effect of immunosuppressive treatment, is highlighted by the course of HBV when immunosuppressive therapy is stopped and by recurrent HBV in grafted livers. The accelerated clinical course after transplantation may lead to a cirrhosis in less than one year. Fibrosing cholestatic hepatitis, may be related to the effect of corticosteroids on the intracellular handling of core antigen within the hepatocyte (Lau et al., 1992).

The most intriguing observation of an association between viral infection and auto-immunity is hepatitis C infection which may shed light on aspects of auto-immunity. This virus is associated with a number of auto-immune phenomena and in particular the appearance of the LKM antibody, reacting with cytochrome oxidase P450 2D6. Anti-HCV antibodies have been reported to be present in between 5 and 80% cases, with auto-antibody positive auto-immune hepatitis. Some of these patients have replicating virus, as demonstrated by the presence of HCV RNA in serum; such patients tend to respond well to interferon and poorly to corticosteroids (Magrin et al., 1991). Of those with anti-LKM positive chronic active hepatitis, patients with HCV tend to be older, male and have lower titres of anti-LKM, whereas those with presumed auto-immune chronic hepatitis tend to have higher anti-LKM-I (greater than 1:10 000), be female and younger. Thus, HCV-associated chronic liver disease may be associated with auto-immune features, but these are not necessarily involved in the pathogenesis of the disease.

Conclusions

Changes in the immune system may occur as a consequence of a direct, toxic effect on the liver, or may be important in either initiating and maintaining disease processes, rather than terminating them. The increasing use of organ transplantation has resulted in a clearer idea of the immune responses to liver antigens, as well as providing a further intellectual and commercial stimulus to research in this area. The use of increasingly sophisticated techniques has allowed greater understanding into the mechanism of immune-mediated processes. Current practice has advanced little in this area in the last decade; however, the greater understanding from recent research will allow more specific and less toxic therapy, such as peptide treatment for auto-immune hepatitis or the development of tolerance in transplantation.

References

Adams, D. & Neuberger, J. (1990). Patterns of liver allograft rejection. *Journal of Hepatology*, **10**, 113–19.

Barry, R. E., McGiven, J. & Hayes, M. (1981). Acetaldehyde binds to liver cell membranes without affecting membrane function. *Gut*, **25**, 412–16.

Butler, P., Valle, F., Hamilton-Miller, D., Brumfitt, W., Baum, I. S. & Burroughs, A. (1993). M_2 mitochondrial antibodies and urinary rough mutant bacterium in patients with PBC and in patients with recurrent bacterium. *Journal of Hepatology*, **17**, 408–16.

Daar, A. S., Fuggle, S., Fabre, J., Ting, A. & Morris, P. (1984). Detailed distribution of MHC class 2 antigens in normal human organs. *Transplantation*, **38**, 293–7.

Day, C. D. & Bassendine, M. (1992). Genetic predisposition to alcoholic liver disease. *Gut*, **33**, 1444–7.

Dustin, M. L., Rothlein, R., Bhan, A., Dinarello, C. & Springer, T. (1986). Tissue distribution, biochemistry and function of a natural adherence molecule – ICAM-1. Induction by IL-1 and Interferon-gamma. *Journal of Immunology*, **137**, 245–54.

Hopf, U., Miller, B., Stermerowicz, R. *et al.* (1989). Relations between E coli R (rough) forms in gut, lipid A in liver and PBC. *Lancet*, **ii**, 1419–21.

Lafay, J., Poupon, R., Legendre, C., Homberg, J. & Darnis, F. (1976). Atteintes hepatiques associées aux anticorps antimicrosumes de foie et de rein (type 2) et à la prise d'acide tienilique. *Gastroenterology and Clinical Biology*, **7**, 523–8.

Lau, J., Bain, V. G., Davies, S. *et al.* (1992). High level expression of hepatitis B viral antigens in fibrosing cholestatic hepatitis. *Gastroenterology*, **102**, 956–62.

Lo, S. K., Chapman, R., Dooley, J. & Fleming, K. (1993). Aberrant HLA-DR expression by bile duct epithelium in primary sclerosing cholangitis is down-regulated by ursodeoxycholic acid. *Gastroenterology*, **104**, A943.

Loeper, J., Descatoire, V., Maurice, M. *et al.* (1993). Cytochrome P450 in human hepatocyte plasma membrane. *Gastroenterology*, **104**, 203–11.

McCaughan, G., Davies, J., Waugh, J. & Bishop, G. A. (1990). A quantitative analysis of T-lymphocyte populations in human liver allografts undergoing rejection. *Hepatology*, **12**, 1305–13.

MacKay, I. & Gershwin, M. (1989). Primary biliary cirrhosis: current knowledge, perspective and future directions. *Seminars in Liver Disease*, **9**, 149–57.

Magrin, S., Craxi, A., Fabiano, C. *et al.* (1991). Hepatitis C virus replication is 'autoimmune' chronic hepatitis. *Journal of Hepatology*, **13**, 364–7.

Mitchison, H. & Bassendine, M. (1993). Rolling review: autoimmune liver disease. *Alimentation Pharmacology Therapy*, **7**, 93–109.

Neuberger, J. & Adams, D. (1993). Newer immunosuppressive agents. In *Immunology of Liver Transplantation*, ed. J. Neuberger & Adams, D. pp. 250–260. London: Edward Arnold.

Pattarroyo, M. & Makgoba, M. (1989). Leucocyte adhesion to cells in immune and inflammatory responses. *Lancet*, **ii**, 1139–42.

Peters, M., Vierling, J., Gershwin, M. *et al.* (1991). Immunology and the liver. *Hepatology*, **13**, 977–94.

Pohl, L. (1990). Drug induced allergic hepatitis. *Seminars in Liver Disease*, **4**, 305–15.

Rubenstein, D., Roska, A. & Lipsky, P. (1987). Antigen presentation by liver sinusoidal lining cells after antigen exposure *in vivo*. *Journal of Immunology*, **138**, 1377–80.

Steinhoff, G. (1989). Major histocompatibility antigens in human liver transplants. *Journal of Hepatology*, **11**, 9–15.

Stricker, B. H. (1992). Drug induced hepatic injury. In *Drug Induced Disorders,* ed. A. N. G. Dukes, vol. 5. London: Elsevier.

Tavoloni, M., Tsuji, T., Matsumuar, K. *et al.* (1987). The intrahepatic biliary epithelium. *Seminars in Liver Disease,* 7, 280–92.

Treichel, V., Poralla, T., Hess, G., Manns, M. & Mayer Zum Buschenfelde, K. (1990). Autoantibodies to the asialoglycoprotein receptor (ASGPR) in autoimmune type chronic hepatitis. *Hepatology,* 11, 606–12.

Tuma, D. & Klassen, L. W. (1992). Immune responses to acetaldehyde protein adducts. *Gastroenterology,* 102, 1969–73.

Yokikawa, M., Tsuji, T., Matsumura, K. *et al.* (1992). Immunomodulatory effects of ursodeoxycholic acid on immune responses. *Hepatology,* 16, 358–64.

Index